Global Midwifery: Principles, Policy and Practice

Joy Kemp • Gaynor D. Maclean
Nester Moyo

Global Midwifery: Principles, Policy and Practice

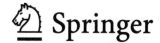 Springer

Joy Kemp
Global Professional Advisor
The Royal College of Midwives
London
UK

Nester Moyo
Global Midwifery Advisor
The Hague, Zuid-Holland
The Netherlands

Gaynor D. Maclean
Maternal and Newborn Health,
Department of Interprofessional Health
Swansea University
Swansea
UK

ISBN 978-3-030-46767-8   ISBN 978-3-030-46765-4   (eBook)
https://doi.org/10.1007/978-3-030-46765-4

This Springer imprint is published by the registered company Springer Nature Switzerland AG
The registered company address is: Gewerbestrasse 11, 6330 Cham, Switzerland

For women around the world and to the midwives who travel with you; may you have courage, strength and joy along a safe and satisfying journey

Foreword

Midwifery is increasingly recognised as a vital solution to the unconscionably high levels of maternal and newborn mortality and morbidity globally. This book—a first of its kind—is timely. It connects together multiple aspects of global midwifery, providing unique insights into and clarity about what is really needed to successfully implement this complex intervention in various contexts. This goes beyond the traditional focus on the curriculum and education and sets out political, geographical, historical and contemporary influences and places midwifery firmly in the context of the Sustainable Development Goals. The content addresses the challenges of education and regulation, as well as the urgency of supporting national midwives associations to ensure future leadership in the profession of midwifery. It provides much needed information on models of care in different settings. In an era where poor quality of care in facilities has become a major cause of mortality and morbidity, guidance on evidence-based practice, research, the role of the midwife in fragile and humanitarian settings, and where to find resources is welcome. Developed and written by midwives with many years of exceptional global experience, this comprehensive and refreshing resource about global midwifery will go a long way in helping all of us to ensure that women, newborns and families of the future will not only survive, but thrive and transform their societies.

Through an engaging mix of presenting information, explaining impact and encouraging reflection and discussion, Global Midwifery brings to life the history and the current day realities of midwifery for women, societies, midwives and other healthcare providers alike. The in-depth presentation of the development of quality midwifery care and the midwifery profession and practice from a number of angles adds to the existing literature on midwifery. Bringing together local, regional and global developments in quality maternal and newborn care and the midwifery philosophy and model of care, Global Midwifery contributes to the strengthening of respectful, safe and woman-centred care for all.

It is becoming clearer by the day, supported by rigorous research, that midwives have a key role to play when it comes to optimising the sexual and reproductive healthcare and rights of women and their families globally. The implementation of midwifery that is '*a unique body of knowledge, skills and professional attitudes… practised by midwives within a professional frame-*

work of autonomy, partnership, ethics and accountability[1] deserves to be given a top priority for high-, middle- and low-income countries alike.

This book therefore comes at an opportune time as it supports a deeper understanding of the broad scope of the practice of midwives as well as the various pathways midwifery has taken befitting different contexts. The global ICM community of one million midwives united in 143 Midwives' Associations in 124 countries will welcome these insights as they will contribute to ICM's vision of a world where every childbearing woman has access to a midwife's care for herself and her newborn.

Fran McConville
Department for Maternal,
Newborn, Child, Adolescent Health
and Ageing & Office of Chief Nurse,
World Health Organization HQ
Geneva, Switzerland

Petra ten Hoope-Bender
UNFPA Office of Geneva,
Geneva, Switzerland

Franka Cadée
International Confederation of Midwives (ICM),
The Hague, The Netherlands

---

[1]International Confederation of Midwives (2017) Definition of midwifery. Cited Sept 2020.   https://www.internationalmidwives.org/our-work/policy-and-practice/icm-definitions.html

Preface

In 2013 I took on a new role as Global Professional Advisor for the Royal College of Midwives (RCM), the largest professional association dedicated to midwives and those who work with midwives in the United Kingdom (UK). The decision to develop such a position signified a change in direction for the RCM as it considered its role in supporting midwives outside of the UK's borders. The RCM had just started its journey in midwifery twinning partnerships and was on a steep learning curve as an organisation, developing the systems and processes needed to support programmes and partners in different countries, managing large numbers of UK-based midwife volunteer 'twins', allowing time for reflection on the reciprocal learning from our international midwife twins and their organisations and being willing to change ourselves. As a midwife, I am fortunate to have had a parallel career in international development; even so, I wished there had been an instruction manual in the first few months and years of the job. With my team, I started talking about developing a toolkit to document the learning as we travelled along, and thus, the idea for this textbook on Global Midwifery was born. We knew the book would be richer with a wider authorship, and so I was delighted when Gaynor D. Maclean and Nester T. Moyo, both highly experienced and respected global midwifery advisors and writers, agreed to join the team.

As a trio we have faced illness, family emergencies and a global pandemic that have challenged our timelines and patience. Midwife means 'with woman'; I believe we have midwifed each other throughout the past two years, one stepping into the breach when another had to step down temporarily. I could not have wished for more generous-natured and hard-working teammates but also for co-authors with such a wealth of expertise and history in global midwifery.

The book is written in six sections. Part I is an overview of the place of midwives on the global scene, exploring evidence for the contribution of midwives to global health and development goals, as well as taking a historical perspective. Midwifery is mapped across the world's continents, identifying the different contexts and systems in which midwives work. Part II examines three foundational pillars for midwives' practice: education, regulation and professional association. This includes the international standards for midwifery education, essential competencies for midwives' practice and the purpose and functions of midwives' associations. Part III centres on midwives' practice and the challenge of providing high-quality, respectful maternity care to women and their newborns. Innovation is also explored, with inspiring examples of how midwives and others are innovating to strengthen global midwifery. Part IV examines midwifery itself, the development of professional identity and the importance of effective leadership and research in driving the profession forward. The penultimate section, Part V, considers midwives and women who cross borders for different reasons and the challenges of midwifery and motherhood in complex settings such as humanitarian emergencies, along with a how-to-guide to global midwifery partnerships. Finally, Part VI looks forward to 2030 and beyond, presenting an in-depth analysis of the current context of midwifery around the world and giving recommendations for future midwifery policy, practice, education and research.

London, UK   Joy Kemp

Acknowledgements

Many people played a part in the conception, development and delivery of this book. We acknowledge the staff of the RCM (past and present) for having the vision and courage for global outreach and for all their support, ideas and encouragement. Mary Dharmachandran (the RCM's librarian) and her colleagues in the Royal College of Obstetricians and Gynaecologists (RCOG) library have conducted countless literature searches and retrieved hundreds of articles and resources with consistent grace and efficiency. We salute the International Confederation of Midwives (ICM) for their example of leadership and for nurturing and supporting Nester during her career, allowing opportunities for experience and for growth and support. This includes the midwives' associations around the world with whom Nester had the privilege to work, providing impetus for many of the achievements shared in this book. Many midwives and friends of midwives have helped to shape the direction of various chapters and given helpful feedback—thanks to everyone for your time, support and commitment. Finally, we gratefully acknowledge our editor Marie-Elia Come-Garry and her team at Springer Nature for inviting us to write this book and for all of their support and encouragement.

London, UK   Joy Kemp
Swansea, UK   Gaynor D. Maclean
The Hague, Zuid-Holland, The Netherlands   Nester T. Moyo

Contents

About the Authors

Joy Kemp is Global Professional Advisor for the Royal College of Midwives (RCM). She is a midwife with a background in clinical practice, education and research. Joy's international career started in 1988 when she worked in a maternal and child health clinic in a Cambodian refugee camp in Thailand. This was followed by further humanitarian work with Kurdish refugees in Iraq after the Gulf War and with refugees from Kosovo in Albania in the 1990s. She has also worked on longer term community development projects in Cambodia and elsewhere and spent 3 years as Tearfund's Southeast Asia Desk Officer. She is a Khmer (Cambodian) language speaker. Since joining the Royal College of Midwives in 2013, Joy's work has focused on building the capacity of midwifery associations in Asia and Africa through twinning. This work has been widely published, and Joy frequently teaches and gives presentations on global midwifery at conferences and events. She is a member of the RCM's Expert Clinical Advisory Group and represents the RCM widely in the global health arena.

Gaynor D. Maclean is an international consultant in maternal and newborn health; a midwife with extensive experience in clinical practice, teaching, research and UK Statutory Body service. She is an honorary fellow of Swansea University (Wales). Having worked for some years in India early in her career, she has acquired skills in the Hindi and Urdu languages. She has since worked with numerous government and non-governmental organisations focusing on promoting safer childbirth, with assignments in many countries where maternal mortality remains high. From 1991, she worked as a consultant to the World Health Organization (Geneva) authoring the first edition of the WHO Safe Motherhood Educational Modules. She has produced online learning modules for the Royal College of Midwives (RCM) to prepare students for international electives and to inform midwives about global issues. She has long been associated with the Africa Midwives Research Network (AMRN) and subsequently with the Lugina Africa Midwives Research Network (LAMRN) through a partnership project with the University of Manchester. She is a member of the RCM Global Advisory Group. Gaynor has carried out numerous literature searches and desk reviews; some of this work was in preparation for the launch of the global skilled attendance initiative and technical consultation at WHO Geneva. Gaynor writes and edits training manuals, professional texts and reports; speaks at national and international conferences and has received several awards in recognition of her contribution to promoting safer childbirth and midwifery worldwide.

Nester T. Moyo is a consultant Global Midwifery Advisor, with specialities in midwifery education, regulation, developing midwives' associations and leadership. She retired from the International Confederation of Midwives (ICM) after 17 years of leading activities on strengthening midwifery globally. She worked closely with Ministries of Health and midwifery programme managers to provide strategic and supportive leadership, technical and programmatic assistance for the design, development and implementation of global-, regional- and country-level programmes in midwifery and SRMNCAH. She has expertise in developing and supporting the implementation of capacity building strategies for midwives; curriculum development and review; developing training manuals and other learning materials for continuing professional development, developing, and conducting tailor-made interventions and trainings. She is an expert trainer of trainers, organisational development and development and implementation of assessment and evaluation tools. She is a resource person for strengthening midwifery globally. Nester has a sound understanding of working in low- and middle-income countries in all regions of the world. In 2014–2016, Nester led the country assessment for the Midwifery Services Framework in Afghanistan, Bangladesh, Kyrgyzstan, Lesotho and Togo. With excellent facilitation skills, Nester has experience in organisational capacity building and the ability to work in diverse, multi-professional and multi-cultural teams and hierarchies.

Abbreviations

AAAQ	Availability Accessibility Acceptability and Quality
ACM	Australian College of Midwives
ACNM	American College of Nurse-Midwives
AEC	Asian Economic Community
AI	Appreciative Inquiry (sometimes known as Appreciative Enquiry)
AIDS	Acquired Immunodeficiency Syndrome
AJM	African Journal of Midwifery
AMA	Afghan Midwives Association
AMRN	African Midwives Research Network
AMU	Alongside Maternity unit
ANC	Antenatal Care
ARC	African Health Professional Regulation Collaborative
ASEAN	Association of South East Asian Nations
BEmONC	Basic Emergency Obstetric and Newborn Care
BMS	Bangladesh Midwifery Society
CAIPE	Centre for Advancement of Interprofessional Education
CAM	Canadian Association of Midwives
CARMMA	Campaign for Accelerated Reduction of Maternal Mortality
CBE	Competency-Based Education
CEmONC	Comprehensive Emergency Obstetric and Newborn Care
CHI	Copenhagen Health Innovation
CONAMA	Confederation of African Midwives Associations
COVID-19	Corona Virus Disease 2019
CPD	Continuing Professional Development
Cradle VSA Device	Cradle Vital Signs Alert Device
CRED	Centre for Research on the Epidemiology of Disasters
CRMA	Caribbean Regional Midwives Association
DFID	Department of International Development
ECSA	East Central and Southern Africa
EEC	European Economic Commission
ELRHA	Enhancing Learning and Research for Humanitarian Assistance
EMA	European Midwives Association
ENAP	Every Newborn Action Network

EOC	Emergency Obstetric Care
ERA	Education Regulation and Association
ESSAE	Empire State Society of Association Executives
EU	European Union
EWEC	Every Woman Every Child
FASFAF	Federation of French Speaking African Midwives' Associations
FCI	Family Care International
FGM	Female Genital Mutilation
FIGO	International Federation of Gynecology and Obstetrics
FLO	Latin American Federation of Midwives
FMA	Freestanding Maternity Unit
FOB	Fear of Birth
G-ANC	Centering Pregnancy (Group Antenatal Care)
GAVI	Global Alliance for Vaccines and Immunisation
GFF	Global Financing Facility
GRMCC	Global Respectful Maternal Health Council
HDI	Human Development Index
HICs	High-Income Countries
HIV	Human Immunodeficiency Virus
HMIS	Health Management Information Systems
HPCAs	Health Care Professions Associations
IARH	Inter-Agency Emergency Reproductive Health
IASC	Inter-Agency Standing Committee
IAWG	Inter-Agency Working Group
ICM	International Confederation of Midwives
ICN	International Council of Nurses
IFRC	International Federation of the Red Cross and Red Crescent Societies
IMC	International Medical Corps
IOM	International Organisation for Migration
IPA	International Paediatric Association
IPE	Inter-Professional Education
JAMA	Japanese Midwives Association
KI	Karolinska Institute (Sweden)
KMC	Kangaroo Mother Care
KNOV	Koninklijke Nederlandse Organisatie van Verloskundigen (Royal Dutch Organisation of Midwives)
LAMRN	Lugina African Midwives' Research Network
Lao PDR	Lao People's Democratic Republic
LGBTI	Lesbian, Gay, Bisexual, Transgender, Intersex
LGH	Laerdal Global Health
LIC	Low-Income country
LMICs	Low- and Middle-Income Countries
LSHTM	London School of Hygiene and Tropical Medicine
M&E	Monitoring and Evaluation
MACAT	Member Association Capacity Assessment Tool
MAMA	Mobile Alliance for Maternal Action

MANA	Midwives Associations of North America
MATE	Midwifery Assessment Tool for Education
MCAT	Midwifery Coordination Alliance Team
MCH Aides	Maternal and Child Health Aides
MCH	Maternal and Child Health
MDGs	Millennium Development Goals
MEAP	Midwifery Education Accreditation Programme
MHTF	Maternal Health Task Force
Midirs	Midwives Information and Resource Service
MIDSON	Midwifery Society of Nepal
MISP	Minimum Initial Services Package
MMHA	Maternal Mental Health Alliance
MMR	Maternal Mortality Ratio
MNCH	Maternal, Newborn and Child Health
MNH	Maternal and Newborn Health
MNR	Maternal Newborn and Reproductive Health
MOHC	Ministry of Health Cambodia
MOMENTUM	Model of Mentorship for Ugandan Midwifery Students
MOOC	Massive Open Online Course
MRA	Mutual Recognition Arrangements
MSF	Médecins Sans Frontières
MSF	Midwifery Services Framework
NAS	National Academy of Science
NCZM	New Zealand College of Midwives
NGO	Non-Governmental Organisation
NHS	National Health Services
NICE	National Institute for Health and Care Excellence
NIHR	National Institute of Health Research
NMBA	Nursing and Midwifery Board of Australia
NMC	Nursing and Midwifery Council
NPEU	National Perinatal Epidemiology Unit
NSPCC	National Society for Prevention of Cruelty to Children
OCHA	Office for the Coordination of Humanitarian Affairs
OU	Obstetric Unit
OXFAM	Oxford Committee for Famine Relief
PA	Professional Association
PAHO	Pan American Health Organization
PESTLE	Political, Economic, Social, Technological, Legal and Environmental
PMNCH	Partnership for Maternal and Newborn Health
PROMPT	Practical Obstetric Multi-Professional Training
PSE	Poverty and Social Exclusion
QI	Quality Improvement
QMNC	Quality Maternal and Newborn Care
RAN	Research Advisory Network
RCM	Royal College of Midwives
RMC	Respectful Maternity Care
SAMA	South Asian Midwives Association

SARS	Severe Acute Respiratory Syndrome
SBA	Skilled Birth Attendant
SC	Save the Children
SDGs	Sustainable Development Goals
SMART	Specific Measurable Achievable Realistic and Time-bound
SME	Small and Medium Enterprises
SMI	Safe Motherhood Initiative
SMS	Short Messaging System
SoWMy	State of the World's Midwifery
SRH	Sexual and Reproductive Health
SRMNCAH	Sexual, Reproductive, Maternal, Newborn, Child and Adolescent Health
SRMNCH	Sexual, Reproductive, Maternal, Newborn and Child Health
SRMNH	Sexual, Reproductive, Maternal and Newborn Health
SWOT	Strengths, Weakness, Opportunities and Threats
TAM	Tanzania Association of Midwives
TBA	Traditional Birth Attendant
TFR	Total Fertility Rate
THET	Tropical Health and Education Trust
UHC	Universal Health Coverage
UK	United Kingdom
UKCISA	United Kingdom Council of International Student Affairs
UKMidSS	United Kingdom Midwifery Study System
UN	United Nations
UNDP	United Nations Development Programme
UNDRR	United Nations Office for Disaster Risk Reduction
UNFPA	United Nations Population Fund
UNHCR	United Nations High Commissioner for Refugees
UNICEF	United Nations Children's Fund
UNOCHA	United Nations Office for the Coordination of Humanitarian Affairs
UNOHCHR	United Nations Human Rights Office of the High Commissioner
UNOOSA	United Nations Office for Outer Space Affairs
UNV	United Nations Volunteers
URC	University Research Company
US MERA	United States Midwifery Education, Regulation and Association
USA	United States of America
USAID	United States Agency for International Development
VAG	Violence Against Women and Girls
WASH	Water Sanitation and Hygiene
WD	Women Deliver
WEF	World Economic Forum
WFP	World Food Programme

WHA	World Health Assembly
WHO AFRO	World Health Organization Africa Regional Office
WHO EMRO	World Health Organization Eastern Mediterranean Regional Office
WHO EURO	World Health Organization European Regional Office
WHO SEARO	World Health Organization South East Asia Regional Office
WHO	World Health Organization
WRA	White Ribbon Alliance
WWF	World Wide Fund for Nature
YML	Young Midwifery Leader
ZICOM	Zimbabwe Confederation of Midwives

Part I

Midwifery on the Global Scene

Midwifery in Global Health

1

Expected Learning Outcomes

By the end of the chapter, the reader should be able to:

1. Appreciate the critical role of midwives in contributing to the global agenda to transform the world by 2030
2. Identify the Sustainable Development Goals as part of the 2030 Agenda and consider why and how these relate to the health and well-being of women and newborns
3. Identify some of the historical landmark achievements in reducing global maternal mortality and morbidity and the role of midwives in these endeavours
4. Discuss the geographical variations in making progress towards safe childbirth and quality care and identify some of the reasons for this
5. Determine the importance of political commitment in providing high-quality maternal and newborn care (QMNC) and consider ways of raising the political visibility of this issue
6. Describe some of the contemporary challenges to achieving QMNC for all, consider the importance of 'leaving no-one behind' and the role of midwives and policymakers in achieving this

1.1 Introduction

Midwives have been acknowledged as critical to achieving the 2030 Agenda (UNFPA 2011, 2014a). This agenda has been described as 'A plan of action for people, planet and prosperity' (United Nations 2015), and currently, amongst numerous global efforts, the world is aspiring towards universal health coverage and promoting good health and well-being for everyone. Embodied in the new agenda, there is the vision to enable women, children and adolescents everywhere not only to survive but also to thrive and contribute to the transformative change anticipated with the realising of the Sustainable Development Goals (SDGs). In reflecting on the Millennium Development Goals (MDGs) and anticipating the SDGs, it has been stated that:

> Midwifery is a vital solution to the challenges of providing high-quality maternal and newborn care for all women and newborn infants, in all countries. Improvements in availability, accessibility, acceptability, and quality of midwifery services, within a functioning health system that is responsive to women's needs and requirements, is crucial…to the development of the post-2015 agenda's goals and targets, in which emphasis on reduction in maternal and newborn morbidity should be even stronger than it has been in the past.
> ten Hoope-Bender et al. (2014:7)

Given the enormous agenda that has been presented to the global community, it would seem appropriate initially to examine these issues in

© Springer Nature Switzerland AG 2021
J. Kemp et al., *Global Midwifery: Principles, Policy and Practice*,
https://doi.org/10.1007/978-3-030-46765-4_1

some detail and the vital contribution of midwifery in this context and then to reflect on the historical, geographical and political issues that have influenced and will continue to influence progress in this critical area of human life, before considering some of the contemporary challenges facing the world of today and tomorrow. In considering the historical as well as the contemporary challenges, it is claimed that well-educated midwives strategically placed, given appropriate support and working within an enabling environment serve as critical catalysts in this anticipated global transformational process.

1.2   The Sustainable Development Goals

The most outstanding global co-operation ever witnessed has been enshrined in the Sustainable Development Goals (SDGs). These were launched by the United Nations (UN) in January 2016 following a global meeting of heads of states held towards the end of 2015. It has been declared that the SDGs are 'the blueprint to achieve a better and more sustainable future for all' (United Nations 2019a). These goals have been designed based on the successes of the Millennium Development Goals (MDGs) which are discussed in Chapter 2. There are 17 SDGs and 169 associated targets which interconnect, addressing issues including poverty, inequality, health, clean water and sanitation, gender equality, climate, prosperity and peace and justice (Fig. 1.1). The interconnection between the goals has been stressed since the achievement of one goal may be dependent on tackling issues more commonly associated with another (UNDP 2019a).

Several partnerships have been developed in the early years of the SDG programme. For example, the European Union (EU) and the United Nations (UN) have embarked on a new, global initiative centring on SDG 5 and spotlights eliminating all forms of violence against women and girls (VAWG). This is especially relevant to the health and well-being of women, children and adolescents. The Spotlight Initiative focuses on women's empowerment and gender

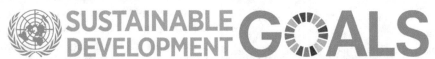

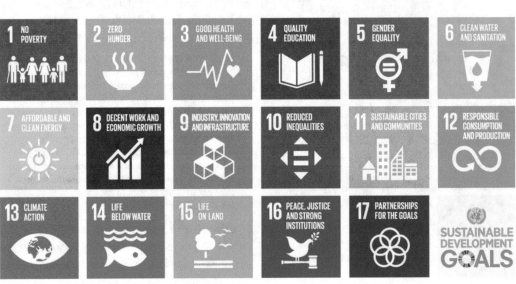

Fig. 1.1 Sustainable development goals (UN 2019a)

equality. Special emphasis has been placed on violence both in the family and within the domestic environment and on sexual and gender-based violence. There is also a focus on harmful practices, female infanticide, trafficking of human beings and sexual and economic labour exploitation (United Nations 2019b). At the launch of the initiative, the deputy Secretary General of the United Nations Organization deplored the 'global pandemic' of VAWG and stated that this initiative was an essential tool to make such violence 'a thing of the past'. It was acknowledged that almost half of the murders of women committed worldwide are carried out by partners or ex-partners. VAWG is often deeply embedded in the accepted practice and norms of some societies. An extreme form of such violence surrounds the killing of female infants (Mohammed 2018), Midwives clearly have a role to play in promoting and achieving a number of these goals.

The SDG relating to health is embedded in SDG 3 'good health and well-being' and specifies the aim to ensure healthy lives and promote well-being for all. It includes targets to reduce the maternal mortality ratio (MMR) and preventable deaths of babies and children under 5 years of age. Universal health coverage is also regarded as integral to achieving SDG 3, ending poverty and reducing inequalities. Furthermore, it has been stressed that gender-sensitive, rights-based approaches are critical to address inequalities across all sectors (UNDP 2019b). Of the 17 SDGs, goals 1 and 6 relating to eliminating poverty and providing clean water and sanitation respectively have been identified along with SDG 3 as being the most important for health services development in vulnerable populations. However, Homer (2018) identifies several key SDGs that are intricately connected to SDG 3 (Fig. 1.2).

The links between these goals may seem fragile at times, but it could well be considered that

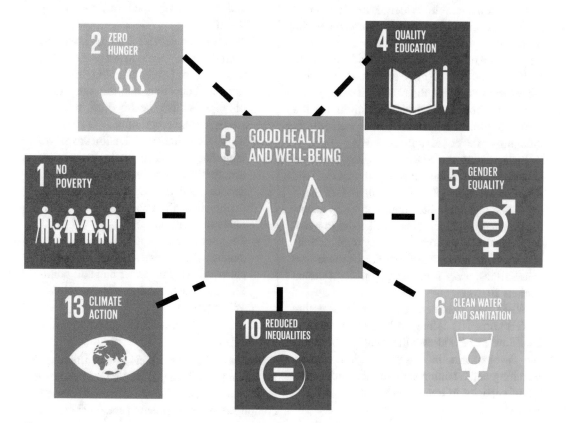

Fig. 1.2 The interdependence of SDGs in relation to health. (Derived from Homer 2017)

midwives provide a network imperceptibly intertwining these global targets. Global midwifery with a woman-centred approach to achieving health and well-being offers both direction and dexterity in a dynamic world drama unfolding in the early twenty-first century.

Debate surrounds the issue as to whether the SDGs are realistic given that low income countries do not always have the resources or the support to achieve these goals (World Economic Forum 2015). Whereas the SDGs can be seen as an unrealistic financial challenge by some, efforts have been made to urge heads of governments and donor countries to invest in funding and policymaking that embraces the vision of universal health coverage (Summers 2015). It is also asserted that investing in 'pro-poor pathways' through realising the SDGs and ensuring universal health coverage has been identified by a world leading economist and Nobel prize winner as 'an affordable dream'. Sen (2015) reckons that there is considerable evidence that universal health care not only powerfully enhances the health of a population but that a strong relationship exists between health and economic performance. It is worthy of note that during the efforts to achieve the MDGs, it was agreed that there should be no poor solutions for the poor. The world may need to reconcile these thoughts in the context of the SDGs.

In launching the SDGs, delegates from the United Nations member states recognised the fundamental principle of the dignity of each individual and committed their nations to ensuring that no one got left behind. The aim to reach all people in all sections of society in all nations was set, with the commitment to reach those who were furthest away from the targets first (United Nations 2016).

WHO has identified specific targets within SDG 3 (Box 1.1). Along with these, underlying issues are to be addressed that include research and development, increasing health financing, recruiting and retaining staff and the strengthening of capacity in low income countries (WHO 2019).

Box 1.1. Global health targets for SDG 3
Targets to be achieved by 2030 unless otherwise stated...

1. To reduce MMR to <70/100,000
2. To end preventable deaths of babies and children under 5 years
3. To end the epidemics of AIDS, tuberculosis, malaria and neglected tropical diseases and combat hepatitis, water-borne diseases and other communicable diseases
4. To reduce by one third premature mortality from non-communicable diseases through prevention and treatment and promote mental health and well-being
5. To strengthen the prevention and treatment of substance abuse, including narcotic drug abuse and harmful use of alcohol
6. To halve the number of global deaths and injuries from road traffic accidents (by 2020)
7. To ensure universal access to sexual and reproductive healthcare services, including for family planning, information and education, and the integration of reproductive health into national strategies and programmes
8. To achieve universal health coverage, including financial risk protection, access to quality essential healthcare services and access to safe, effective, quality and affordable essential medicines and vaccines for all
9. To substantially reduce the number of deaths and illnesses from hazardous chemicals and air, water and soil pollution and contamination
WHO (2019)

Research into the critical issues affecting the health and well-being of women and babies has traditionally attracted the funding and focused on complication management (Tuncalp et al. 2015).

However, Kennedy et al. (2016) purport that in undertaking research, midwives may be asking different questions. They suggest that:

> …studying ways of providing such care has the potential to improve the provision of quality care for all, enhance women's and infants' own capabilities, and maximise the health promotion potential of midwives.
> Kennedy et al. (2016: e778)

Midwifery research and the identified priorities are discussed in some detail in Chapter 12.

1.3 Early Historical Landmarks

There are numerous global issues that impact the lives of women, newborns and families. Midwifery, with the emphasis on supporting women through childbirth has always played an important part in contributing to global health, though until comparatively recently, recognition of this fact has been very limited. For several centuries, making childbirth safer has challenged generations of communities, professionals and politicians across the world. During the eighteenth and nineteenth centuries, Sweden led the way in markedly reducing maternal mortality by the early twentieth century. Norway and the Netherlands soon improved their outcomes, and like Sweden, the achievements were largely accounted for by extensive collaboration between physicians along with midwives known to be very competent and who were available in the local communities. Between 1751 and 1900, the Swedish maternal mortality ratio (MMR) fell from 900 to 230 (Högberg 2004). By contrast, the MMR in England and Wales was 440 at the beginning of the twentieth century, and in the United States, it was estimated to be between 520 and 850 at that time (Loudon 1992). Landmark achievements in northern Europe have served as important pointers in the battle against maternal and perinatal mortality. The significant achievements in Sweden were realised in a country challenged by scattered populations beset by poverty, with many living in remote rural areas; this was prior to the introduction of medical, pharmaceutical and techno-logical advances. Blood transfusion, antibiotics and reliable communication networks were non-existent, but progress was real and sustained. In considering the unprecedented progress in Sweden, Högberg (2004) asserts the impact of 'midwife-assisted deliveries' on the outcome of maternal and child survival to be of 'major historical importance' and maintains that progressive reduction of maternal mortality in these countries would not have been as significant if it were not for the establishment of welfare states. In his comprehensive review of the decline of maternal mortality, Loudon (2000) states that since the causes of death in countries with high MMRs today reflect the situation in the global north more than 50 years ago, it is therefore reasonable to assume that the measures that were effective in the former would currently be valuable in the latter. In reviewing the critical historical issues, confidential enquiry into every maternal death has also been highlighted as an indispensable approach to preventing avoidable mortalities (Loudon 2000; Högberg 2004).

1.4 Geographical Variations

Historical achievements cannot be reviewed in isolation from geographical factors. Where a woman is domiciled and gives birth is as relevant as the timing of her lifespan. It was acknowledged towards the end of the twentieth century that the rates of maternal mortality showed greater disparity between the rich and poor nations than any other public health indicator. It was also recognised that most of the women who die live in remote areas and are poor (Royston and Armstrong 1989). Undoubtedly geographical location can be critical in determining whether a woman will survive childbirth and whether her baby will be born alive. It has long been recognised that 99% of maternal deaths occur in low income countries and that most of them are preventable (WHO 2018). Midwives working within a supportive healthcare system are deemed to be best able to provide the solution to this global burden of death and disability (UNFPA 2014a, b). It has been stated that:

…midwives, when educated and regulated to international standards, have the competencies to deliver 87% of this service need.
(UNFPA 2014a:iv).

However, in most cases, midwives comprise just 36% of the midwifery workforce, and it is a fact that many countries do not have 'a dedicated professional cadre focused on supporting women and newborns' (UNFPA 2014a, b:iv). Midwives, as primary care providers, work closest to where women live, and therefore, this would not have to be an issue if the world promoted and retained well-educated and regulated midwives in all geographical settings. Issues relating to education and regulation are discussed in Chapters 4 and 5.

There are indeed wide geographical inequities in maternal and newborn health outcomes. This has been identified at regional, national and subnational levels in countries of varying economic status. The location of relevant health services is a crucial determinant of whether women can access care (Thaddeus and Maine 1994; Gabrysch and Campbell 2009; Ravelli et al. 2011; Okwaraji et al. 2012). Therefore, where a woman lives and where health facilities are located can be a matter of life and death in many communities across the world if there is no means of covering the distance between these two focal points.

In China, although substantial economic growth had been reported by the turn of the millennium, a vast geographical difference remained in the numbers of maternal deaths, and this has been related to inequity in socio-economic development between urban and rural areas (Gao et al. 2002; Rudan et al. 2010; Wang et al. 2010).

Survival can undoubtedly be shown to vary depending on geographical location, since it had been reported that in sub-Saharan Africa as many as 1 in 16 women may die from pregnancy-related complications, in Asia this decreased to 1 in 94 and in Europe the risk had been reduced to 1 in 4000 (Sibbald 2007). By 2015, it was declared that in sub-Saharan Africa, the lifetime risk of dying in childbirth was 1 in 36, in the European Union it was 1 in 8400 and in 'fragile and conflict affected areas' it was 1 in 46 (World Bank 2019). However, there is also evidence of considerable variation

in MMR between different racial and ethnic groups in high-income countries. For example, in the United States, there has been a higher MMR reported amongst African-American women than amongst white women (Lang and King 2008). In the Netherlands (Schutte et al. 2010) and in Germany (Razum et al. 1999), there has been a higher incidence of maternal death amongst the immigrant populations by comparison with the indigenous populations. So, it would seem that in attempting to survive childbirth, who you are in relation to the ability to access health care, is as relevant as where you are, in addition to the timing of your lifespan. The issue is likely to be complex. It could relate to inaccessibility disadvantaging some ethnic groups, to racial discrimination, educational and linguistic limitations or economic hardship where equitable access to free health care is not available.

1.5   Political Issues

The location of a family's habitat and the maternal and neonatal outcomes will inevitably be greatly influenced by the political environment in which they currently reside. It has been stressed that there is considerable evidence that the most reliable predictors of health outcomes across the lifespan are the societal or structural causes of ill health (Navarro 2004; Raphael 2009). In considering issues surrounding maternal and newborn mortality, McGibbon (2011:343) maintains that these 'structural causes are best articulated within the realm of the political economy of health'. She also suggests that it is imperative to consider 'the societal context within which women live' because it is the societal causes of maternal mortality that become the 'causes-of-the-causes' underlying the deaths of these women. McGibbon therefore proposes using a 'political economy lens' in order to attempt to understand and confront these issues, maintaining that the growing inequities in health outcomes are related to such matters as class distinction, racism and sexism. These, she maintains, are 'the structural determinants of health'.

In considering why some global health initiatives achieve political visibility whereas others do not, Shiffman (2008) asserts that several factors are involved. These include the existence of credible evidence proving the severity of the problem. Whether or not there is appropriate leadership which can offer 'effective global champions for the issue' has been highlighted and whether a set of institutions exist whose members are able to advance the matter successfully through advocacy. Shiffman admits that more research is needed to uncover ways of achieving further political visibility but offers pointers which are more likely to lead to success in achieving this (Box 1.2).

Box 1.2. National health advocates are more likely to succeed if they…

1. Coalesce into unified policy communities, translating their potential moral and knowledge-based authority into political power and pressing national political officials to act
2. Bring into their communities respected and well-connected national political entrepreneurs with track records in placing public health issues on national agendas
3. Develop credible measures that mark the severity of this problem and make political leaders aware of these measures so that they cannot plausibly deny that a problem exists
4. Organize large-scale focusing events such as national forums to generate widespread attention to the issue.
5. Present leaders with clear policy alternatives proven to be effective, so that policymakers come to believe the problem can be surmounted and know what they are expected to do.

Shiffman (2008)

Nanda et al. (2005) underline the importance of evidence-based advocacy in order to promote an enabling policy environment and enhance political commitment. Shiffman (2007) conducted case studies in five countries to examine the level of political commitment apportioned to reducing maternal mortality. The studies were carried out in Guatemala, Honduras, India, Indonesia and Nigeria. He discovered that there was considerable variation in the political priority accorded to this matter in these countries. Shiffman identified three criteria which he used to assess the situation in each country (Box 1.3).

Box 1.3. Shiffman's criteria for assessing the level of national political priority

1. National political leaders publicly and privately express sustained concern for the issue
2. The government, through an authoritative decision-making process, enacts policies that offer widely embraced strategies to address the problem
3. The government allocates and releases public budgets commensurate with the problem's gravity

Shiffman (2007:796)

Using these criteria, Honduras rated 'very high' in the level of political priority afforded to reducing maternal mortality. The priority in Indonesia was high, whilst in India it was rated as moderate at the time, but low in Guatemala and Nigeria. Honduras managed to reduce maternal mortality by 40% during a 7-year period from 1990. With QMNC becoming a high political priority, Honduras demonstrated one of the most significant reductions in MMR in the shortest time span ever observed amongst low-income countries (Meléndez et al. 1999, Koblinsky 2003, Shiffman et al. 2004). The example of Honduras well illustrates the effect that political commitment can have in reducing mortality.

However, maternal mortality is a complex subject demanding attention to a number of issues. In acknowledging Nigeria's situation with one of the highest numbers of maternal deaths across the world, it has been asserted that in Nigeria advocates of maternal mortality reduction:

...will need to focus more attention on developments in the educational sector and not just on making direct improvements to the healthcare system.
(Mojekwu and Ibekwe 2012:135)

This reverberates established epidemiological findings that claim that improving the education of women has been influential in improving maternal outcomes (WHO 2012). Multifactorial it may be, but there are strong indications that without political commitment little will change in the aspiration to achieve safe childbirth for all. At a global conference in Mexico City in 2015, it was stressed that political leadership acting on scientific evidence was a priority and that the public should be empowered to make demands that would improve maternal and newborn survival. Furthermore, it was agreed there that governments and societies were obliged to embrace and implement an evidence-based maternal and newborn health agenda and monitor its progress (Momentum 2015).

1.6   Contemporary Challenges

Building on the lessons learned historically, giving cognizance to geographical location and emphasising the importance of political commitment, there remain an ever-increasing number of contemporary challenges. Commitment by the global community to promote maternal and newborn health is a solid foundation upon which to build a better future. However, the numerous contemporary challenges which constantly arise can frustrate the purposes and delay achievement. Amongst others, these can include epidemiological, demographic, socio-economic and political factors which are liable to change, particularly in fragile states and typically affecting those who are most vulnerable.

In an examination of the social epidemiological issues surrounding QMNC, Cwikel (2008) asserts that a review of Semmelweiss' study of hand washing to prevent puerperal sepsis could act as a benchmark from which contemporary women and QMNC advocates could identify salient issues today. She stresses that marginality

and social exclusion still dictate who can access a safe birthing experience and identify which women risk their lives in giving birth. The Covid-19 pandemic has added new dimensions to this problem in 2020.

Cwikel argues that when health researchers critically use the tools of social epidemiology in research and practice, there is a good chance that public health goals can be achieved. This can bring about valuable behavioural change, evidence-based medicine and community-based participatory action research. Such an approach can also be beneficial in reducing maternal mortality and morbidity as well as improving other areas of women's health. Cwikel stresses that the current epidemiological practice in women's health can help to promote public health predominantly benefiting women who are marginalised and most particularly those in low-income countries. Several of these basic approaches may well have alleviated some of the devastation caused by the Ebola outbreak in more recent times. It has been claimed that the advances that had been made in achieving QMNC in West Africa were largely wiped out during that epidemic (UNFPA 2014a).

In 2016 the World Health Organization (WHO) declared the Zika virus and its complications a public health emergency of international concern. This was decided because 84 countries, territories or national areas were identified as having evidence that this mosquito-borne infection was being transmitted (WHO 2017a). The infection was related to foetal abnormalities with numerous babies being born in affected areas with microcephaly. This problem cast a shadow over the 2016 Olympic Games in Brazil with many top athletes declining to travel to the region (Attaran 2016) and again the novel coronavirus Covid-19 has caused cancellation of the 2020 Olympic Games in Tokyo.

It is fitting to consider at this point not only what the world has learned from these experiences but to reflect on how midwives were able to contribute to addressing such international crises. These catastrophes have sorely affected the progress of QMNC and fundamental issues of perinatal and sexual and reproductive health. If the world's midwives were not critically involved in seeking and assisting in delivering solutions, then the question why must be asked. Midwifery needs to be on the global agenda for such times as these which inevitably reverberate across the continents with alarming frequency at times.

Malaria continues to be a global epidemiological challenge and can result in maternal illness with considerable risk to the newborn child (WHO 2017b). The advent of the human immunodeficiency virus and acquired immune deficiency syndrome (HIV/AIDS) shocked the world in the early 1980s, and it was not until 1997 that an antiretroviral therapy became available which reduced the death rate in the United States by 47% (Nall 2018). In 2018 it was estimated that this global epidemic affected 36 million people worldwide (Cichocki 2018).

The effect that the movement of populations can have has been illustrated above in respect of the Zika and Covid-19 viruses. However, numerous issues have caused mass migration challenging health and threatening the possibility of providing QMNC. In the early twenty-first century war, civil unrest and natural disasters have caused massive evacuations from some parts of the world and many women give birth in refugee camps or even when travelling to escape conflict, danger, abuse or persecution. These issues which cannot be separated from some of the socio-economic challenges and political matters are discussed further in Chapter 14. In celebrating the seventieth anniversary of the founding of the United Nations Organization, a new agenda was agreed. It was acknowledged that it was the first time ever that the world leaders had pledged their commitment to such a broad and universal policy agenda, the 2030 Agenda. It was from this that the SDGs described above were generated (UNDP 2019c).

1.7   The 2030 Agenda

In looking forward, it is pertinent to remember that the world is challenged by a new Agenda. This has been introduced at the beginning of this chapter and is guided by the purposes and principles of the Charter of the United Nations (1945a, b). It encompasses total respect for international law and is grounded in the Universal Declaration of Human Rights, international human rights treaties, the Millennium Declaration and the 2005 World Summit Outcome Document (United Nations 1948, 2000, 2005). Additionally, the 2030 Agenda is informed by other instruments such as the Declaration on the Right to Development (United Nations 1986). The new agenda recognised that the targets for some of the Millennium Development Goals were not reached, particularly those relating to maternal and child health, and these are discussed in see Chapter 2. The SDGs would prompt recommitment to achieving these goals and a new commitment to giving focused and scaled up assistance to those nations most needing support (United Nations 2015). In order to achieve the health-related targets of the 2030 Agenda, 12 international organisations (Box 1.4) have committed to

---

Box 1.4. The international organizations committed to the Global Action Plan

GAVI (Vaccine Alliance Lead Global Vaccine Marketing)

GFF (Global Financing Facility)

Global Fund (to fight AIDs, tuberculosis and malaria)

UNAIDS (a joint programme of 11 UN organisations fighting HIV/AIDs)

UNDP (United Nations Development Programme)

UNFPA (United Nations Population Fund)

UNICEF (United Nations Children's Emergency Fund)

Unitaid (an international drug purchasing facility)

UN Women (the global champion for gender equality)

World Bank Group (five international organizations that make leveraged loans to low income countries)

WFP (World Food Programme)

WHO (World Health Organization)

WHO (2019)

developing a Global Action Plan. This Plan reflects an historic commitment by global health and development agencies to increase joint action and hasten progress (World Health Organization 2019).

1.8   Conclusion

In looking back and looking forward, there are clearly challenges and opportunities. History offers lessons that should have been learned; a diversity of geographical situations and political issues both confront and offer prospect for progress. Nevertheless, many challenges remain. By 2019 it had already been acknowledged that 'the world is off-track to achieve the health-related SDGs'. Although there had been progress, it has been uneven, within and between countries. Whilst some countries have made remarkable gains, when examining just the national averages, it is not immediately apparent that many countries are being left behind (UNDP 2019b). A deeper analysis is required in order to perceive the true picture. This matter is discussed further in Chapters 2 and 3.

By the end of 2017, there were 21.7 million people with the human immunodeficiency virus (HIV) who were receiving antiretroviral therapy. However, in 2019 more than 15 million people with HIV were stated to be still waiting for this treatment (UNDP 2019b). Mass migration, national crises and natural disasters have shown no sign of abating. New challenges create new opportunities. Within this complex global situation, the midwife is beginning to be recognised as a valuable resource. It has been estimated that 83% of all maternal deaths, stillbirths and newborn deaths could be averted with the full package of midwifery care that includes family planning (Homer et al. 2014). There is no shortage of opportunity, the challenge remains as to whether the global community will rise to it, recognising the importance of midwifery in global health can never be overstated.

Key Messages
Principles
   The principles identified from historical evidence which have been instrumental in reducing maternal mortality and progress achieved in contrasting geographical areas can be used as a basis to promote continuing progress across the globe. QMNC is evident where midwifery exists within an environment of mutual respect and cooperation between midwives, medical professionals and communities.
   Policy
   Political commitment to QMNC is a critical component of effective midwifery care. Midwives are the professionals best suited to advocate for enabling policies at each level and across every strata of society. This is in order to enable them to practice effectively and for women to be able to access skilled care which is appropriate and acceptable.
   Practice
   Well-educated midwives who are highly skilled, respectful and enabled to provide evidence-based care are key to achieving the targets of SDG3 in the context of sexual, reproductive, maternal and newborn health care (SRMNH).

Questions for Reflection or Review
1. Loudon (2000) asserts that since the causes of death in countries with high MMRs today reflect the situation in the global north decades ago, it is reasonable to assume that the measures that were effective in the former would be effective in the latter. What measures have been influential historically in reducing MMR and how practical would it be to introduce these in countries still struggling with high levels of MMR today? How might the skill of the pro-

fessional midwife in global health contribute to such progress?

2. Consider the reasons why geographical location can be a matter of life and death for women and newborns. It has been stated above that 'Midwives, as primary care providers, work closest to where women live and therefore this would not have to be an issue if the world promoted and retained well educated and regulated midwives in all geographical settings'. What needs to change in order to offer the most vulnerable the same chances of health and survival as others?

3. Think about specific areas with which you are concerned. Identify practical ways of raising the political visibility of QMNC within an identified community (see Box 1.1) and consider approaches to using 'evidence-based advocacy' (Nanda et al. 2005) in order to achieve this.

4. Reflect on the role of midwives in promoting global health in general and safe childbirth in particular.

Additional Resources for Reflection and Further Study

Look at the website about the Sustainable Development Goals and download the app offered at: https://www.sdgsinaction.com/. Identify goals that are important to you; get updates from around the world and become actively involved in promoting actions

The International Confederation of Midwives (ICM) '… envisions a world where every childbearing woman has access to a midwife's care for herself and her newborn'. Visit the ICM website and reflect on the Bill of Rights for Women and Midwives. https://www.internationalmidwives.org/assets/files/general-files/2019/01/cd2011_002-v2017-eng-bill_of_rights-2.pdf

The following resources may offer some further perspectives for reflection and action: Maclean GD (2017) Achieving safe motherhood globally: an historical overview. Lambert Academic Publishing, Germany

United Nations Population Fund (2014) State of the world's midwifery: a universal pathway to women's health. A United Nations publication

United Nations (2015) Transforming our world: the 2030 Agenda for Sustainable Development. United Nations, New York: A/RES/70/1. https://sustainabledevelopment.un.org/content/documents/21252030%20Agenda%20for%20Sustainable%20Development%20web.pdf

References

Attaran A (2016) Zika virus and the 2016 Olympic games. Lancet 16(9):1001–1003

Cichocki M (2018) A brief history of HIV: key moments in the fight against the world's greatest global epidemic. Verywellhealth. https://www.verywellhealth.com/the-history-of-hiv-49350. Accessed 27 April 2019

Cwikel J (2008) Learning from Semmelweiss – a social epidemiologic on safe motherhood. Soc Med 3(1):19–35

Gabrysch S, Campbell OM (2009) Still too far to walk: literature review of the determinants of delivery service use. BMC Pregnancy Childbirth 9:34. https://doi.org/10.1186/1471-2393-9-34

Gao J, Qian J, Tang S et al (2002) Health equity in transition from planned to market economy in China. Health Policy Plan 17(suppl 1):20–29. https://doi.org/10.1093/heapol/17.suppl_1.20

Högberg U (2004) The decline in maternal mortality in Sweden: the role of community midwifery. Am J Public Health 94(8):1312–1320. https://doi.org/10.2105/AJPH.94.8.1312

Homer C (2018) Maternal health and sustainable goals – a new focus for the world and for our region. Pac J Reprod Health 1(7):344–345. https://doi.org/10.18313/pjrh.2018.900

Homer C, Friberg I, Dias M et al (2014) The projected effect of scaling up midwifery. Lancet 384:1146–1157

ten Hoope-Bender P, de Bernis L, Campbell J et al (2014) Improvement of maternal and newborn health through midwifery. The Lancet series. https://www.komora-primalja.hr/datoteke/Improvement%20of%20health.pdf. Accessed 18 May 2020

Kennedy H, Yoshida S, Costello A et al (2016) Asking different questions: research priorities to improve the quality of care for every woman, every child. Lancet Glob Health 4(11):E777–E779. https://www.thelancet.com/journals/langlo/article/PIIS2214-109X(16)30183-8/fulltext. Accessed 31 Oct 2019

Koblinsky MA (2003) Reducing Maternal Mortality: Learning from Bolivia, China, Egypt, Honduras, Indonesia, Jamaica, and Zimbabwe. Health, Nutrition, and Population. Washington, DC: World Bank. © World Bank. https://openknowledge.worldbank.org/handle/10986/15163. License: CC BY 3.0 IGO." URI. http://hdl.handle.net/10986/15163 [last accessed 05.11.2020]

Lang CT, King JC (2008) Maternal mortality in the United States. Best Pract Res Clin Obstet Gynaecol 22:517531. https://doi.org/10.1016/j.bpobgyn.2007.10.004

Loudon I (1992) Death in childbirth. Clarendon Press, Oxford

Loudon I (2000) Maternal mortality in the past and its relevance to developing countries today. Am J Clin Nutr 72(1):241S–246S

McGibbon EA (2011) Political economy of maternal and newborn mortality: focusing on the 'causes-of-the-causes'. Br Med J 343:d4993. https://doi.org/10.1136/bmj.d4993. Accessed 26 April 2019

Meléndez J, Ochoa J, Villanueva Y et al (1999) Investigation on maternal mortality and women of reproductive age in Honduras: final report corresponding to the year 1997 [in Spanish]. Pan American Health Organization/World Health Organization, Tegucigalpa/Geneva

Mohammed A (2018) Spotlight initiative can make violence against women a thing of the past. European Development Days Forum, Brussels. https://www.un.org/sustainabledevelopment/blog/2018/06/spotlight-initiative-can-make-violence-against-women-a-thing-of-the-past-says-un-deputy-chief-2/

Mojekwu JN, Ibekwe U (2012) Maternal mortality in Nigeria: examination of intervention methods. Int J Humanit Soc Sci 2(20 special issue):135–149

Momentum (2015) Momentum for maternal newborn health. In: Global maternal newborn health conference, Mexico City, 18–21 Oct. https://cdn2.sph.harvard.edu/wpcontent/uploads/sites/44/2016/02/GMNHC_MomentumforMNH_momentum-poster-print-NObleeds3.pdf. Accessed 27 April 2019

Nall R (2018) The history of HIV/AIDS in the United States. Healthline Newsletter. https://www.healthline.com/health/hiv-aids/history#cultural-response. Accessed 27 April 2019

Nanda G, Switlik K, Lule E (2005) Accelerating progress towards achieving the MDG to improve maternal health: a collection of promising approaches. Health, Nutrition & Population Discussion Paper. The International Bank for Reconstruction and Development/The World Bank, Washington, DC, p 20433

Navarro V (2004) The political and social contexts of health. Baywood Publishing, New York

Okwaraji Y, Cousens S, Berhane Y et al (2012) Effect of geographical access to health facilities on child mortality in rural Ethiopia: a community based cross sectional study. PLoS One 7(3):e33564. https://journals.plos.org/plosone/article?id=10.1371/journal.pone.0033564. Accessed 15 May 2019

Raphael D (2009) Social determinants of health, 2nd edn. Canadian Scholar's Press, Toronto

Ravelli A, Jager K, de Groot M et al (2011) Travel time from home to hospital and adverse perinatal outcomes in women at term in the Netherlands. Br J Obstet Gynaecol 118(4):457–465. https://doi.org/10.1111/j.1471-0528.2010.02816.x

Razum O, Jahn A, Reitmaier P et al (1999) Trends in maternal mortality ratio among women of German and non-German nationality in West Germany, 1980-1996. Int J Epidemiol 28:919–924. https://doi.org/10.1093/ije/28.5.919

Royston E, Armstrong S (1989) Preventing maternal deaths. World Health Organization, Geneva

Rudan I, Chan K, Zhang J et al (2010) Causes of deaths in children younger than 5 years in China in 2008. Lancet 375:1083–1089

Schutte J, Steegers E, Schuitnmaker N et al (2010) The Netherlands maternal mortality committee: rise in maternal mortality in the Netherlands. Br J Obstet Gynaecol 117:399–406

Sen A (2015) Universal health coverage – the affordable dream. The Guardian, The Long Read: Health, 6 Jan 2015. https://www.theguardian.com/society/2015/jan/06/-sp-universal-healthcare-the-affordable-dream-amartya-sen

Shiffman J (2007) Generating political priority for maternal mortality reduction in 5 developing countries. Am J Public Health 97:796–803

Shiffman J (2008) Why do some global health initiatives receive political priority while others don't? A conversation with professor Jeremy Shiffman about political advocacy for maternal, newborn and child health. The Partnership for maternal, newborn and child health. https://www.who.int/pmnch/topics/advocacy/jshiffmaninterview_090908/en/. Accessed 26 April 2019

Shiffman J, Stanton C, Salazar AP (2004) The emergence of political priority for safe motherhood in Honduras. Health Policy Plan 19(6):380–390

Sibbald B (2007) The struggle to reduce maternal mortality. Can Med Assoc J 177:243–245

Summers LH (2015) Economists' declaration on universal health coverage. Viewpoint on behalf of 267 signatories. Lancet. https://doi.org/10.1016/S0140-6736(15)00242-1. Accessed 01 May 2019

Thaddeus S, Maine D (1994) Too far to walk: maternal mortality in context. Soc Sci Med 38(8):1091–1110

Tuncalp W, Were W, MacLennan C et al (2015) Quality of care for pregnant women and newborns-the WHO vision. BJOG 122:1045–1049

United Nations (1945a) Charter of the United Nations and statute of the International Court of Justice, San Francisco. https://www.un.org/en/charter-united-nations/. Accessed 30 April 2019

United Nations (1945b) Universal Declaration of Human Rights. United Nations, New York: https://www.un.org/en/universal-declaration-human-rights/index.html. Accessed 30 April 2019

United Nations (1986) Declaration on the right to development. In: United Nations General Assembly, 97th plenary meeting, 4 December. United Nations, New York. https://www.un.org/documents/ga/res/41/a41r128.htm. Accessed 30 April 2019

United Nations (2000) The Millennium Declaration. In: United Nations General Assembly, eighth plenary meeting, 55/2. United Nations, New York. https://www.un.org/millennium/declaration/ares552e.htm. Accessed 30 April 2019

United Nations (2005) 2005 World Summit outcome. In: United Nations General Assembly, eighth plenary meeting, 60/1. United Nations, New York. https://www.un.org/womenwatch/ods/A-RES-60-1-E.pdf. Accessed 30 April 2019

United Nations (2015) Transforming our world: the 2030 agenda for Sustainable Development. In: United Nations General Assembly, fourth plenary meeting, 70/1. United Nations, New York

United Nations (2016) The Sustainable Development Goals report 2016 leaving no one behind. United Nations, New York. https://unstats.un.org/sdgs/report/2016/leaving-no-one-behind. Accessed 29 April 2019

United Nations (2019a) About the Sustainable Development Goals. United Nations, New York. https://www.un.org/sustainabledevelopment/sustainable-development-goals/. Accessed 29 April 2019

United Nations (2019b) Sustainable development goals: partnerships. United Nations, New York. https://www.un.org/sustainabledevelopment/partnerships/. Accessed 29 April 2019

United Nations Development Programme (2019a) Sustainable Development Goals. United Nations Development Programme, New York. https://www.undp.org/content/undp/en/home/sustainable-development-goals.html. Accessed 29 April 2019

United Nations Development Programme (2019b) SDG 3: good health and wellbeing. United Nations Development Programme, New York. https://www.undp.org/content/undp/en/home/sustainable-development-goals/goal-3-good-health-and-well-being.html. Accessed 29 April 2019

United Nations Development Programme (2019c) Transforming our world: the 2030 Agenda for sustainable development. United Nations Development Programme, New York. https://sustainabledevelopment.un.org/post2015/transformingourworld. Accessed 30 April 2019

United Nations Population Fund (2011) State of the world's midwifery: delivering health, saving lives. A United Nations publication

United Nations Population Fund (2014a) State of the world's midwifery: a universal pathway to women's health. A United Nations publication

United Nations Population Fund (2014b) Ebola wiping out gains in safe motherhood. Press release 17 October. https://esaro.unfpa.org/news/ebola-wiping-out-gains-safe-motherhood. Accessed 27 April 2019

United Nations Universal Declaration of Human Rights (1948) https://www.jus.uio.no/lm/en/pdf/un.universal.declaration.of.human.rights.1948.portrait.letter.pdf [last accessed 05.11.2020]

Wang YP, Lei M, Li D et al (2010) A study on rural-urban differences in neonatal mortality rate in China, 1996-2006. J Epidemiol Community Health 64:935–936

World Bank (2019) Lifetime risk of maternal death. The World Bank, New York. Derived from WHO, UNICEF, UNFPA, World Bank Group, and the United Nations Population Division. Trends in Maternal Mortality: 1990 to 2015. World Health Organization, Geneva, 2015 https://data.worldbank.org/indicator/SH.MMR.RISK. Accessed 01 May 2019

World Economic Forum (2015) Are the new health development goals realistic? World Economic Forum. https://www.weforum.org/agenda/2015/09/are-the-new-health-development-goals-realistic. Accessed 01 May 2019

World Health Organization (2012) Trends in maternal mortality: 1990–2010. World Health Organization, Geneva

World Health Organization (2017a) Zika virus and complications: 2016 public health emergency of international concern. World Health Organization, Geneva. https://www.who.int/emergencies/zika-virus-tmp/en/. Accessed 27 April 2019

World Health Organization (2017b) Malaria in pregnant women. World Health Organization, Geneva. https://www.who.int/malaria/areas/high_risk_groups/pregnancy/en/. Accessed 27.04.2019

World Health Organization (2018) Maternal mortality: key facts. World Health Organization, Geneva. https://www.who.int/en/news-room/fact-sheets/detail/maternal-mortality. Accessed 25 April 2019

World Health Organization (2019) The goals within a goal: Health targets for SDG3. World Health Organization, Geneva. https://www.who.int/sdg/targets/en/. Accessed 29 April 2019

Global Maternal and Newborn Health

2

Expected Learning Outcomes

By the end of the chapter, the reader should be able to:

1. Describe the global initiatives which have contributed to making childbirth safer
2. Discuss issues surrounding stillbirth and perinatal morbidity which need to be addressed
3. Discuss some of the successes and challenges engendered by Millennium Development Goals 4 and 5
4. Identify the key approaches which have enabled some countries to make considerable progress in reducing avoidable deaths and disability
5. Discuss the importance of the increasing evidence placed on mental health in the context of childbirth

2.1 The Launch of the Safe Motherhood Initiative

Although progress had been made in many high-income countries, it was not until the latter part of the twentieth century that the persistently appalling levels of maternal mortality worldwide gained acknowledgement on the international agenda. At an interregional meeting of the World Health Organization (WHO) in 1985, Dr. Mahmoud Fathalla brought the avoidable tragedy of maternal mortality into focus as he related the story of 'Mrs X' and considered various strands of inquiry into her death. He questioned why this woman, who could have represented women in many countries across the world, had died. Fathalla emphasised that the causes of maternal mortality were complex but that there were several places along the 'Road to Maternal Death' where the eponymous Mrs. X could have been helped during her journey to access 'exits' from that fatal road; her life could have been saved (WHO 1986) (see Fig. 2.1).

Following an analysis of maternal deaths in nine countries, when investigators evaluated whether maternal deaths could be prevented, it was concluded that from 88 to 98% of all such fatalities could probably have been avoided. This was established using standards deemed realistic in the circumstances and not through any aspirations towards idealism. A firm conviction emerged from this interregional meeting that a major new initiative should be instigated to prevent maternal deaths (WHO 1986). So, the Safe Motherhood Initiative (SMI) was launched at a conference in Nairobi, Kenya (WHO 1987). This agenda escalated across continents, and by 1992, every region had held a Safe Motherhood confer-

---

© Springer Nature Switzerland AG 2021
J. Kemp et al., *Global Midwifery: Principles, Policy and Practice*,
https://doi.org/10.1007/978-3-030-46765-4_2

Fig. 2.1 The road to
maternal death. (Derived
from WHO 1986)

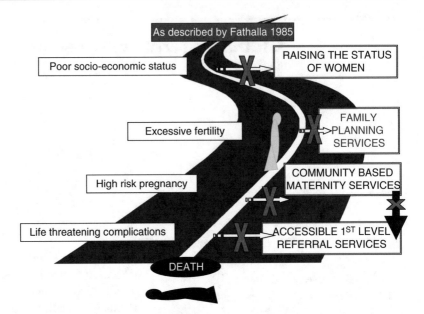

ence (Otea 1992). The story of Mrs. X has been
updated (Fathalla 2012), but the road to maternal
death still exists in every country, and there are
women who will always need to be able to access
its exits.

As the SMI gained momentum, a range of
low-income countries offered considerable evidence, suggesting that discernible decreases in
maternal deaths were attainable through simple,
cost-effective interventions made in environments experiencing political support (Danel
1999; Koblinsky 2003). Examples include
Bolivia, China, Egypt, Honduras, Jamaica and
Zimbabwe. Evidence of similar improvements
starting even earlier than the launch of the SMI
was identified. From as early as 1930 up until
1995, progress was observed in Malaysia and Sri
Lanka. The success of the national plans in both
these countries has been attributed to some strategic approaches. In particular, political commitment demonstrating continued support was
deemed crucial, along with a comprehensive
reinforcement of national infrastructure. Poor,
underserved areas became priorities in this process. Significant investments were made in
improving maternal health services, and expansion of the roles of nurse-midwives facilitated
increased access to skilled care (Pathmanathan
et al. 2003; Shiffman and Smith 2007). During
this time, the total fertility rate (TFR) fell signifi-

cantly in both these countries (Martins et al.
2003). In Sri Lanka, improving the status of
women which resulted in their high standing in
society was a key factor in improving maternal
health outcomes. This comprised free education
for all, equality in access to education for girls,
improving female literacy and increasing the age
of marriage (Liljestrand and Gryboski 2002).

It soon became apparent that progress was
unlikely without the commitment of national
governments. In less than two decades from the
launch of the SMI, Fathalla had challenged the
world again by stating that not only *could* wom-
en's lives be saved but whether they *should* be
saved rested on the principle as to whether their
lives were considered worth saving (Fathalla
2006). By the turn of the millennium, safe motherhood had evolved not only as a medical, obstetric or social matter but increasingly as a human
rights issue (Magowe 1995; Cook 1997;
Liljestrand and Gryboski 2002; AbouZahr 2003;
Fathalla 2006). It was stressed that:

> A human rights strategy can help increase the
> long-overdue emphasis on women's right to choose
> when to have a child and to experience safe moth-
> erhood, by increasing government accountability
> to provide adequate reproductive health services.
> (Liljestrand and Gryboski 2002:122)

Gradually the world began to realise how
potent was the question raised by Fathalla and

cited above. Women's lives *should* be saved; they have a right to survive their most natural function, and they have a right to health and well-being. However, it was not until 2014 that it was formally recognised that midwives were the key to saving lives (UNFPA 2014). It took until 2019 for the world to commit to strengthening midwifery education for this specific purpose (WHO 2019a), and this is further discussed in Chapter 4. The inability to recognise the critical role of midwives in reducing maternal mortality no doubt frustrated efforts to achieve MDG 5 and this is discussed below.

2.2   The Millennium Development Goals

At the turn of the century, the Millennium Development Goals (MDGs) were initiated (Fig. 2.2) (UN 2000). These goals provided a comprehensive approach to the dilemma of maternal mortality as well as addressing numerous other issues that impede progress in low-income countries. MDG 5 aimed to 'improve maternal health', and two targets were identified: firstly to 'reduce by three quarters, between 1990 and 2015, the maternal mortality ratio' and sec-

ondly to 'achieve by 2015 universal access to reproductive health' (WHO 2015). The identified target of MDG 4 was to reduce child mortality by three quarters, between 1990 and 2015.

It was soon recognised that attempts to improve maternal health and reduce mortality (MDG 5) were linked to other MDGs, particularly MDGs 1, 3, 4 and 6 (Filippi et al. 2006). The goals associated with reducing poverty, empowering women and addressing infections such as HIV/AIDS and malaria could not be separated from MDG 5 and improving the health of women would without doubt improve child health and survival (MDG 4). Hence, MDG 5 was considered pivotal in moving towards the other global goals at this time (Maclean 2010) (Fig. 2.3).

So much was yet to be achieved as the target date for the attainment of the MDGs approached in 2015. At that time undoubtedly the 'Road to Maternal Death' still existed in every country. As the new millennium dawned women in the poorest parts of the world still had no means or 'exits' to facilitate their escape from this distressing road that terminated in death.

In 2005, more than half a million women were still estimated to lose their lives giving birth; 99% of these were living in low-income countries. Fourteen countries reported MMRs of at least

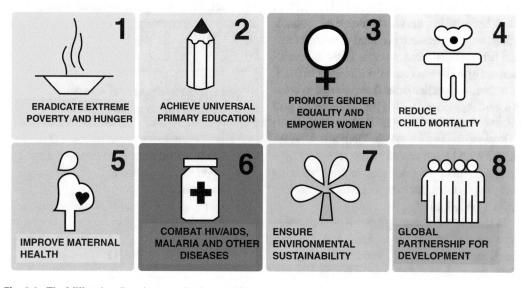

Fig. 2.2 The Millennium Development Goals (UN 2000)

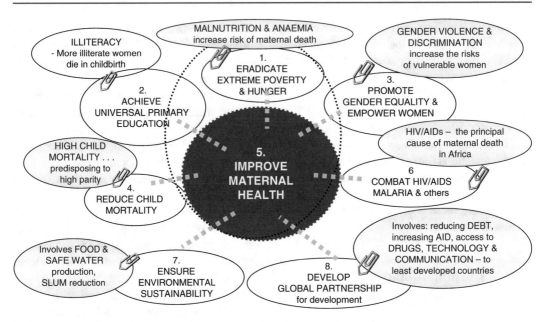

Fig. 2.3 MDG 5 plays a pivotal role in global development. (Maclean 2010 derived from UN 2000; Save the Children 2009; UNICEF 2009)

1000, and 13 of these were in sub-Saharan Africa. Sierra Leone topped the list with an MMR of 2100, and Niger and Afghanistan were close behind with 1800 (WHO 2007). It was estimated that a third of the total numbers of maternal deaths across the world took pace in India and Nigeria, and ten countries accounted for two-thirds of all maternal deaths. Between 1990 and 2005, an analysis of trends showed that globally, MMR decreased at an annual average rate of less than 1%. However, in sub-Saharan Africa, the area burdened by the highest figures, this decrease occurred at a rate of less than 0.1%. It had been estimated that an annual decrease of 5.5% was crucial in achieving MDG 5. Therefore, this decline would have needed to occur at a much greater rate if the fifth millennium goal was to be realised (WHO 2007).

Representatives of WHO, UNICEF, UNFPA and the World Bank vowed in September 2008, to strengthen their support to countries showing least progress in order to hasten efforts to achieve MDG 5 (WHO 2008).

In spite of the daunting overall picture, there were success stories in maternal and newborn health too. Between 1990 and 2012, the global MMR decreased by 47%, and in the decade preceding 2012, the number of births attended by skilled health professionals increased from 55 to 63%. During this period, the percentage of women who received antenatal care increased from 63 to 80%. The annual decline in MMR exceeded 5.5% in some countries during the first decade of the twenty-first century (WHO 2016a). In a systematic analysis of the progress made towards MDG 5, four 'powerful drivers' of maternal mortality have been observed to influence improvement (Hogan et al. 2010) (Box 2.1).

Box 2.1. The four powerful drivers influencing improvement in MMR

- Reduction in total fertility rate (TFR)
- Rising income per head of population
- Improving maternal educational attainment
- Increase in coverage of skilled attendance at delivery

Hogan et al. (2010:11)

In 2015 in preparation for the launch of the Sustainable Development Goals (SDGs), it was claimed that there were 15 million success stories related to the MDGs which could be measured in lives saved. Furthermore, although these victories were global victories, the majority occurred in sub-Saharan Africa (McArthur 2015). The SDGs were designed based on the successes of the MDGs (UNDP 2019), and these latest global goals are discussed in Chapter 1.

2.3 The Launch of Skilled Attendance Initiatives

Whether a woman experienced skilled attendance at birth was one of the process indicators used to measure progress towards achieving MDG 5 (UN 2000). Along with other recommendations coming out of a Technical Consultation in Sri Lanka in 1997, 'skilled attendance at delivery' was high on the list of priorities to be addressed if childbirth was to become safe for women across the globe (Box 2.2) (FCI 1999).

Box 2.2. Recommendations of the 1997 Technical Consultation on Safe Motherhood, Sri Lanka
Ensure skilled attendance at delivery
    Delay marriage and first birth
    Realise the power of partnerships
    Prevent unwanted pregnancy and address unsafe abortion
    Measure progress
    Improve access to good quality maternal health services
    Recognise that every pregnancy faces risks
    FCI (1999)

At the beginning of the twenty-first century, therefore, the Safe Motherhood Initiative (SMI) of 1987 was followed by a new initiative to promote skilled attendance at birth. This specified professionally skilled birth attendants, to practise within an 'enabling environment'. The definition of these birth attendants has been revised several times; they are health professionals who must be able to provide quality care, identify and manage complications or refer these women and/or their newborns to a higher level of care (Box 2.3) (WHO 2018a).

Box 2.3. Definition of skilled birth attendants
Skilled health personnel, as referenced by SDG indicator 3.1.2, are competent maternal and newborn health (MNH) professionals educated, trained and regulated to national and international standards. They are competent to:

(a) Provide and promote evidence-based, human rights–based, quality, socio-culturally sensitive and dignified care to women and newborns
(b) Facilitate physiological processes during labour and delivery to ensure a clean and positive childbirth experience
(c) Identify and manage or refer women and/or newborns with complications

In addition, as part of an integrated team of MNH professionals (including midwives, nurses, obstetricians, paediatricians and anaesthetists), they perform all signal functions of emergency maternal and newborn care to optimize the health and well-being of women and newborns. Within an enabling environment, midwives trained to International Confederation of Midwives (ICM) standards can provide nearly all of the essential care needed for women and newborns.[1]
    WHO (2018a)

---

[1]In different countries, these competencies are held by professionals with varying occupational titles.

Significant reductions in maternal mortality have been noted in countries where women have gained access to skilled attendance at birth with available Emergency Obstetric Care (EOC) facilities and access to family planning. Examples of such successes are evident in several countries including China, Cuba, Jamaica, Malaysia, Sri Lanka, Thailand and Tunisia. Many of these countries managed to reduce their maternal deaths by half during the decade preceding the end of the twentieth century. It has been contended that professionally trained midwives have been central to this progress and that a dearth of skilled midwives had impeded progress in many regions (UNICEF/WHO/UNFPA 1997). It became evident that the 73 countries that carried the major burden of maternal and perinatal mortality were served by less than 42% of the world's physicians, midwives and nurses (UNFPA 2014).

It had been observed in the late twentieth century that MMR fell to <200 where skilled attendance was evident at >80% of births (World Bank 1999). However, traditional birth attendants (TBAs) continued to provide an essential service in many parts of the world. It became very evident that in spite of the ideal, achieving skilled care for all was an impracticable goal in many countries. In low-income countries, rural neighbourhoods and the urban poor were obliged to depend on TBAs as their only source of assistance when giving birth (Bergström and Goodburn 2001). Demographic health survey analyses from 22 countries in sub-Saharan Africa provide evidence that only one country, Botswana, provided skilled care during >75% of births (Stanton et al. 1997). Eight categories of healthcare workers have been acknowledged as providing sexual, reproductive, maternal and newborn health care (SRMNH) (Box 2.4) and accurately estimating the level of skilled attendance which these personnel provide has proved challenging (UNFPA 2014).

- Nurse-midwives
- Nurses
- Auxiliary (midwives)
- Auxiliary (nurses)
- Associate clinicians
- Physician generalists
- Obstetric-gynaecologists
- Nurse-midwife technicians
- Maternal and Child Health Aids

HSSE (2009), Holman (2012), UNFPA (2014:9), UNICEF (2016)

The word 'skilled' replaced the categorisation of 'trained' as it was agreed that the latter could not necessarily be equated with the former (Starrs 1997). For some considerable time, it has been questioned how 'skilled' the skilled attendants actually are (Harvey et al. 2007), and so much is needed to be done to ensure quality as well as quantity in educating competent professionals for safe practice. In some countries, it was discovered that some of the individuals termed 'skilled' were actually not skilled at all (Kruk et al. 2018; Radovich et al. 2019). Hence, the need to specify that 'skilled' refers to those educated to competency in specific life-saving midwifery competencies.

However, the skilled attendant has been clearly defined (Box 2.3) and TBAs have never been included in the official definition (WHO 2018a).

Some countries have demonstrated progress where TBAs and midwives collaborate in order to provide safer outcomes for women and newborns. In the Democratic Republic of Congo, the collaboration between midwives and TBAs in health centres in rural districts has produced considerable change in maternal health outcomes. Specifically, more women attend health facilities and are assisted by midwives; TBAs have received basic training, and they support midwives sharing their workload, thus enabling them to focus on providing quality care (Baba 2018). In Guatemala, the collaboration has received mixed reviews, some TBAs reporting increased confidence and others perceiving the

Box 2.4. Ten broad categories of healthcare workers providing sexual, reproductive, maternal and newborn health (SRMNH) care
- Midwives

skilled workers in their community with suspicion (Fonesca-Becker et al. 2004). Since 1973, collaborative working between TBAs and skilled birth attendants in Malaysia was apparent and resulted in improving poor relationships as the role of TBAs was gradually modified to become 'a more exclusively family supportive role' (Koblinsky et al. 1999:402). In a number of countries, TBAs have been made to feel unwelcome in health facilities (Fonesca-Becker et al. 2004). However, in Mexico and Peru, relationships between the two cadres were seen to improve when culturally appropriate models of care were used along with a broad participatory approach, TBAs functioning as birth companions, providing massage and ensuring the labouring women received adequate fluids (Braine 2008; Gabrysch et al. 2009). Clearly education of the skilled birth attendants as well as the TBAs and communities has been found to be instrumental in removing barriers and enabling effective collaboration (Miller and Smith 2017).

Although the MDG and skilled attendance objectives had not been realised globally, by 2015 the number of births attended by skilled healthcare professionals had increased to 79%, and the global MMR had decreased to 216 per 100,000 live births (UNFPA 2019). There were clearly achievements, but challenges remained.

2.4   Change of Focus

Increasingly during the twenty-first century, emphasis has been laid not only on reducing maternal mortality but also on the reduction of morbidity, stillbirth and perinatal morbidity. Whilst there have been measures of success in reducing maternal mortality, it had been recognised that for every death there are a number of severe morbidities or 'near misses' (WHO 2010). Maternal mortality has often been described as 'Just the Tip of the Iceberg', so that there is a vast base representing maternal morbidity remaining largely *un-described'* (Marwah and Sharma 2017:1703).

In high-income countries, changing demographics and demands have contributed to co-morbidities with hypertension, diabetes, cardiac disease and increased caesarean section rates due in part to the increase in advanced maternal age, obesity and multiple pregnancies (Shamshirsaz and Dildy 2018). In low-income countries, the process of analysing 'near misses', namely those who have recovered from life-threatening complications, has become a useful instrument in developing evidence-based protocols in providing care for these women (Say et al. 2004; Marwah and Sharma 2017; Adulojo et al. 2018). Morbidities can be associated with prolonged and obstructed labour resulting in ruptured uterus, vesico-vaginal fistula and postpartum haemorrhage, conditions rarely seen in high-income countries (Mcgeady and Mutabingwa 2014). Thromboembolic and hypertensive complications (Cromwell and Paidas 2018) and those associated with unsafe abortion (WHO 2019b) also threaten the lives of women worldwide.

It has been acknowledged that the 'neglected tragedy of stillbirths' which was not addressed specifically in the Millennium Development Goals (MDGs) remains absent from the Sustainable Development Goals (SDGs) (WHO 2016b). More than two and a half million stillbirths occur each year, the highest proportion of these (98%) occur in low- and middle-income countries, with sub-Saharan Africa and South Asia accounting for 75% of these deaths. It is estimated that at the present rate, 160 years will elapse before a woman in Africa has the same chance of her baby being born alive as her counterpart in a high-income country, and even in the latter stillbirth rates vary and are far from acceptable. Furthermore, like maternal mortality, stillbirths are deemed to be largely preventable and appropriate key interventions could save 1.5 million lives a year (Frøen et al. 2016; WHO 2019b).

A global strategy for women's, children's and adolescents' health has been identified in order to address the post 2015 agenda. The strategy aspires that this significant proportion of the world population should, as a human right, be enabled to survive, to thrive and to transform. This initiative seeks to unlock human potential across the life course through improvements in health and well-being and is central to the 'every woman every child' drive (WHO 2018b:40). In

Fig. 2.4 Addressing the challenges. (Derived from WHO 2018b)

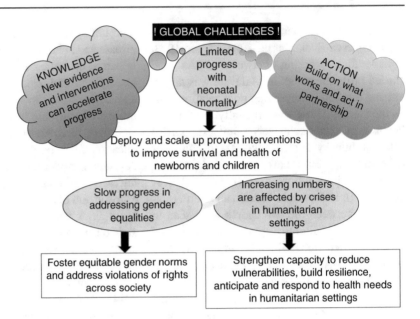

launching the strategy, Dr. Ban Ki Moon on behalf of the United Nations maintained that:

> No woman, child or adolescent should face a greater risk of preventable death because of where they live or who they are. (UN 2015:5)

There remain many challenges that confront the global community, but it is purported that these can and must be addressed using available knowledge and taking appropriate action. Some examples of pertinent issues which challenge the 2030 agenda and impact on maternal and perinatal health are summarised in Fig. 2.4.

2.5 A Further Shift in Emphasis

Making childbirth safer has thus experienced several transitions until the emphasis on well-being rather than mortality and morbidity has emerged during the early decades of the twenty-first century. The Sustainable Development Goals (SDGs) with their aspiration towards 'good health and well-being' (Chapter 1) have caused a further modification in the focus of achieving safe and satisfying birthing experiences. The endeavour that women, children and adolescents should not only survive but thrive and furthermore experience and facilitate transformation

(UN 2015) has helped lift the target beyond mortality and morbidity to health and well-being.

The organisation 'Women Deliver' has emerged as one global advocate for the health, rights and well-being of girls and women. With the establishment of its Young Leaders Programme in 2010, there have been efforts to 'elevate the incredible potential and passion of young advocates by providing them with skills-building training and access to platforms for them to share their voices and experiences' (WD 2019). The topic of leadership is further developed in Chapter 11.

A global well-being index of women and children has been compiled annually by Save the Children from 2000 until 2015. It is estimated using five indicators, namely maternal and children's health, along with educational attainment, economic well-being and political participation (SC 2015). The index identified Sweden at the top of the list in 2009 with Norway in the second place followed by Australia, whilst Niger rated the lowest of all. Chad preceded Sierra Leone at the lowest end of the list (Save the Children 2009). By 2015, Scandinavian countries had procured the top five places in the Index. Somalia was placed last preceded by Niger, Mali, Central African Republic and the Democratic Republic of Congo (SC 2015:9) (Fig. 2.5).

Top 10: Best places to be a mother	Lowest 10: Worst places to be a mother
1. Norway	169. Haiti, Sierra Leone
2. Finland	171. Guinea-Bisseau
3. Iceland	172. Chad
4. Denmark	173. Cote d'Ivore
5. Sweden	174. Gambia
6. Netherlands	175. Niger
7. Spain	176. Mali
8. Germany	177. Central African Republic
9. Australia	178. DR Congo
10. Belgium	179. Somalia

Fig. 2.5 Mothers' index 2015 rankings (Save the Children 2015)

By the early part of the twenty-first century, greater emphasis had been placed on maternal mental health as well as physical well-being. Worldwide it has been estimated that 10% of women experience mental health issues during pregnancy and 13% in the early postnatal period. However, in low-income countries, these figures rise to 15.6% and 19.8%, respectively. Depression is the predominant problem in most of these cases with suicide presenting a real risk and serious impairment of children's growth and development, resulting from maternal mental ill health (WHO 2019c). WHO published a comprehensive mental health action plan 2013–2020 which was adopted by the 66th World Health Assembly. The initiative focuses international attention on a problem that has been neglected for centuries and is resolutely embedded in human rights principles. It calls for changes in the attitudes that isolate sufferers, propagating discrimination and stigmatising them. There is a call to expand services promoting more effective and efficient use of resources to this end (WHO 2019d).

2.6 Conclusion

The attainment of maternal and perinatal physical and mental health and well-being continues to challenge the international community. Addressing maternal morbidity and perinatal mortality and morbidity is becoming a key issue alongside maternal health. Much progress has been made, but much remains to be done. Enshrined in the principles of human rights and

underpinned by political commitment, women and families should be able not only to survive but thrive and transform their own communities. Midwives are critical to the process of promoting and maintaining maternal and newborn health across the globe.

Key Messages

Principles

The shift away from the focus on mortality towards the principles of good health and well-being as a human right which extends to every person, even the most vulnerable, continues to emerge. Midwives can be instrumental in promoting the principles that address preventable deaths and so contribute significantly towards transforming the global community in the context of the 2030 agenda.

Policy

Maternal and neonatal healthcare policies should be enshrined in the human rights agenda. Policies should promote and enable a woman's right to choose and a midwife's right to practice in an enabling clinical and political environment.

Practice

Midwifery care should provide holistic physical and mental/emotional woman-centred care. Whilst evidence-based practice provided by skilled midwives should above all be safe; it should also be satisfying and supportive in order to promote optimum maternal and newborn health and well-being.

Questions for Reflection or Review
1. Look again at Box 2.1. What issues lie beneath these 'powerful drivers' that need to be considered by clinicians and policymakers in implementing a local or national strategy for change?
2. Consider some of the examples of collaboration between midwives and TBAs

cited in this chapter. What needs to be done so that such partnerships could best contribute to effective SRMNH care in an area with which you are familiar?

3. Reflect on the WHO mental health action plan 2013–2030 (WHO 2019d). What basic changes need to be made in order to improve attitudes towards those suffering the stigma of mental ill health? Consider ways of making practical changes in an area with which you are familiar.

Additional Resources for Reflection and Further Study

Look at the UNFPA website: https://www.unfpa.org/swop-2019 regarding 'Unfinished business'. Consider some of the questions posed and suggest how the obstacles of women still not reaching the full potential in their lives could be removed? Are these the same obstacles that prevented Mrs. X cited above from exiting the Road to Maternal Death (see Fig. 2.1)?

Go to the WHO website and download the WHO safe childbirth checklist at https://www.who.int/patient-safety/topics/safe-childbirth/childbirth/en/. Then look at the WHO report on 'Learning from implementation of the WHO safe childbirth checklist'. https://www.who.int/patientsafety/topics/safe-childbirth/consultation2017/en/

Review the experiences shared by the participants, looking particularly at the lessons learned and the barriers to implementation and success. Consider how this learning could be transferred to an area with which you are familiar. Go to the 'Women Deliver' website and consider the 'Deliver for Good' initiative which is 'an evidence-based advocacy and communications push to promote the health, rights, and wellbeing of girls and women'. Identify at least one of the 'investment areas' and consider how the call to action could be initiated in an area with which you are familiar. https://womendeliver.org/deliver-for-good/view-briefs/

Liljestrand J and Gryboski K (2002) Women who die needlessly: maternal mortality as a human rights issue. Article 12, p 122. Reproductive Health and Rights—Reaching the Hardly Reached. pp 121–128

UN (2015) The Global Strategy for Women's, Children's and Adolescents' Health 2016–2030, Every Woman, Every Child, United Nations https://www.who.int/life-course/partners/global-strategy/ewec-globalstrategyreport-200915.pdf?ua=1

References

AbouZahr C (2003) Safe motherhood: a brief history of the global movement 1947-2003. Br Med Bull 67(1):13–25

Adulojo AP, Aduloju T, Oluwadare MI (2018) Profile of maternal near miss and determinant factors in a teaching hospital in Southwestern Nigeria. Int J Obstet Gynaecol Res 5(1):598–617

Baba A (2018) A midwives and traditional birth attendants collaboration in rural north eastern DR Congo: a complementing strategy where there are few qualified midwives. Rebuild Consortium: research for stronger health systems during and after crisis. https://rebuildconsortium.com/blog-news/blogs/2018/midwives-and-traditional-birth-attendants-collaborate-in-dr-congo/. Accessed 18 April 2019

Bergström S and Goodburn E (2001) The role of traditional birth attendants in the reduction of maternal mortality. In: DeBrouwere V, Van Lerberghe W (eds). Safe Motherhood strategies: a review of the evidence, vol. 17. Studies in Health Services Organization & Policy, pp 77–96.

Braine T (2008) Mexico's midwives enter the mainstream. Bull World Health Organ 86(4):244–245

Cook R (1997) Advance safe motherhood through human rights. Presentation at the Safe Motherhood Technical Consultation, Sri Lanka, 18–23 October. The Safe Motherhood Action Agenda: priorities for the next decade. Family Care International, New York

Cromwell C, Paidas M (2018) Haematologic changes in pregnancy, chap. 151. In: Haematology, 7th edn. Elsevier, Amsterdam

Danel I (1999) Maternal mortality reduction, Honduras, 1990-1997: a case-study. The World Bank, Washington, DC, p 566

Family Care International (1999) Report on the safe motherhood technical consultation (18–23 October 1997, Colombo, Sri Lanka). Final report on the program to mark the tenth anniversary of the Safe Motherhood Initiative. Safe Motherhood Inter-Agency Group. Family Care International, New York

Fathalla MF (2006) Human rights aspects of Safe Motherhood. Best Prac Res Clin Obstet Gynaecol 20(3):409–419

Fathalla MF (2012) On Safe Motherhood at 25 years: looking back, moving forward. Hands on for mothers and babies. https://www.birmingham.ac.uk/Documents/heroes/on-safe-motherhood-fathalla.pdf. Accessed 14 April 2020

Filippi V, Ronsmans C, Campbell OM et al (2006) Maternal health in poor countries, the broader context and a call for action. Maternal survival 5. Lancet 368:1535–1541

Fonesca-Becker F, Ainslie R, Borda M et al (2004) Impact Evaluation: Community Mobilization and Behavior Change, Maternal and Neonatal Health Component, Ministry of Health and Public Assistance. Baltimore: Johns Hopkins Bloomberg School of Public Health Center for Communication Programs.

Frøen JF, Friberg IK, Lawn JE et al (2016) Stillbirths: progress and unfinished business. Lancet Ending Preventable Stillbirths Series study group. https://doi.org/10.1016/S0140-6736(15)00818-1. Accessed 08 April 2019

Gabrysch S, Lema C, Bedrinana E et al (2009) Cultural adaptation of birthing services in rural Ayacucho, Peru. Bull World Health Organ 87(9):724–729

Harvey S, Ayabaca P, Bucagu M et al (2007) Are skilled birth attendants really skilled? A measurement method, some disturbing results and a potential way forward. Bull World Health Organ 85(10):733–820

Health System Strengthening for Equity (HSSE) (2009) Who is doing what? Performance of the emergency obstetric signal functions by non-physician clinicians and nurse midwives in Malawi, Mozambique and Tanzania. Health System Strengthening for Equity; Global Resource Center. https://www.hrhresourcecenter.org/node/4113.html. Accessed 17 July 2020

Hogan MC, Foreman KJ, Naghavi M et al (2010) Maternal mortality for 181 countries 1980–2008: a systematic analysis of progress towards Millennium Development Goal 5. Lancet 375(9726):1609–1623

Holman J (2012) The role of nurse midwife technicians in task shifting in Malawi. MPH thesis, University of Washington

Koblinsky M (ed) (2003) Reducing maternal mortality: learning from Bolivia, China, Egypt, Honduras, Jamaica, and Zimbabwe, vol 567. The World Bank, Washington, DC

Koblinsky MA, Campbell O, Heilchelheim J (1999) Organizing delivery care: what works for safe motherhood? Bull World Health Organ 77(5):399–406

Kruk ME Gage A, Arsenault C et al (2018) High-quality health systems in the Sustainable Development Goals era: time for a revolution. The Lancet Global Health Commission. https://www.thelancet.com/action/showPdf?pii=S2214-109X%2818%2930386-3. Accessed 14 April 2020

Liljestrand J, Gryboski K (2002) Women who die needlessly: maternal mortality as a human rights issue. Article 12, p 122. Reproductive Health and Rights—Reaching the Hardly Reached, pp 121–128

Maclean GD (2010) An historical overview of the first two decades of striving towards Safe Motherhood. Sex Reprod Healthcare 1(1):7–14

Magowe M (1995) Using a human rights framework to promote Safe Motherhood. Paper presented at an ICM regional conference for Africa

Martins JM, Pathmanathan I, Liljstrand J et al (2003) Investing in maternal health; learning from Malaysia and Sri Lanka. World Bank. ISBN: 0-8213-5362-4

Marwah S, Sharma M (2017) Maternal near miss review: a brief appraisal. Int J Reprod Contracep Obstetr Gynaecol 6(5):1703–1706

McArthur J (2015) 15 million success stories under the Millennium Development Goals. Brookings Institution, Washington, DC. https://www.brookings.edu/blog/up-front/2015/09/24/15-million-success-stories-under-the-millennium-development-goals/. Accessed 05 April 2019

Mcgeady R, Mutabingwa T (2014) Obstetrics in the tropics, chap 79. In: Farrer et al (eds) Manson's tropical infectious diseases, 23rd edn. Elsevier, Amsterdam, pp 1170–1196

Miller T and Smith H (2017) Establishing partnership with traditional birth attendants for improved maternal and newborn health: a review of factors influencing implementation. BMC Pregnancy Childbirth. BMC series 17:365. https://doi.org/10.1186/s12884-017-1534-y. Accessed 18 April 2019

Otea K (1992) Progress and prospects: the Safe Motherhood Initiative 1987-1992. Family Care International, New York

Pathmanathan I, Liljestrand J, Martins J et al (2003) Investing in maternal health: learning from Malaysia and Sri Lanka, vol 568. The World Bank, Washington, DC

Radovich E, Benova L, Penn-Kekana L et al (2019) 'Who assisted with the delivery of (NAME)?' Issues in estimating skilled birth attendant coverage through population-based surveys and implications for improving global tracking. BMJ Glob Health. https://gh.bmj.com/content/bmjgh/4/2/e001367.full.pdf. Accessed 14 April 2020

Save the Children (2009) Mothers index 2009. Connecticut: Save the Children.

Save the Children (2015) The urban disadvantage: state of the World's Mothers 2015. Save the Children, London

Say L, Betran AP, Villar J et al (2004) WHO systematic review of maternal morbidity and mortality: the prevalence of severe and acute maternal morbidity (near miss). Reprod Health 1(1):3. https://doi.org/10.1186/1742-4755-1-3

Shamshirsaz AA, Dildy GA (2018) Reducing maternal mortality and severe maternal morbidity: the role of critical care. Clin Obstet Gynaecol 61(2):359–371. https://doi.org/10.1097/GRF.0000000000000370. Accessed 08 April 2019

Shiffman J, Smith S (2007) Generation of political priority for global health initiatives: a framework and case study of maternal mortality. Lancet 370(9595):1370–1379

Stanton C, Abderrahim N and Hill K (1997) DHS Maternal Mortality Indicators: An Assessment of Data Quality and Implications for Data Use. DHS Analytical Reports No. 4. Calverton, Maryland: Macro International Inc.

Starrs A (1997) The Safe Motherhood Action Agenda: priorities for the next decade. Inter-Agency Group for Safe Motherhood and Family Care International, New York

UNICEF/WHO/UNFPA (1997) Guidelines for monitoring the availability and use of obstetric services. UNFPA, New York

UNICEF (2009) The State of the World's Children 2009. UNICEF, New York

United Nations (2000) UN millennium declaration. United Nations, New York

United Nations (2015) The global strategy for women's, Children's and Adolescents' Health 43-2030, Every Woman, Every Child, United Nations

United Nations Children's Fund (2016) At a glance: Sierra Leone. https://www.unicef.org/infobycountry/sierra-leone_89966.html. Accessed 22 May 2019

United Nations Development Programme (2019) Transforming our world: the 2030 Agenda for sustainable development. United Nations Development Programme, New York. https://sustainabledevelopment.un.org/post2015/transformingourworld. Accessed 02 May 2019

United Nations Population Fund (2014) State of the world's midwifery: a universal pathway to women's health. A United Nations publication

United Nations Population Fund (2019) World population. https://www.unfpa.org/data/world-population-dashboard. Accessed 24 April 2019

Women Deliver (2019) Women Deliver. http://womendeliver.org/about/our-history/. Accessed 12 April 2019

World Bank (1999) Safe motherhood and the World Bank: Lessons from 10 Years of Experience. Washington: The World Bank.

World Health Organization (1986) Maternal mortality: helping women off the road to death. WHO Chron 40(5):175–183

World Health Organization (1987) Safe Motherhood Initiative (SMI). Preventing the tragedy of maternal deaths. A report of the international Safe Motherhood conference, Nairobi, Kenya. WHO, Geneva

World Health Organization (2007) Maternal mortality in 2005. Estimates developed by WHO, UNICEF, UNFPA & the World Bank. WHO, Geneva

World Health Organization (2008) Joint statement on maternal & newborn health by WHO, UNICEF, UNFPA, WB, 25 Sept 2008

World Health Organization (2010) Maternal near miss and maternal death in the World Health Organization's 2005 global survey on maternal and perinatal health. Bull World Health Organ 88(2):81–160

World Health Organization (2015) MDG 5: improve maternal health. Reviewed 2015. https://www.who.int/topics/millennium_development_goals/maternal_health/en/. Accessed 05 April 2019

World Health Organization (2016a) Maternal mortality fact sheet: key facts. World Health Organization, Geneva. http://apps.who.int/mediacentre/factsheets/fs348/en/index.html. Accessed 24 April 2019

World Health Organization (2016b) The neglected tragedy of stillbirths. World Health Organization, Geneva. https://www.who.int/reproductivehealth/topics/maternal_perinatal/stillbirth/Lancet-series/en/. Accessed 10 May 2019

World Health Organization (2018a) Definition of skilled health personnel providing care during childbirth: the 2018 joint statement by WHO, UNFPA, UNICEF, ICM, ICN, FIGO and IPA. Department of Reproductive Health, World Health Organization, Geneva

World Health Organization (2018b) Survive, thrive, transform global strategy for women's, children's and adolescents' health (2016–2030) 2018 monitoring report: current status and strategic priorities. https://www.who.int/life-course/partners/global-strategy/global-strategy-2018-monitoring-report.pdf. Accessed 14 April 2020

World Health Organization (2019a) Strengthening quality midwifery education for Universal Health Coverage 2030: framework for action. https://www.who.int/maternal_child_adolescent/topics/quality-of-care/midwifery/strengthening-midwifery-education/en/?fbclid=IwAR3MxPIdgIbRAhzFn1c9-kbIagvp-WUY7VRgdAlMKI0FYHEg7W8eJ-k11WY. Accessed 22 May 2019

World Health Organization (2019b) Preventing unsafe abortion. Sexual and Reproductive Health, World Health Organization, Geneva. https://www.who.int/reproductivehealth/topics/unsafe_abortion/hrpwork/en/. Accessed 08 April 2019

World Health Organization (2019c) Maternal mental health. Sexual and Reproductive Health, World Health Organization, Geneva. https://www.who.int/mental_health/maternal-child/maternal_mental_health/en/. Accessed 12 April 2019

World Health Organization (2019d) Comprehensive mental health action plan 2013-2020. World Health Organization, Geneva. https://www.who.int/mental_health/action_plan_2013/en/. Accessed 12 April 2019

The Contribution of Midwifery to Global Health and Development

3

Expected Learning Outcomes

By the end of this chapter, readers should be able to:

1. Position and profile midwifery onto the global health agenda
2. Demonstrate the relationship between midwifery services, global health and development
3. Explain the critical nature of the contribution of midwives and midwifery to the strategies for the achievement of the global health agenda
4. Describe some successful evidence-based midwifery pathways for the enhancement of global health
5. Outline the challenges to the contribution of midwives to the global health agenda
6. Map out midwives and midwifery across the globe and the variety of health systems in which midwifery functions

3.1 Evidence on the Value of Midwives' Contribution

Evidence abounds on the critical importance of midwives' contribution to achievement of better health outcomes for women, newborn and their families (Renfrew et al. 2014; UNFPA 2011, 2014a, b). It is therefore reasonable to postulate that without the contribution of midwives providing quality midwifery care, the achievement of the global health agenda for women and newborn would be difficult.

3.2 Positioning and Profiling Midwifery into the Global Health Agenda

During the MDG era (2000–2015), three goals in particular were most relevant to midwives and midwifery. These were Goal 3: to promote gender equality; Goal 4: to reduce child mortality and Goal 5: to reduce maternal mortality. The achievement of these goals relied on quality midwifery services. Hence, the focus on rapid production of midwives and other cadres who were intended to fill in the gap for serious shortages of midwives where they were needed most and the introduction of skilled attendants at birth (see Chapter 2). Some of the said 'skilled attendants' were actually not skilled (UNFPA 2014a, b; WHO 2015a, b, c, d), and this posed a problem. The evidence further demonstrated that to get the best out of midwives' contributions, the midwives had to be well educated, regulated, supported and work within a well-functioning health system. Numbers alone were not enough. Management systems, infrastructure and other logistic issues had to be addressed (UNFPA 2011, 2014a, b; Renfrew et al. 2014; WHO 2015a, b, c, d).

The Global Health Agenda (2016–2030) focuses on ensuring that everyone everywhere has access to basic health care at a cost that does not leave the individual impoverished (WHO 2017a, b, c, d). The global strategy for women's, children's and adolescents' health (2016–2030), launched to operationalise the 2016–2030 agenda, envisions a world in which every woman, child and adolescent in every setting realises their rights to physical and mental health and well-being, has social and economic opportunities and is able to participate fully in shaping prosperous and sustainable societies (WHO 2015a, b, c, d). In a world that is becoming more connected through globalisation, with advances in technology and innovation, it would be tempting to think that Universal Health Coverage (UHC) is easy to achieve. Yet evidence shows that women and children are still disproportionately affected by issues like poverty, environmental vulnerability, hunger, conflict, discrimination and violence (The World Bank 2017). To address these inequalities, initiatives like the UHC, Every Woman Every Child (EWEC) and Every Newborn Action Plan (ENAP) were launched to ensure that in the post 2015 global health agenda no one was left behind. The Sustainable Development Goals (SDGs) provide focus to all these initiatives, specifically SDGs 3.8; 3.8.1 and 3.8.2 which cover women and newborns (Box 3.1). Through the operationalisation of these strategies, midwives' contributions lead to improvement in equity, empowerment of women and, ultimately, strengthening the health system because strengthening midwifery services positively impacts on the health system.

Box 3.1. SDG targets 3.8, 3.8.1 and 3.8.2

SDG target 3.8: Achieve universal health coverage, including financial risk protection, access to quality essential healthcare services and access to safe, effective, quality and affordable essential medicines and vaccines for all.

SDG indicator 3.8.1: Coverage of essential health services (defined as the average coverage of essential services based on tracer interventions that include reproductive, maternal, newborn and child health; infectious diseases; noncommunicable diseases; and service capacity and access; amongst the general and the most disadvantaged population).

SDG indicator 3.8.2: Proportion of population with large household expenditures on health as a share of total household expenditure or income.

Source: World Bank, World Health Organization (2017). Tracking Universal Health Coverage: 2017 Global Monitoring Report

---

In the majority of low- and middle-income countries, 73 of them surveyed during the State of the World's Midwifery study (UNFPA 2011, 2014a, b) where the highest burden of maternal and newborn mortality and morbidity occur, midwives were the care providers closest to where women live. And yet it was in these same countries where midwifery was not perceived as a distinct profession. The practising midwifery workforce was not easily identifiable by country data. There were deficits in both numbers and competencies amongst the workforce. Coverage of births by a competent workforce and quality care was limited. Regulation and regulatory processes were insufficient to promote the professional autonomy of a midwife and to fulfil government obligations to protect the public; educational pathways and capacity required strengthening, and policy coherence and adherence were disjointed (UNFPA 2011:30). Midwifery services were, therefore, not able to take their position as a critical aspect of healthcare services because of prevailing socioeconomic and gender issues. Hence, in the SDG era, focus on improvement of midwifery education and services took centre stage (WHO 2016a, b, 2017a, b, c, d, 2018a, b, 2019a, b). Midwives were still the key to the achievement of global maternal and newborn health.

3.3 Midwifery Services, Global Health and Development

According to the Merriam Webster Dictionary (2018), *development* is 'a process that creates growth, progress, positive change or the addition of physical, economic, environmental, social and demographic components'. That is what midwifery does for women. Midwives provide comprehensive sexual and reproductive health services, including family planning counselling and services, post-abortion care, treatment of malaria in pregnancy and the prevention of mother-to-child transmission of HIV (UNFPA 2014a, b). Through their community education services, they contribute to the creation of awareness of non-communicable diseases and the value of families to seek care. Midwifery, by its very nature, when provided by midwives who are well educated, regulated and supported within a functioning healthcare system will lead to a reduction of up to 80% of maternal deaths, still births and neonatal deaths (WHO 2019a, b). Further evidence demonstrated that besides reduction of deaths and disability, there are 50 more advantages of quality midwifery services provided by qualified midwives the most important of which is health and well-being of women, newborn and their families (WHO 2019a, b), so that women and newborn do not only survive but thrive and transform. Healthy families constitute a healthy nation. A healthy nation is the prerequisite to economic growth and development of a nation. However, Saraki (2017) suggests that there is a perception gap between midwifery and development that must be addressed, citing the example of midwives in Africa who often make the difference between life and death in their communities.

For effective provision of safe, accessible midwifery services, there is a need for water, electricity, effective and efficient communication and transport systems and purpose—built health facility infrastructure to ensure efficient and respectful care for women. Respectful care of the care providers includes the provision of respectable and safe housing with adequate water and sanitation, security, methods of connectivity with the rest of the world, relevant amenities such as schools for the children, recreation and shopping facilities for families and any other amenities that add comfort to life. All these contribute to the general development of a community. In this light, midwifery services, when well supported by a government become a conduit for development. When governments invest in midwifery, they get a 16-fold return on investment in terms of lives saved and interventions prevented (UNFPA 2014a, b). It is therefore in every country's advantage to invest in midwifery. Thus, global health and development are closely intertwined with each facilitating the other.

3.4 Emphasising the Critical Nature of Midwifery and Midwives' Contribution

Global health initiatives are about ensuring that every woman everywhere has access to care—'Leaving No One Behind' (The World Bank 2017). In many countries, up to 80% of the population live in rural areas, some of which are inaccessible for various reasons and considered 'remote' or 'hard to reach' (The World Bank 2017). To achieve UHC and therefore *leave no one behind*, services must be available, accessible physically and psychologically to this large segment of the population irrespective of the changing demographic, epidemiological and technological trends occurring globally. Despite these changes, midwives continue to constitute the numerical bulk of the care providers providing services in difficult settings in low- and middle-income countries including in crisis situations (UNFPA 2016; FCI 2014; WHO 2016a, b). According to the 'Midwives Realities' report, 'Midwives are deeply committed to providing the best quality of care for women, newborns and their families' (WHO 2016b:2). As a result, midwives, continue to offer comprehensive services and promote woman-centred care and the well-being of women and newborns across the continuum of sexual, reproductive, maternal, newborn and child health (SRMNCH) (UNFPA 2014a, b). The WHO Regional Office for Europe

(2015b) in 'Health 2020'[1] described midwives as 'a vital resource for health' and provided evidence that midwives contribute to improving health and preventing disease, empowering individuals and communities. They contribute to developing evidence-based practice, conducting health research and developing innovative practices; have expertise and potential to improve population health and that with effective policies and workforce planning, regulatory frameworks, educational standards and supportive managerial practices, as part of an interdisciplinary team, midwives provide safe, high-quality and person-centred care, improve the coverage and integration of health services and reduce the costs of healthcare organisations and health systems (WHO European Region 2015b). Even in Europe, midwives comprise the majority of healthcare professionals providing maternity care, have close contact with many people and use every opportunity to influence health outcomes, influence social determinants of health and the policies necessary to achieve change (WHO 2015a, b, c, d; WHO, World Bank 2017; UNFPA 2017).

3.5 Some Successful Evidence-Based Midwifery Pathways

Global bodies have developed creative and innovative ways of enhancing the contribution of midwives and midwifery to the global health agenda and to operationalise the concepts of survive, thrive and transform. The selected frameworks and pathways below support and enable governments who wish to invest in the development and promotion of midwifery services in their countries based on evidence-based tools and frameworks.

3.5.1 The ICM Midwifery Services Framework[2] (MSF)

At the advent of the SDGs, despite consensus having been reached about their value in SRMNCH, midwives and midwifery were not part of the regular healthcare system in many countries. ICM exists to strengthen midwifery globally, so it developed a tool that allows systemic and systematic approaches to strengthening midwifery services and the quality of midwives a country could produce. The tool allows a wholistic approach to the scrutiny of healthcare systems and services and places midwives and midwifery services into their rightful place in the healthcare system. It presents a step-by-step approach for developing and strengthening midwifery (Annex 3.1).

3.5.2 The Midwifery Pathway 2030

The Midwifery Pathway 2030 envisions that all women of reproductive age and adolescents have universal access to midwifery care by 2030. The Pathway outlines key planning and policy measures that increase maternal and newborn survival leading to healthy communities (Annex 3.2).

3.5.3 The Framework for Quality Maternal and Newborn Care (QMNC)

Described in detail in the Lancet Series on Midwifery (2014), the QMNC demonstrates that midwifery care covers 100% of the greater part of the health needs of women and newborns, and they continue to contribute to care even when other care providers get involved during complications (Renfrew et al. 2014). Annex 3.3 provides a detailed description of the framework.

---

[1] For the aims of WHO European Region's objectives for Health 2020, see Chapter 11, Box 11.6.

[2] For a more detailed description, see Annex 3.1.

3.5.4   State of the World's Midwifery Reports 2011 and 2014

The State of the World's Midwifery Reports 2011 and 2014 describe in great evidence-based detail the situation of midwifery in high burden countries and what needs to be done to improve the situation (UNFPA 2011, 2014a, b). These reports elucidate the impact of scaling up midwifery in individual countries under different scenarios. The scenarios are excellent frameworks for decision-making for countries. An evaluator process was in progress starting 2019 for the production of the State of the World's Midwifery Report 2021 which will include data from all countries, not just from those with a high burden of maternal and newborn mortality.

3.6   Challenges to Effective Full Potential Midwifery Contribution to These Initiatives

For effective and optimum benefit from midwives' contributions, policymakers and governments globally need to listen to midwives because midwives have an in-depth awareness of what is needed to improve the quality of care. Yet, according to the 'Midwives Realities' report (2016), midwives' voices are rarely heard. As a result, key issues are absent from policy dialogue at all levels. Additionally, the understanding of midwives and midwifery has been restricted by a failure to apply consistent definitions, resulting in professional and non-professional staff being seen as midwives (Renfrew et al. 2014). Not all countries use the globally accepted definition of midwifery (Renfrew et al. 2014) (Box 3.2) and of a midwife (ICM 2014) (Box 3.3). In some settings, the understanding of midwifery is confined to pregnancy, birth and post-partum care. The broader, more diverse contributions are not known. As a result, other care providers take responsibility for the SRMNCH of women leading to an increased medicalisation of birth and the confinement of midwives in closed institutions (Ruiz-Berdun et al. 2016). There needs to

---

Box 3.2. Definition of midwifery

Midwifery is 'skilled, knowledgeable and compassionate care for child-bearing women, newborn infants and families across the continuum from pre-pregnancy, pregnancy, birth, post-partum and the early weeks of life'. Core characteristics include optimizing normal biological, psychological, social and cultural processes of reproduction and early life, timely prevention and management of complications, consultation with and referral to other services, respecting women's individual circumstances and views and working in partnership with women to strengthen women's own capabilities to care for themselves.

Source: Renfrew et al. (2014) in the Lancet Series on Midwifery (2014)

Box 3.3. Definition of a midwife

A midwife is a person who has successfully completed a midwifery education programme that is based on the ICM Essential Competencies for Basic Midwifery Practice and the framework of the ICM Global Standards for Midwifery Education and is recognized in the country where it is located; who has acquired the requisite qualifications to be registered and/or legally licensed to practice midwifery and use the title 'midwife' and who demonstrates competency in the practice of midwifery.

Source: International Confederation of Midwives website. Accessed 2 March 2020

---

be better recognition of midwives and midwifery, better understanding of what midwifery is and does and a clearer definition of who is a midwife and what midwifery is through better regulatory frameworks, clearer job descriptions and strengthened midwives' associations. The matters of professionalisation and professional identity of midwifery are discussed in some detail in Chapters 10 and 18. The need for better and stronger pre-service education and continuing professional development cannot be over-emphasised. Neither can the need for more representation of midwives in decision-making circles at all levels. Hence, WHO dedicated 2020 as '*the year of the nurse and the midwife*' for the recognition, improvement and support for the contribution of midwives and nurses to global health.

Inconsistencies are perpetuated by the variety of pathways to becoming a midwife. SoWMy 2011 describes three main pathways followed in 57 countries: direct entry, combined with nursing and post nursing. Education is provided by either private or public institutions. The duration and content of programmes vary widely with programmes ranging from 6 months to 5 years. There are also variations across and within pathways and between public and private institutions (UNFPA 2011:21). Details and examples of various midwifery education programmes are discussed in Chapter 4.

Professionally, because of lack of opportunities for leadership, especially at national level, midwives are absent from policy dialogue and thus unable to contribute to policy decisions. In some countries, midwives' professional competence is either unknown or not recognised, leading to inappropriate restrictions on practice. In situations of severe midwife shortages, midwives are compelled to work for the government for a fixed period of time. Most frustratingly, in many low- and middle-income countries, midwives are expected to provide services with minimal or no equipment. The net effect is that some midwives suffer moral distress and burn out. In general, midwives often suffer from overall poor human resource policies and management within health systems (WHO 2016a, b).

Economic challenges are experienced mainly in low- and middle-income countries where the midwife's salary is so low that midwives are unable to meet the family expenses and are forced to look for other sources of income. In some situations, salaries are not paid regularly or they are not paid at all. This puts midwives into a very difficult situation and creates room for unscrupulous practices where midwives are forced to ask for under-the-table payments from women and families. In some settings, midwives are so few that those available are not able to take a break or can only do so after a long period. In other settings, housing is poor and not safe, and midwives experience security risks including sexual assaults (WHO 2016a, b). Gender inequality predisposes midwives to physical and sexual violence.

In many countries, midwives feel disrespected despite being empowered through their education and training. There are unequal power relations within the health system and within communities. When hierarchical power is wielded by other health professionals, the authority and decision-making ability of midwives are undermined, negatively impacting on the ability of midwives to offer quality care. There is also lack of or limited social capital, solidarity and organisational power because many midwives' associations do not have the resources to provide support to the profession and to individual midwives. In other countries, there are social norms, legal and regulatory environments that encourage gender inequality and low public opinion of midwives and midwifery (WHO 2016a, b).

Some barriers are systemic and beyond the reach of midwives. These include social inequalities where maternal and child health services are not evenly distributed across population groups; poverty, in some cases extreme poverty which makes populations unable to afford care; and shifting demographics due to massive population movements, natural disasters, civil unrest and conflicts. In other settings, the practice environments militate against the provision of quality care. The status of midwifery and that of women is low (WHO and World Bank 2017). The whole issue of quality in midwifery care is discussed in Chapter 8.

All these barriers make provision of effective quality midwifery care difficult and in some cases impossible. Midwives alone are not able to change such situations. They need support through professional associations, collaboration with other healthcare providers and development partners to optimise their value and take their position in care provision. With strong associations, midwives can negotiate, persuade and dialogue with the policymakers and other stakeholders including the community they serve and can add their voice at the decision-making table.

3.7   Mapping Midwifery Across the Globe

According to the World Bank database (2019), the global average distribution of nurses and midwives is 3.4 per 1000 people. (Not many countries distinguish or are willing to separate midwives from nurses. As a result, it is difficult to obtain data on midwives only. All the same, the distribution of midwives is influenced by the same factors that influence the distribution of other health care providers especially nurses.) According to SoWMy (UNFPA 2014a, b), the 73 countries profiled account for 96% of all maternal deaths, 91% of all still births and 93% of all newborn deaths but have 42% of the world's midwives, nurses and doctors, suggesting that, for a variety of reasons, the global distribution of midwives is not directly related to where the need is greatest (UNFPA 2014a, b). Figure 3.1 presents averages across the globe. It is important to note

that distribution of healthcare providers differs between and within countries, and these differences are not usually visible on national averages.

3.8   Regional Distribution of Midwives

Figure 3.2 presents the distribution of midwives like other care providers in different regions with the same observation that even within a region, there are factors that impact on where midwives are found.

3.9   Across Different Economic Groupings

The World Bank database (2019) further shows that economic groupings and collaboration amongst countries and other social factors such as population movements, human development and a country's income level also impact on the distribution of healthcare providers. Figures 3.3 and 3.4 present these data.

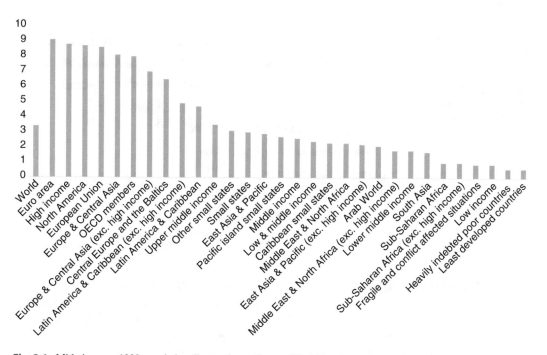

Fig. 3.1   Midwives per 1000 people by all groupings. (Source: World Bank Database 2019. Accesses 1 March 2020)

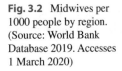

Fig. 3.2 Midwives per 1000 people by region. (Source: World Bank Database 2019. Accesses 1 March 2020)

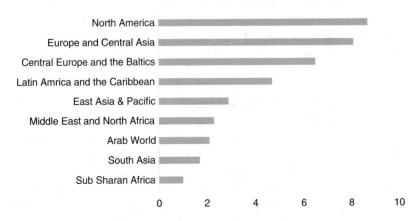

Fig. 3.3 Midwives per 1000 people by income level. (Source: World Bank Database 2019. Accesses 1 March 2020)

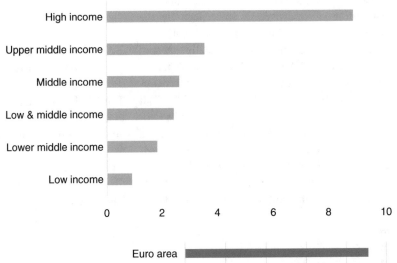

Fig. 3.4 Midwives per 1000 people by economic groupings, development and other social factors. (Source: World Bank Database 2019. Accesses 1 March 2020)

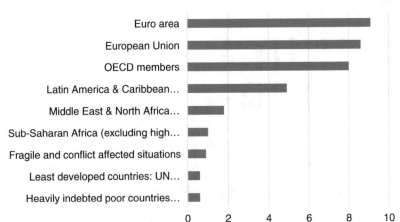

3.10   Midwifery in High-Income Countries

In most high-income countries, midwifery is an autonomous protected profession and midwives practise their full scope and more at all levels of care across the whole continuum from primary care to tertiary care (Ruiz-Berdun et al. 2016). Midwives are in administration and management, academia and research. In administration, midwives hold posts ranging from managing a hospital and/or a family health centre to carrying out auditing tasks for public and private providers and insurers. Additionally, midwives work in research and teaching at undergraduate and postgraduate levels in public and private universities and professional institutions.

In Norway, midwives are authorised to lead in the care of pregnant women who want to see a midwife. Midwives can be individual consultants, work in obstetric units or in midwife led units. Women have a choice. In Ireland, studies showed that midwifery-led care was as safe as consultant-led care, resulted in less intervention, was viewed by women with greater satisfaction in some aspects of care and was more cost-effective (Ruiz-Berdun et al. 2016).

With migration of health workers from low- and middle-income countries, immigrant midwives complement the staffing levels in high-income countries. Service coverage is high with a coverage index of 77 for North America, Europe and East Asia (UHC Report 2017), and in 2005–2015, 74% of mothers and infants in the richest households received at least six of the seven basic maternal and child health services (see Box 3.4).

Box 3.4. The seven basic maternal health and child services

- Four or more antenatal care visits
- At least one tetanus vaccination during pregnancy
- Skilled birth attendance (birth attended by skilled health personnel)
- Bacillus Calmette-Guerin vaccination
- The third dose of diphtheria–tetanus–pertussis containing vaccine
- Measles vaccination
- Access to improved drinking water

Source: WHO and World Bank (2017). Tracking Universal Health Coverage: 2017 Global Monitoring Report

---

The greatest challenges in high-income countries are rising intervention rates, the over-use of technology and the increasing use of the right to choose by women with no professional explanation and support. For example, in Norway in 2013, 99.2% of births took place in big institutions (Ruiz-Berdun et al. 2016). Because births take place in big institutions, technology takes over and compromises the human touch of the midwife. More interventions mean that less women benefit from the care of a midwife. Additionally, because of the easy access to varieties of care, and the ability and the right to choose, women choose interventions like epidural as they see it as their legal right to have it. Because of these rights, many women will request or receive interventions without professional assessment or questioning if it is the best for them (Ruiz-Berdun et al. 2016). Medicalisation is therefore a threat to both women and midwives, and this issue is discussed further in Chapter 10.

3.11   Midwifery in Low- and Middle-Income Countries

The situation is very different in low- and middle-income countries where numbers of midwives are low, sometimes dangerously low; the profession is not recognised, the education programmes and processes are weak and the recruitment, deployment and retention mechanisms are missing or weak. Midwives work in rural areas and hard to work environments with minimal or no incentives, no support and poor remuneration (UNFPA 2011, 2014a, b; Renfrew et al. 2014; WHO 2017a, b, c, d, 2019a, b). Midwives are not always permitted to practise to their full scope. Regulation is weak, and job descriptions and definitions are missing or not clear, leading to non-professional staff being seen as midwives (Renfrew et al. 2014).

The massive population movements and migration from low- and middle-income countries to countries where work conditions and remuneration are perceived as better have exacerbated the deficit of midwives where they are most needed. Hence, the International Confederation of Midwives focuses on strengthening midwifery by creating and strengthening national midwives' associations. The Midwifery Map shows where ICM has members. The map can be accessed on the ICM website.

The distribution of midwives differs greatly between and within countries with the richer receiving considerably more than the poorer segments of populations. Large inequalities in basic maternal and child health services persist (Box 3.4). The UHC service coverage index is lowest in sub-Saharan Africa (42) followed by South Asia (53); and, between 2005 and 2015, only 17% of mothers and infants in households in the poorest wealth quantile received at least six of the seven interventions compared to 74% in the richest quantile. It is feared that, unless interventions are designed to promote equity, efforts to attain UHC may lead to improvements in the national average of service coverage while inequalities worsen at the same time. This reinforces the importance of restructuring health services so that no one is left behind (WHO and World Bank 2017:2, 4).

The age-old issues of poverty, poor leadership and management of health systems, lack of political will and low socio-economic status and human development persist. Encouragingly, the UHC Report (2017) observed that,

> never before has there been as much political momentum for universal health coverage as there is right now. And never before has there been greater need for commitment to health as a human right to be enjoyed by all, rather than a privilege for the wealthy few. (p.xii)

3.12   Impact of Global Movements, Epidemics and Pandemics on Distribution of Midwives

3.12.1 Migration

Emigration of healthcare workers to higher-income countries within North America and Europe (Aluttis et al. 2014) led to up to 70 and 75% of the physicians originally from Angola and Mozambique, respectively, practising abroad (Clemens and Pettersson 2008). Approximately, 65,000 doctors and 70,000 nurses from sub-Saharan Africa, which is equal to approximately 28% of the region's medical workforce, work internationally (Clemens and Pettersson 2008). The outward flow related to low salaries, poor working environments, underfunded healthcare facilities and the lack of opportunities for career advancement (Eastwood et al. 2005) and political instability appear to worsen the outflow.

3.12.2 Epidemics and Pandemics

It is estimated that diseases and infections such as HIV, AIDS and Ebola outbreaks caused a 20% decrease of frontline health workforce especially in sub-Saharan Africa (Chen et al. 2004) in countries with the highest maternal and newborn mortality (Gerein et al. 2006). The WHO indicated a growing deficit of approximately 4.3 million health workers, including midwives, in almost every region of the world. Forty six out of the 47 sub-Saharan countries had significantly less than the required minimum threshold of 2.28 physicians or nurses per 1000 people, to deliver basic health services (WHO 2006) despite the region carrying nearly 24% of the world's disease burden with only 3% of its healthcare workforce and only 1% of its financial resources for health care (Anyangwe and Mtonga 2007).

In 2019 the Corona Virus Disease 2019 (COVID-19) pandemic killed hundreds of healthcare workers, creating crises in almost every facet of public health systems as well as changing the contexts within which midwifery care is provided. Midwifery, by its very nature, makes the social distancing[3] required to prevent the disease spreading impossible.

---

[3] Social distancing = it was required that individuals keep a distance of one and half metres from each other to prevent the spread of the disease (WHO 2020).

3.13 Where There Is No Midwifery

In their report, 'Making a case for midwifery' (2014), Family Care International and the International Confederation of Midwives (ICM) stated that midwives promote woman-centred care and the well-being of women and newborns across the continuum of sexual, reproductive, maternal, and newborn health (SRMNH) including HIV prevention (UNFPA 2014a, b). Midwives act as a hub of information and education for women, giving guidance on everything from nutrition to contraception, educating women on the value of breastfeeding, tackling the information gap amongst women in the immediate lead-up to and aftermath of birth. In thousands of communities, the midwives' role transcends birth. Midwives are a focal point for community inquiries and information and an entry point for many women to the wider primary healthcare system, including informing women about their sexual and reproductive health rights. Women and families are deprived of all these services or receiving them at less than optimum level when there are no midwives (Saraki 2017).

3.14 Health Systems and the Identity of Midwives

Midwives function in different health systems. The health systems impact on the level at which midwives are perceived to function within the power dynamics enabled by the healthcare system. In medically led systems, it is difficult for midwives to be allowed to function as autonomous professionals who will collaborate on equal footing with other healthcare providers. Society has tended to view the doctor as the most senior healthcare provider with the rest, including midwives, being subservient to them (Puras 2019). There are power gradients and turf wars as a result of these power gradients. Unfortunately, in low- and middle-income countries, because of the quality of education for midwives, this perception of a senior–junior relationship between obstetricians and midwives is perpetuated leading to loss of confidence and identity amongst midwives.

In health systems which are based on midwife-led care,[4] the midwife is perceived and recognised as a specialist in normal childbirth and the obstetrician as a specialist when child birth is complicated. There is mutual trust amongst professional groups. Roles and job descriptions are clear. Midwives are perceived as autonomous practitioners. There is mutual support and eye-level collaboration amongst midwives and other healthcare providers. This amicable relationship in general tends to lead to provision of quality care to women and their families.

3.15 Conclusion

All in all, midwives are crucial, if not vital for the achievement of global health. All the health-related SDGs heavily assume and rely on the effective contribution of well-educated, regulated, supported midwives in a functioning health system. But it has to be acknowledged that no one healthcare profession can do it alone. There is a need for respectful collaboration, mutual support amongst care providers and the effective addressing of health system issues in order to get the best out of midwives and midwifery services as they contribute to global health and development.

3.15.1 Principles

Providing adequate financial and material support to midwifery enhances the capacity of a country to get the best out of midwives and midwifery services. Because midwives are closest to where women live whether in urban or rural areas. Policymakers and managers should listen to midwives in order for them to include all the relevant issues important to women and their families for the reduction of maternal and newborn mortality.

---

[4]In midwife-led care, the midwife is the 'lead healthcare professional responsible for the planning, organisation and delivery of care given to a woman from initial booking of antenatal visits through to the postnatal period' (WHO).

3.15.2 Policy

Midwives must be represented at decision-making tables by midwife leaders in order for countries to focus investment on issues that lead to a country's development and the improvement of midwifery services.

3.15.3 Practice

Governments and development partners must work together to ensure that midwives are integrated into the health systems of nations and that midwifery services are well resourced for the provision of quality care.

Questions for Reflection

1. The text suggested that midwifery is critical for the achievement of the objectives of the global health agenda. Based on your knowledge of midwifery in your own country or region, how far do you think this is true?
2. Critically analyse the concept of universal health coverage. Discuss the possibilities of its achievement or lack thereof in low- and middle-income countries given the current status of midwifery globally.
3. Scrutinise midwifery services in high income countries. How far do you think the global health agenda and the contribution of midwives and midwifery are applicable in these countries?

Annex 3.1: The International Confederation of Midwives Midwifery Services Framework (MSF)

Published in 2015, the Midwifery Services Framework (MSF) is a framework that provides a step-by-step approach for developing or strengthening midwifery services in all countries irrespective of income level and brings together existing global evidence-based tools, approaches and guidelines in its steps. The tool has specific components (Box 3.2) which enable a country to examine the services that women and their families receive in comparison to the globally accepted minimum benefits package of care and identify gaps in its healthcare system. The country can then develop evidence-based approaches to fill in the gaps. It was the only tool at the time of writing which starts off with what women need and thus avoids turf wars amongst MNCH healthcare providers.

The MSF acknowledges the complexity of issues involved in maternal and newborn deaths and disability. It allows for a detailed, collaborative, examination of the breadth and depth of all these issues and creates a platform where all stakeholders involved in preventing these come together and discuss solutions. The tool pinpoints the areas that need improvement, not only in the care provision, but also in the healthcare system, the education process of midwives and other healthcare providers, the management and leadership process and policies which determine the deployment, recruitment and retention of care providers. Thus, countries which use the tool, besides coming to a clearer and deeper understanding of their healthcare system, own both the problems and their solutions and develop momentum and willingness to implement the solutions.

The ICM implemented this tool in six countries, and an evaluation conducted in 2019 demonstrated some improvement in SRMNCH services. The lessons learnt from the evaluation were used to review the tool and implementation process. Countries wishing to use this tool can contact the International Confederation of Midwives on info@internationalmidwives.org.

Annex 3.2: Steps of the Midwifery Service Framework, Under Review, at the Time of Writing

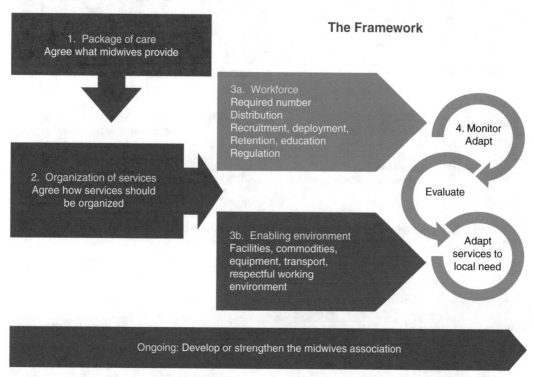

The Framework

1. Package of care
Agree what midwives provide

3a. Workforce
Required number
Distribution
Recruitment, deployment,
Retention, education
Regulation

4. Monitor
Adapt

2. Organization of services
Agree how services should
be organized

Evaluate

3b. Enabling environment
Facilities, commodities,
equipment, transport,
respectful working
environment

Adapt
services to
local need

Ongoing: Develop or strengthen the midwives association

Source: https://www.internationalmidwives.org/icm-publications/midwifery-services-framework.html

Annex 3.3: Midwifery 2030

The Midwifery 2030 vision sets out that all women of reproductive age, including adolescents, have universal access to midwifery until 2030. The global number of pregnancies per year between now and 2030 is expected to remain constant at 166 million. To compensate for the shortage of midwives, countries need to strengthen their policies and planning to extend the reach of midwifery. Midwifery 2030, A Pathway to Health, outlines key planning and policy measures that will increase maternal and newborn survival and healthy communities. These are summarised in Fig. 3.5 and the foundations that are considered essential if the pathway is to be realised are set out in Fig. 3.6.

Further information can be found on this topic in at: https://reader.elsevier.com/reader/sd/pii/ S0266613   815002855?   token= 7FBA7457625268886DAFC0440CF83EB D71D1529F641BD78D292A6F5FFFAEE4D9 E7D86DC3986C88E103FC9B976B026424 [last accessed 30.09.2020]

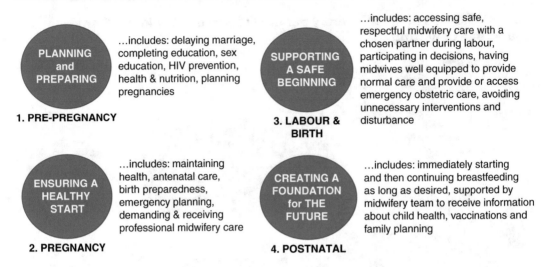

Fig. 3.5 Midwifery 2030: the key components contributing to a 'pathway to health' during the four stages of a woman's reproductive life. (Derived from State of the World's Midwifery 2014:46–7)

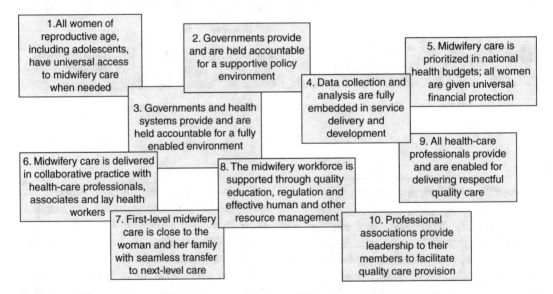

Fig. 3.6 Ten foundations are considered essential if the 2030 vision is to become a reality. (Derived from State of the World's Midwifery 2014:46–7)

Annex 3.4: Quality Maternal and Newborn Care Framework

The framework demonstrates the aspects where midwifery care addresses 100% of the needs of women and newborn (shaded in green). The parts shaded pink, midwifery care complements the care provided by other care providers as indicated. Hence, midwifery care is required throughout the continuum of care from home (primary) to the tertiary level of care.

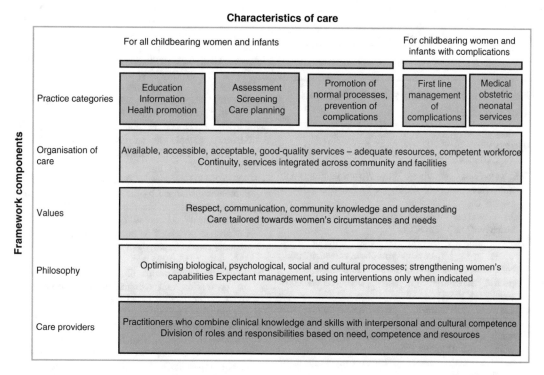

The Lancet Series on Midwifery: Framework for Quality Maternal and Newborn Care (QMNC) (Renfrew et al. 2014). Source: The Lancet Series on Midwifery: https://www. researchgate.net/publication/305418621_Midwifery-led_antenatal_care_models_Mapping_a_systematic_review_to_an_evidence-based_quality_framework_to_identify_key_components_and_characteristics_of_care

With earlier Ebola and HIV (Haseeb 2018), several countries made efforts to address the shortage mainly through international policy implementations and regional programmes such as task shifting, skilled attendants at birth, bonding of new graduates and an attempt to comply with policies that minimise migration based on the Global Code of Practice on the International Recruitment of Health Personnel for the ethical recruitment of healthcare workers. The complexity and scope of the issue made it extremely difficult to resolve. The Code was as a policy framework for the ethical recruitment of health professionals (Aluttis et al. 2014; WHO 2017a, b, c, d) intended to address the health worker shortage on the international level. Compliance is voluntary. In regions where public health systems were weak, the rates of disease and mortality were extremely high as in sub-Saharan Africa. A large fraction of the population lacked access to basic healthcare services (WHO 2017a, b, c, d).

Key Messages

Midwives contribute to the development economic and social development of a country.

Midwives are crucial to the achievement of global health initiatives.

Where there are no midwives, women and their families are deprived of critical services and information.

Additional Resources for Reflection and Further Study

Videos

The value of midwives. https://www.youtube.com/watch?time_continue=20&v=2TF4FsQnBOs&feature=emb_logo

Health workers count. https://www.youtube.com/watch?v=QXpp4kmUCLU

What would the world be like without midwives. https://www.youtube.com/watch?time_continue=3&v=d5Mo-5qNmIs&feature=emb_logo

Respectful maternity care. https://www.youtube.com/watch?v=K105F9o3HtU

Causes of disrespect. https://www.youtube.com/watch?v=83FYPFbNFCo

Women's reproductive rights. https://www.youtube.com/watch?v=R5gDnnPTK7Q

Person centred care. https://www.youtube.com/watch?v=pj-AvTOdk2Q

Map

The Midwifery Map. https://www.internationalmidwives.org/icm-publications/map.html.

Further Reading

Christoph A, Bishaw T, Frank MW (2014) The workforce for health in a globalized context – global shortages and international migration. Glob Health Action 7. https://doi.org/10.3402/gha.v7.2361

Clark PF, James B, Stewart JB et al (2006) The globalization of the labour market for health-care professionals. Int Labour Rev 145(1–2):37–64. https://doi.org/10.1111/j.1564-913X.2006.tb00009.x

Every Woman Every Child (2015) Global strategy for women's, children's and adolescents' health. https://www.everywomaneverychild.org/global-strategy/. Accessed 10 March 2020

Health Sciences and Medicine (2018) The critical shortage of healthcare workers in Sub-Saharan Africa: a comprehensive review by Saud Haseeb. https://ysjournal.com/the-critical-shortage-of-healthcare-workers-in-sub-saharan-africa-a-comprehensive-review/. Accessed 2 March 2020

Homer C, Friberg IK, Dias BA et al (2014) The projected impact of scaling up midwifery. Lancet 384(9948):1146–1157

International Confederation of Midwives (2019) State of the world's midwifery 2021. https://www.internationalmidwives.org/assets/files/general-files/2019/10/sowmy-official-letter-for-icm-mas_english.pdf. Accessed 2 March 2020

Lemiere CH, Jahanshahi C, Smith N et al (2010) Reducing geographical imbalances of health Workers in sub-Saharan Africa. World Bank Working Papers. The World Bank. https://doi.org/10.1596/978-0-8213-8599-9

Mullan F, Frehywot S, Omaswa F et al (2011) Medical schools in sub-Saharan Africa. Lancet 377(9771):1113–1121. https://doi.org/10.1016/S0140-6736(10)61961-7

UNICEF (2015) Levels and trends in child mortality 2015. Estimates developed by the UN Inter Agency Group for child mortality estimation. UNICEF, New York

Van Lerberghe W, Matthews Z, Achadi E et al (2014) Country experiences with strengthening of health systems and deployment of midwives. Lancet 384(9949):1215–1225

World Health Organization (2015) WHO statement on the prevention and elimination of disrespect and abuse during facility based childbirth. World Health Organization, Geneva

WHO – Global Burden of Disease (2017) WHO. http://www.who.int/topics/global_burden_of_disease/en

World Health Organization (2019) State of the World's nursing report 2020; State of the World's Midwifery report 2020. https://www.who.int/hrh/nursing-midwifery/state-of-the-worlds-nursing-and-midwifery-2020-get-engaged.pdf. Accessed 2 March 2020

Yang YT, Kozhimannil KB (2015) Making a case to reduce legal impediments to midwifery practice in the United States. Elsevier. Womens Health Issues 25(4):314–317. https://doi.org/10.1016/j.whi.2015.03.006

References

Aluttis C, Bishaw CT, Frank MW, et al (2014) The workforce for health in a globalized context – global shortages and international migration. Glob Health Action 7. https://doi.org/10.3402/gha.v7.23611

Anyangwe SC, Mtonga C (2007) Inequities in the Global Health Workforce: the greatest impediment to health in Sub-Saharan Africa. Int J Environ Res Public Health 4(2):93–100

Chen L, Evans T, Anand S, et al. (2004) Human resources for health: overcoming the crisis. The

Lancet 364(9449):1984-90. https://doi.org/10.1016/S0140-6736(04)17482-5

Clemens MA, Pettersson G (2008) New data on African health professionals abroad. Hum Resour Health 6:1. https://doi.org/10.1186/1478-4491-6-1

Eastwood JB, Conroy RE, Naicker S et al (2005) Loss of health professionals from sub-Saharan Africa: the pivotal role of the UK. Lancet 365(9474):1893–1900. https://doi.org/10.1016/S0140-6736(05)66623-8

Family Care International (2014) Making the case for midwifery: a toolkit for using evidence from the state of the World's midwifery report 2014 to create policy change. file:///C:/Users/Gebruiker/Documents/Book%20poposal/Book%20content/Part%201/Chapter%203/AdvocacyToolkit-English%20Making%20a%20case%20for%20Midwifery.pdf. Accessed 15 Jan 2020

Gerein N, Green A, Pearson S (2006) The implications of shortages of health professionals for maternal health in sub-Saharan. Afr Reprod Health Matters 14(27):40–50. https://doi.org/10.1016/S0968-8080(06)27225-2

Haseeb S (2018) The critical shortage of healthcare workers in sub Saharan Africa: a comprehensive review. Health Sci Med. https://ysjournal.com/the-critical-shortage-of-healthcare-workers-in-sub-saharan-africa-a-comprehensive-review/. Accessed Jan 2020

Pura D (2019) Human rights-based approaches to health workforce education: preparing the health workforce for a more just, equitable and sustainable future. United Nations Human Rights Office of the High Commissioner. Fact sheet. https://www.ohchr.org/EN/Issues/Health/Pages/SRRightHealthIndex.aspx. Accessed 5 Nov 2019

Renfrew M, McFaden A, Bastos MH et al (2014) Midwifery and quality care. Findings from a new evidence-informed framework for maternal and newborn care. Lancet 384(9948):1129–1145

Ruiz-Berdun L, Escuriet R, Leon-Larios F et al (2016) In maternity care in different countries. Midwife's Contribution Publisher: Consell del Collegis d'Infermeres de Catalunya. ISBN: 978-84-608-7254-2

Saraki T (2017) Midwifery: the hidden hero of development. Financial Times, 19 June 2017

The World Bank (2017) Sub-Saharan Africa – data. Data.worldbank. https://data.worldbank.org/region/sub-saharan-africa

The World Bank (2019) Nurses and midwives (per 1 000 people). World Bank Data. https://data.worldbank.org/indicator/SH.MED.NUMW.P3. Accessed 7 March 2020

United Nations Population Fund (2011) State of the World's midwifery 2011. Delivering health, saving lives. United Nations Population Fund, New York

United Nations Population Fund (2014a) Midwives are key to a healthy and safe pregnancy and childbirth. http://unfpa.org/public/home/pid/16021. Accessed 11 March 2020

United Nations Population Fund (2014b) State of the World's midwifery 2014: a universal pathway. A woman's right to health. United Nations Population Fund, New York

United Nations Population Fund (2016) Quality midwifery care in the midst of crisis. Midwifery capacity building strategy for northern Syria 2017–2021. United Nations Population Fund, New York

United Nations Population Fund (2017) Quality midwifery care in the midst of crisis. Midwifery capacity building strategy for northern Syria 2017–2021. UNFPA Cross Border Operations 2017

World Health Organization (2006) The world health report 2006: working together for health

World Health Organization (2015a) UN global strategy for women's, children's and adolescents' health 2016 – 2030. World Health Organization, Geneva

World Health Organization (2015b) Nurses and midwives: a vital resource for health. European compendium of good practices in nursing and midwifery towards health 2020 goals. World Health Organization Regional Office for Europe, Copenhagen

World Health Organization (2015c) Skilled attendants: management systems and other logistics need to be addressed. World Health Organization, Geneva

World Health Organization (2015d) Trends of maternal mortality: 1990 – 2015 estimates by WHO, UNICEF UNFPA, World bank and the United Nations population division. World Health Organization, Geneva

World Health Organization (2016a) Global strategy for human resources for health: workforce 2030. WHO Library I. World Health Organization. ISBN: 978-92-4-151113-1

World Health Organization (2016b) Midwives voices, midwives realities: findings from a global consultation on providing quality midwifery care. WHO Library I. World Health Organization. ISBN: 978-92-4-151611-2 (Originally published under ISBN: 978-92-4-151054-7)

World Health Organization (2017a) Global Health Observatory Data Repository – maternal mortality – data by WHO region. WHO. http://apps.who.int/gho/data/view.main.1370?lang=en

World Health Organization (2017b) Global burden of disease. WHO, Geneva. http://www.who.int/topics/global_burden_of_disease/en

World Health Organization (2017c) Global health observatory data repository – density of healthcare workforce Per 1000. WHO. http://apps.who.int/gho/data/node.main.A1444?lang=en&showonly=HWF

World Health Organization (2017d) Strengthening quality midwifery education. WHO Meeting report July 25–26, 2016. In support of Global Strategy for Women's, Children's and Adolescents' Health 2016–30; Global Strategy for Human Resources for Health: Workforce 2030. World Health Organization, Geneva

World Health Organization (2018a) Definition of skilled health personnel providing care during childbirth. The 2018 joint statement by WHO, UNFPA, UNICEF, ICM, ICN, FIGO, IPA. WHO/RHR/18.14 © World Health Organization

World Health Organization (2018b) Survive, thrive and transform. Global Strategy for women's, children's and adolescents' health (2016–2030). 2018 monitoring report: current status and strategic priorities. WHO/FWC/18.20 © World Health Organization

World Health Organization (2019a) 2020 International year of the nurse and the midwife: a catalyst for a brighter future for health around the globe. https://www.who.int/news-room/campaigns/year-of-the-nurse-and-the-midwife-2020. Accessed 30 April 2020

World Health Organization (2019b) Strengthening quality midwifery education for universal health coverage 2030: framework for action. ISBN: 978-92-4-151584-9 © World Health Organization

World Health Organisation (2020) Corona Virus Disease 2019: Advice to the public. https://www.who.int

World Health Organization and International Bank for Reconstruction and Development/The World Bank (2017) Tracking universal health coverage: 2017 global monitoring report. World Health Organization and the International Bank for Reconstruction and Development/The World Bank 2017. ISBN: 978-92-4-151355-5. Licence: CC BY-NC-SA 3.0 IGO

Part II

Midwifery Education, Regulation and Association Development

1.1   Section Summary

This section discusses the aspects of education, regulation and association development in relation to global midwifery. The International Confederation of Midwives (ICM) has identified what they called the three pillars of a strong professsion (ICM 2011). Though there have been some informal undocumented discussions suggesting the addition of research evidence and workforce as additional pillars, this section discusses these three fundamental pillars. They are:

1. *Education*: The preparation of members of a profession through an academically sound educational process and an educational programme that enables individuals to acquire all the competencies they require to effectively perform the job for which they are being educated. The educational programme must meet the global standards for midwifery education (ICM 2013a, b) and cover all the essential competencies for basic midwifery practice.
2. *Regulation*: A profession's education and practice must be well regulated to ensure that only competent care providers who can demonstrate safe practice are certified (ICM 2011). These professionals are able to provide quality care, and the regulatory mechanism serves to protect the public.
3. *Association*: Members of a profession thus educated and regulated should be brought together into a well-run, well-managed professional association which aggregates the efforts of the individual professionals. The association will then represent the interests of the profession, of its members and of the population they serve and be a physical representation of the existence of the profession. A midwives' association represents the interests of women, newborn, children, families and midwives.

The next three chapters describe each pillar in detail. The three pillars are represented diagrammatically below.

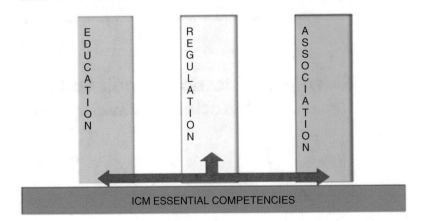

The three pillars of a strong profession. (Reproduced courtesy of the International Confederation of Midwives)

References

International Confederation of Midwives (2011) Young Midwifery Leaders Curriculum for Latin America and the Caribbean. www.internationalmidwives.org

International Confederation of Midwives (2013a) Essential competencies for basic midwifery practice (2010) revised in 2013 and 2019. www.internationalmidwives.org. Accessed 15 May 2019

International Confederation of Midwives (2013b) Global standards for midwifery education (2010) amended in 2013. www.internationalmidwives.org. Accessed 14 May 2019

Midwifery Education

4

Expected Learning Outcomes
By the end of the chapter, readers should be able to:

1. Provide a brief outline of the history of midwifery education
2. Outline the development of midwifery education programmes across different cultures
3. Critically analyse factors impacting on midwifery education globally
4. Outline the opportunities, challenges and threats that exist to the provision of midwifery education in different countries
5. Offer evidence-based suggestions on actions required to offset the challenges and threats and optimise the opportunities
6. Point to available resources to assist in building up quality midwifery education programmes
7. Suggest policy considerations, research and practice to enhance and facilitate provision of quality midwifery education in different settings

4.1 Impact of Qualified Midwives

Global consensus was reached that qualified midwives are the most appropriate, primary care providers for women, newborn and their families (Renfrew et al. 2014). Studies have shown that in countries such as Sweden and the Netherlands, investing in professionalising midwives in the sixteenth and seventeenth centuries led to rapid reduction in maternal and neonatal mortality even before antibiotics, caesarean sections and other technological interventions were available (Högberg 2004). Yet in many countries especially in the low-income countries (LIC), midwifery was and still is perceived as women's work for women and the status of midwifery matches the low status of women (Peabody et al. 2006). In 2007, Masden Wagner highlighted that in those countries where most physicians and obstetricians were men, power dynamics entered the workplace and led to midwives, who are predominantly women, feeling paralysed and powerless in the presence of their male colleagues. The relationship was not an active collaboration based on mutual respect between health professionals of equal standing responding to different needs of women and their families (Chipeta 2016).

© Springer Nature Switzerland AG 2021
J. Kemp et al., *Global Midwifery: Principles, Policy and Practice*,
https://doi.org/10.1007/978-3-030-46765-4_4

4.2   History of Midwifery Education

The development of midwifery education differed from continent to continent. Colonialism, gender issues, social status, perceptions of other health-care professionals and women's needs all had an impact. The global health agenda and governments' understanding of the value of midwives also exerted strong influences (Finerty et al. 2013).

4.2.1   Africa

In Africa, childbirth care was provided by older women introduced to the 'trade' by their parents. In some settings, the training of midwives became a method of extending colonial domination and a way of rewarding the contribution of Africans to the First World War (Turrittin 2002). Western midwifery education was established in some countries by the French, the British and the Dutch and, to a very small extent, the Portuguese during the colonial and missionary era. Western medicine was provided for the settlers and their families (Magobe and Ncube 2006). In South Africa, from 1652, Dutch certified and licensed midwives independently provided maternity care. In the 1960s, women were encouraged to give birth in hospitals. Midwives were no longer allowed to practise independently. They assumed the role of obstetric nurses. Midwifery students had to be registered nurses.

Earlier training focused on the production of assistants to work in rural areas, in most cases as the only care providers there. They could conduct normal delivery, recognise complications and refer (Speirs 1985; Magobe and Ncube 2006). In Zimbabwe, Zambia and Malawi, the students were traditional birth attendants (TBAs), mature women, married, well respected in their families and literate (Speirs 1985). By the 1950s enrolled midwives' training was introduced with entry qualification of 6 years of primary education. From the 1970s, the entry requirements were raised to 4 years secondary school and nursing. By the end of the 1990s, midwifery went into the universities as part of nursing.

4.2.2   Asia

After passing the Midwives Act in 1902 to restrict practice by unlicensed midwives in England, the Victoria Memorial Scholarship Fund was established in British India to restrict the practice of untrained birth attendants. In 1918, Dr. Ida Sophia Scudder started training midwives in South India as part of missionary work and expanded it to China and Japan as an experiment in interdenominational enterprise, in spite of the scepticism and consistently pessimistic attitude of the doctors. There was mutual distrust amongst the doctors and the indigenous traditional birth attendants or 'dais' (Welcome Trust 2005).

Meanwhile in Japan, midwives were autonomous practitioners revered as 'the grannies who delivered life'. Westernisation of Japanese midwifery began 1868 and official training of 'medical midwives' began under the auspices of obstetricians, imposing the first restrictions on midwives' practice and introducing nursing into midwifery through the Midwives Ordinance of 1899. By the 1930s, friction between the female profession of medical midwives and the male profession of obstetricians saw midwives receive further restriction. Midwifery education changed from 2 years direct entry prior to the Second World War to all midwifery students being required to be licensed nurses (Limura 2015).

4.2.3   Europe

In Europe midwifery education started way before caesarean sections, antibiotics and other technologies in the sixteenth and seventeenth centuries in the Scandinavian countries, leading to dramatic drops in maternal and neonatal mortality. In Turkey, midwifery moved from a profession passed from mother to daughter in the 1800s to a graduate programme in the twenty-first century. In the nineteenth century, junior midwives were trained under the supervision of recognised midwives (Apay et al. 2012). In 1880, midwifery lost its autonomy through formal training spearheaded by an obstetrician in Istanbul, and in 1924, it came under the faculty of medicine. In

1978, entry requirements were raised. After 1996, midwifery education became an undergraduate programme at universities in line with a number of European Directives on the education of health workers.

Meanwhile, according to Mivsec et al. (2016), changes were taking place in midwifery education in Slovenia, the Slovak Republic and the Check Republic, starting in the eighteenth century. Midwives were autonomous. The education evolved from short courses in the university in Prague to a 2-year programme following secondary education, and in 1925, doctors required that midwifery education be a 3-year programme. With ascension into the European Union, midwifery education had to comply with the European Union Directives.

In Norway, in 1952, a nursing qualification became a requirement for admission into midwifery education. The Bologna process of harmonisation of higher education in Europe led to the implementation of a common degree structure and qualification framework. In 2012, midwifery, already a postgraduate course, became a master's programme with an increased focus on research (Lukasse et al. 2017). Reports reveal that though the graduates felt theoretically strong, they did not feel competent to practise especially managing complicated situations (Hagtvedt 2008; Hughes and Fraser 2011; Schytt and Waldenstrom 2013).

4.2.4   The Americas

Midwifery and nurse-midwifery education started in response to the 'midwife problem' of the early 1900s in the face of interprofessional rivalries and gross misunderstanding of what midwifery is and does, because midwifery was generally perceived as an extension of nursing. Midwifery education was offered in Schools of Nursing with the content integrated into nursing (Cassells 2000; Varney et al. 2004; Burst 2005). Physicians wanted to call nurse-midwives 'obstetric assistants' until the 1960s (Hellman 1971). The early midwifery advocates, whilst understanding that nursing and midwifery were

separate professions, also understood that to survive and thrive, nurse-midwifery had to compromise at a time when the word 'midwife' conjured up derogatory images (Burst 2005). The profession was allowed to exist only attached to nursing and under medical supervision and control. The autonomy of midwives was sacrificed for credibility and access to the healthcare system.

4.2.4.1   Why Focus on Midwifery Education?

Midwives when educated to global standards, regulated, supported and integrated into a functional health system, can provide 87% of the 46 essential interventions for maternal and newborn health care (Partnership for Maternal Newborn and Child Health 2011) leading to an 83% reduction of maternal and newborn deaths and disability and 80% reduction of still births rate (UNFPA 2014; Ten Hoope-Bender et al. 2014; Castro-Lopes 2016; Renfrew et al. 2014). In addition, besides survival, quality midwifery care improves over 50 additional health outcomes including reduction of preterm labour and birth by 24%, improving breastfeeding rates and psychosocial outcomes and reducing the use of interventions especially caesarean sections (WHO 2019). Figure 4.1 presents 50 additional outcomes from quality midwifery education.

4.3   Factors Impacting on Midwifery Education

4.3.1   The Global Health Agenda

Between 2000 and 2015, aspirations to achieve MDGs 4, 5 and 6 impacted on midwifery education curricula as countries attempted to produce adequate numbers of 'Skilled Attendants at Birth' (SBAs) (Chou 2015). In the post MDG period, global health focused on the 2030 Agenda for Sustainable Development Goals (SDGs) (Campbell et al. 2016). Achievement of two of the SDG strategies 'The Global Strategy for Human Resources for Health: Workforce 2030' and 'The Global Strategy for Women's Newborn's and Adolescents' Health 2016–2030 heavily rely

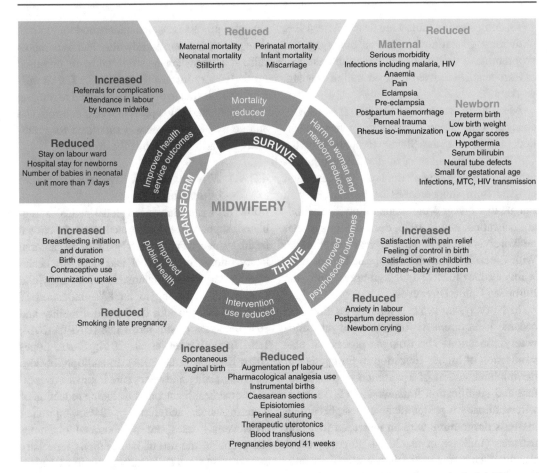

Fig. 4.1 50 additional outcomes from quality midwifery education. Source: WHO (2019): Framework for action: Strengthening quality midwifery education for Universal Health Coverage 2030. https://apps.who.int/iris/bitstream/handle/10665/324738/9789241515849-eng.pdf Accessed October 2019. (Reproduced with permission)

on the availability of a quality midwifery workforce, specifically midwives, and thus led to revitalisation of WHO focus on midwifery education. A series of global meetings and consultations were hosted between July 2016 and December 2018 to develop global consensus on how best to strengthen midwifery education. The meetings culminated into, amongst other things, a seven-step global action plan to strengthen midwifery education (Fig. 4.2) (WHO 2019).

maternal and newborn deaths and stillbirths occur (UNFPA 2014). Out of the 73 countries surveyed, only four had enough midwives for adequate coverage and 22% had serious shortages (UNFPA 2014). These statistics stimulated countries to develop mechanisms for educating midwives, sometimes educating them 'fast' in order to meet targets for the Millennium Development Goals (MDGs) (Renfrew et al. 2014).

4.3.2 Individual Country Needs

Encouraged by the evidence, countries perceived the need to accelerate the production of midwives especially in low-income countries where 90% of

4.4 Midwifery Education Programmes Accross The Globe

Midwifery education has developed at varying paces and in different forms across cultures and sometimes within countries (UNFPA 2011, 2014).

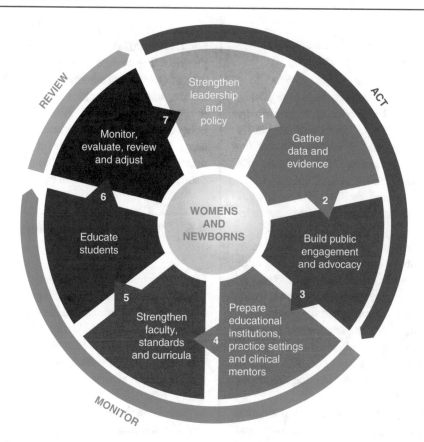

Fig. 4.2 The seven step action plan to strenghten quality midwifery education. Source: WHO (2019): Framework for action: Strengthening quality midwifery education for Universal Health Coverage 2030. https://apps.who.int/ iris/bitstream/handle/10665/324738/9789241515849-eng.pdf Accessed October 2019. (Reproduced with permission)

Many countries responded to the desire to reach MDG targets by increasing the number of education programmes (Nove 2018). Some of these lasted only a matter of weeks or months (Renfrew et al. 2014; WHO 2016) with no qualified faculty and some lacked in practical application (WHO 2016) and in such important areas as infection prevention and respectful care. This led to a possible link between poor education, poor clinical care, sepsis and mistreatment of women (Filby et al. 2016). Mere numbers were not enough to achieve the desired results (Van Lerberghe et al. 2014; Measure 2016). Only when midwives are equitably distributed, educated to international standards and possess the right competencies, will death rates be reduced (WHO 2013, 2016; Renfrew et al. 2014). Additionally, lack of resources, poor infrastructure,

weak health systems and lack of capacity to respond to the needs in some countries were persistent problems (Renfrew et al. 2014) as countries strove to produce 'Skilled Birth Attendants' (SBAs).

4.5   The Skilled Birth Attendants

The WHO and its global partners advocated for skilled attendance, and in 2004, in a joint statement, they defined a skilled attendant (Box 4.1). This care provider was to provide a *continuum* of care to meet the needs of women starting from their homes to the most complex referral facility.

To increase SBA coverage, countries introduced 'task shifting' (Box 4.1) through training 'skills and drills' (Fulton et al. 2011; McPake and

Box 4.1. Definitions: skilled attendance, skilled attendant and task shifting

Skilled attendance: 'Care provided to a woman and her newborn during pregnancy, childbirth and immediately after birth by an *accredited and competent* healthcare provider who has at her/his disposal the necessary equipment and the support of a functioning health system, including transport and referral facilities for emergency obstetric care' (Making Pregnancy Safer 2004).

Skilled attendant: 'an accredited health professional—such as a midwife, doctor or nurse—who has been educated and trained to proficiency in the skills needed to manage normal (uncomplicated) pregnancies, childbirth and the immediate postnatal period, and in the identification, management and referral of complications in women and newborns' (Making Pregnancy Safe 2004:1).

Task shifting: 'A rational redistribution of tasks among health workforce teams and involves a process of delegation whereby tasks are moved, where appropriate, to less specialized health workers' (WHO 2008).

Mensah 2008), but it later became apparent that providing additional training increased knowledge and skills but did not guarantee application of the new knowledge and skills acquired (McPake and Mensah 2008; Evans et al. 2009; Grady et al. 2011). Other countries introduced lower-level cadres to provide antenatal and intrapartum care (Deller et al. 2015) with no standardised or evaluated content and requirements of training programmes due to lack of the capacity and infrastructure needed to adhere to global recommendations (Buttler 2018). Many cadres considered skilled did not meet the internationally agreed criteria set in the 2004 joint statement (Harvey et al. 2007; Adegoke et al. 2012; Harvey 2007), rendering measurement of progress difficult (Hobbs 2019). The SDGs provided an opportunity for reflective analysis of the definition. WHO and

partners redefined SBAs as *skilled health personnel* (WHO 2018) to improve measurement of progress. The revised definition (Chapter 2 Box 2.3) was explicit on who the skilled health personnel are, what they are able to do and how they are to be educated (WHO 2019). This definition obliged countries to revise curricula, revisit and adapt international standards of education and practice. For detailed description of skilled attendance and skilled attendant at birth, see Chapter 2.

4.6   Pre-service Midwifery Education

Graduates' nomenclature is related to the type of programmes undertaken by graduates. Post nursing programmes produce *nurse-midwives*. Direct entry programmes produce midwives whose title suggests the level at which the qualification was acquired—*certificate midwives*, *diploma midwives* and *graduate midwives* (ACNM 2017; SANC 2017). In countries where nurse-midwives rotate to general nursing and midwifery settings, the title *midwife* describes those working in the maternity facilities at that point in time and those who self-identify as midwives (Castro-Lopes et al. 2016).

The entry qualifications, curriculum content and duration of midwifery education programmes vary greatly across and within regions and countries (Buttler 2018). In 2011 and 2013, the ICM published global reference documents for the development of midwifery education programmes (see Annex 4.3 on resources available). But not all countries have the desire, the resources and the know-how to implement these global recommendations (Renfrew et al. 2014; UNFPA 2014 and WHO 2017, 2018, 2019). Wide inconsistencies remained in the nature, content and quality of midwifery education programmes (Van Lerberghe et al. 2014; Bharj et al. 2016).

4.6.1   The Teachers of Midwives

In many LICs, teaching methodologies used do not always facilitate acquisition of competencies (Bharj et al. 2016). Political, social and cultural restrictions to full-scope midwifery practice pose problems. Educators are challenged in providing learning opportunities that ensure acquisition of globally recommended competencies (Bharj et al. 2016). Faculty members are neither educated to teach (Renfrew et al. 2014) nor oriented to the use of competency-based education (CBE) methodologies (ICM 2014). They do not always have access to practice nor do they stay connected with midwifery practice. The role and contribution of preceptors and mentors is not always appreciated and also differs across and between countries (Magge 2015; Manzi 2014; Way 2016; Vitale 2018).

4.6.2 Direct Entry Midwifery

Direct entry midwifery is when students enter the midwifery education programme without a nursing background and become 'independent practitioners educated in the discipline of midwifery' (National Midwifery Institute of California 2019). In many countries, schools and universities set their own entry requirements but generally a minimum of 4 years secondary education is expected. The recommended global standard is 12 years of schooling (ICM 2013a, b), but not all countries adhere to this standard (WHO 2018; Renfrew et al. 2014). Annex 4.1 shows the global distribution and duration of the programmes amongst the 114 ICM member countries at the time of writing.

Advantages of a direct entry programme include clarity of professional identity, clarity of the midwifery care philosophy, ease of deployment (only to maternity settings), stability and retention of the midwifery workforce and improved population health outcomes (Rosskam 2011; Global Health Workforce Alliance 2010). However, it is considered impractical where the midwife is the only care provider and is expected to deal with nursing situations (Rosskam 2011; Global Health Workforce Alliance 2010). Additionally, in some countries, there is no direct career path for this cadre as a nursing qualification is

demanded for promotion and for some senior midwifery positions. This is gradually changing (Ford 2010).

4.6.3 Midwifery Post-Nursing

In many countries, even where once autonomous (Limura 2015; Lukasse et al. 2017), midwifery education is perceived as a post-basic course after nursing (Hellman 1971; Burst 2005; Varney et al. 2004). When midwifery came under the control of nurses, obstetricians, physicians and paediatricians (Apay et al. 2012; Limura 2015; Mivsec et al. 2016; Lukasse et al. 2017; SANC 2017), a nursing qualification became a requirement to enter a midwifery education programme (Midwifery Alliance 2011). Out of 114 ICM member countries, 59 offer post-nursing midwifery education with duration of the programmes varying from 3 to 48 months; 42 offer at the global standard of 18 months and above (ICM Map 2017). But as in direct entry, not many countries are either willing or able to adhere by this global standard (Renfrew et al. 2014).

Nurse-midwives are versatile, a useful characteristic in LMICs where there are serious shortages of staff (Stones and Arulkumaran 2014). They can rotate between departments and can be posted to peripheral areas where they are capable of offering both nursing and midwifery care. They enter midwifery as professionals and are able to handle the stresses of the rapid decision-making demanded by midwifery care settings (Ceschia and Horton 2016).

This versatility is a double-edged sword because when rotated, care providers experience serious emotional distress as they try to fit into the various settings. They fail to develop a professional identity and have difficulties in deciding the direction of their professional development (Ceschia and Horton 2016). They also do not receive relevant in-service training. When there is a shortage of nurses, they are used to fill in nursing positions. Evidence has shown that more nurses were observed to migrate to urban areas and richer countries (Rosskam 2011). Hence de-linking nursing and midwifery education might improve workforce retention.

4.6.4   Midwifery Integrated into Nursing

Some countries like South Africa, Nigeria, Kenya and USA have programmes where midwifery content is integrated into a nursing curriculum. Such programmes run for 3–4 years. Graduates come out with more than one qualification. This poses a problem of quality and ensuring that all competencies for each field have been acquired at the end of the programme (SANC 2017).

4.6.5   Short Programmes

Some countries offer short programmes ranging from 6 months to 2 years duration, which do not meet the global standards. Examples of these include Nurse Midwife Technicians in Malawi and Zimbabwe, Lady Health Visitors in Pakistan and Family Welfare Volunteers in Bangladesh. The content of the programmes and the titles of the graduates vary and are peculiar to the country. When deployed, these health workers are also called midwives, causing confusion amongst women and their families, mirroring the experience in Japan in the 1950s (Limura 2015).

4.6.6   Lifelong Learning in Midwifery

Midwifery education should be designed to prepare graduates for lifelong learning. Bridging courses should be offered to enable short course graduates to attain midwifery education according to global standards. Continuing professional development is a must for the maintenance of competence, and ideally, each country should develop a continuing professional development strategy for its midwives. When midwifery moved into universities in the twentieth century, this enhanced midwifery capacity for leadership, and besides midwifery emerging as an evidence-based profession, it now stands shoulder to shoulder with other

professions, able to develop its own body of knowledge and to depend on its own researchers. It is however paramount to ensure that competencies in clinical midwifery are not lost but rather enhanced with new knowledge identified through midwifery research (Rumsey 2017).

4.7   The Impact of Technological Advnaces

By the early twenty-first century, midwifery education and practice were taking place in an era of progressive technological advances which supported transformational outcomes of safe, integrated, high-quality, knowledge-driven, evidenced-based care and educational approaches (World Health Assembly WHA64.72011). With increased availability and growing capabilities of information and communication technologies off-campus, blended learning programmes became possible. Midwifery could be learnt through a variety of applications without leaving home or workstation. Self-study, self-assessment and self-directed learning in both theory and practice have become an integral part of teaching approaches in many countries, enabling networking and information sharing amongst schools, faculty and students. Virtual and enhanced realities have entered into midwifery education where technology is being used to make situations as close to real as possible (see video clip from Australia in the section Additional Resources for Reflection and Further Study).

4.8   Opportunities, Challanges and Threats to Midwifery Education

4.8.1   Opportunities

The global health agenda provided a huge opportunity for midwifery education as it galvanised key global agencies to focus on improvement of midwifery education. Technological advancement made it possible for individuals who might not have been able to access midwifery education to embark on it from a distance. The desire of countries to reduce preventable deaths and the availability of evidence on the positive impact of quality midwifery services have provided great advocacy tools (WHA 2013; Scotish Government 2017).

4.8.2   Challenges and Threats

Underinvestment remains persistent. Despite the evidence on the major, positive and proven impacts of midwifery care on women and children's health, there has remained startling underinvestment in midwifery education and training at all levels (WHO 2016). A lot of countries where the need for midwives is greatest are not able to finance the midwifery education process (Renfrew et al. 2014). The global standard of a 3-year direct entry programme (ICM 2011) had to be reconsidered as some countries are not able to meet the necessary expenditure (WHO 2016) despite the clear understanding that the duration of a programme is linked to quality and depth of study (UNFPA 2014).

Population movements due to conflicts, civil unrests and other humanitarian disasters which disproportionately affect women and children continue to rapidly change the demography of countries. More midwives are needed in such circumstances. Midwifery education programmes do not change that frequently and easily. Hence, midwifery education curricula need to be flexible enough to accommodate these sudden changes and be robust enough to provide clear and firm guidelines to the production of midwives who meet global standards and provide quality care including in humanitarian crises.

A lack of common understanding about the role and responsibility of a midwife remains. In some situations, midwifery is confused with obstetrics, for example in Kyrgyzstan and China (ICM 2013a, b). In some countries, midwives are considered less educated than obstetricians, and so all the midwifery education is led by obstetricians and physicians. In other situations, midwifery content is integrated into nursing content as described above, and midwives are educated by nurses as midwifery is perceived as part of nursing (Fullerton and Johnson 2011). There is convincing evidence that the poor-quality education and poor-quality educators are exacerbated by lack of mentors and preceptors for students and newly qualified midwives (Gherrisi et al. 2016; Luyben et al. 2017; WHO 2019).

4.9   Cross-Cutting Issues Impacting on Midwifery Education Globally

4.9.1   Gender

Most midwives are women, and the status of midwifery is closely related to the status of women in different countries (March 2019; Newman 2016; Jhpiego 2019). Gender analysis will facilitate the identification of gender transformative action that will help overcome the professional, economic and sociocultural barriers to the provision of quality midwifery care (WHO 2016).

4.9.2   Leadership

It is difficult to separate midwifery education from leadership, management, governance, health system issues and political developments on the global scene. Lack of leadership means lack of advocacy and policy influence (Rumsey 2017). Because midwives tend to be perceived as less educated, they are not always placed in leadership positions. Instead, other professionals are placed to lead and educate midwives to the detriment of care provision (Magge 2015). Hence, leadership development amongst midwives is an urgent requirement.

4.10   Protecting the Title 'Midwife'

A midwife is the prototype of a skilled person to provide midwifery care. It is acknowledged that other professional groups are also involved (Renfrew et al. 2014). Other professionals provide maternity care (ICM 2017) (see Box 2.4).

The title 'midwife' has been clearly defined and internationally agreed (see Box 4.2).

Though not all countries have either the capacity

Box 4.2. The international definition of a midwife

A midwife is a person who has successfully completed a midwifery education programme that is based on the ICM Essential Competencies for Basic Midwifery Practice and the framework of the ICM Global Standards for Midwifery Education and is recognized in the country where it is located, who has acquired the requisite qualifications to be registered and/or legally licensed to practice midwifery and use the title 'midwife' and who demonstrates competency in the practice of midwifery.

International   Confederation   of Midwives (2017)

---

or the resources to provide such education, this should not jeopardise the health of women and newborn. Hence, in some countries, other types of care providers with some midwifery skills provide maternity care. Protecting the title 'midwife' does not ignore these situations. Ideally, those providers should be called by other titles until they have acquired all the midwifery competencies through continuing professional development (CPD). This would be a strong motivator for countries to develop a series of CPD programmes with which to build the capacity of their care providers up to global standards. Title protection would be a positive move towards harmonising midwifery globally.

4.11   Enhancing Quality

Education programmes and processes should enhance the development of positive qualities in the learner and eliminate disrespectful and abusive maternity care (Homer et al. 2014). Faculty should remain connected with midwifery practice and aware of all the changes taking place in care provision in order to guide students. The majority of faculty should be midwives who hold recognised education qualification. Mentors, preceptors and supervisors are essential to enhance high-quality education and effective support in the practice as well as the academic areas. The education processes should enable the students to experience continuity of care with women during their training. There need to be adequate physical facilities for accommodation and learning as well as adequate water and sanitation in the midwifery schools (WHO 2017).

4.12   Strengthening Partnerships in the Provision of Midwifery Education

Political partnerships with regulatory and professional bodies, partnerships with other professional disciplines, amongst different midwifery schools, regions, countries and between women and their care providers can contribute to the development of effective midwifery education (O'Connell and Bradshaw 2016). The New Zealand experience illustrates how a transformation in midwifery education took place as a result of midwives partnering with women in the 1980s, leading to the separation of midwifery education from nursing education as well as giving midwives autonomy through legislation (Gilkison et al. 2016).

4.13   Conclusion

Midwifery education has struggled with pressures from society including gender issues, colonialism and class distinctions, from fellow health professionals including nurses, physicians and obstetricians. Yet, midwifery acquired status, value and importance from its effectiveness in reducing maternal and neonatal deaths as well as improving the health outcomes of women and their families (AbouZahr 2003).

Until the 1950s, midwives were respected, revered and autonomous. In Africa and Asia, midwifery exemplified a local knowledge system controlled by women—TBAs, colonial midwives and wives of missionaries (Turrittin 2002). Whilst in France and England in the 1930s obstetricians controlled obstetrics, women controlled midwifery education in Africa and Asia but when midwifery education was being developed and structured into curricula, the local knowledge was never captured.

As midwifery education was delivered at a higher academic level so did the opposition and control from other professionals and loss of midwifery autonomy in Japan (Limura 2015), Norway (Lekasse et al. 2017), the Czech Republic (Mivsec et al. 2016), Turkey (Apay et al. 2012) and the Americas (Mallot 2009; Burst 2005). Moving midwifery education into universities was a huge strengthening aid to produce competent practitioners, strong leaders and researchers and to restore midwifery autonomy wherever possible (Beran et al. 2019). By the 2020s, midwifery education was in a vantage position not only to contribute to global agendas but also to reclaim much of what the profession had lost on the way. Learning from the Norwegian experience, higher education should not be a double-edged sword so that the quest for higher education should not lead to midwifery losing some of its grounding in clinical practice (Lukasse et al. 2017).

Evidence shows that proposing education as an intervention to fix service delivery problems does not always achieve the desired results (Renfrew et al. 2014; UNFPA 2014; Bharj et al. 2016) because education is only a piece of the puzzle (WHO 2019). Other support parameters are involved. Without addressing these, education alone is likely to fail. Occasionally, there is a tendency to focus too narrowly on the perinatal period to the omission of rapidly changing social, political and legal environments that endanger women's health.

4.13.1 Principles

Only persons interested in midwifery should be educated as such to maximise resources. Countries should be supported to develop programmes which meet global standards.

4.13.2 Policy

Midwives should be educated primarily by midwives. Those teachers who have not been formally educated as teachers should be supported through continuing professional development on the job.

4.13.3 Practice

Midwifery education institutions must be adequately resourced with enough educators and comply with suggested teacher: student ratios for theory and clinical teaching.

Key Messages

The effective education of midwives is critical to the provision of quality maternal and newbron care. Quality midwifery education is the first step to quality maternity care.

Midwifery education has come a long way, all the time fending off oposition and distratcion. Now that midwives are educted to the level of producing their own body of knowledge through the inscresinf number of midwife researchers, it is time to reclame midwifery's position in the health system both at the point of care and at the level of policy making.

Questions for Reflection

1. According to the ICM, only midwives practise midwifery. Other care professionals provide maternity care. What is your opinion on this?
2. The text explains that in many LICs midwifery is post nursing because of the needs of the country. Discuss the merits and demerits of perceiving midwifery as a part of nursing and the pros and cons of having a professional who can rotate between two fields, i.e. midwifery and nursing settings.
3. The World Health Organization produced the seven-step plan for strengthening midwifery education. Critically analyse this strategy and outline the possible challenges and threats to the implementation of this plan.

Annex 4.1: Distribution of Midwifery Programmes According to Type Amongst 114 ICM Member Countries as of 2017

Type of programme	Number of countries	Brief description	Entry qualification in years of schooling		Duration in months		Comments
			Global standard	Range in countries	Global standard	Range in countries	
Direct entry	82	Students enter the midwifery education programme without a nursing background to become independent practitioners educated in the discipline of midwifery. Graduates can only work in midwifery settings including in rural areas closest to where women live, thus reclaiming the midwifery turf lost as the profession developed. Advantages include clarity of professional identity However, it is not practical in those settings where the midwife is the only care provider in the community and is expected to deal with nursing situations. Additionally in some countries direct midwifery graduates had no career pathway as a nursing qualification was demanded for promotion even for some senior midwifery positions. This is gradually changing	12	12–16	36	10–60	Students range from high school and pre-university graduates to include mature individuals who may have been in other professions In 62 countries, programme duration matches or exceeds global standard Schools and universities set their own entry requirements in some countries Direct entry midwifery was related to stability and retention of the midwifery workforce compared to nurse midwifery (Rosskam 2011). Results of 57 country surveys indicated that direct entry was the most favoured midwifery education method (Global Health Workforce Alliance 2010), resulting in improved population health outcomes
Post nursing	59	A nursing qualification is required to enter a midwifery education programme Graduates can work in both nursing and midwifery settings. Very useful in situations of shortage of staff as graduates can be rotated between departments. Graduates can be posted alone in the periphery to offer both nursing and midwifery care, e.g. in Bangladesh, the severe shortage of nurses limited nurse midwives from being entirely utilised for midwifery activities. 'Primarily, serving as hospital staff nurses fulfilling vacancies and continually rotating throughout the hospital, registered nurse-midwives often lack specialised in-service training' (Masoom 2017)	12 + nursing qualification	12 + nursing	18	3–48	42 countries offer the programme at the global standard of 18 months and above The versatility of nurse midwives is a double-edged sword. Studies showed that rotated care providers experienced serious emotional distress as they tried to fit into the new setting, and it was difficult for them to develop in any one particular direction as they failed to develop a professional identity and to receive relevant in-service trainings Observations showed that nurse midwives were amongst the most significant groups of healthcare workers who migrate to urban areas and richer countries. Hence, the recommendation was to de-linking nursing and midwifery education for countries to improve workforce retention and reduce migration

Type of programme	Number of countries	Brief description	Entry qualification in years of schooling		Duration in months		Comments
			Global standard	Range in countries	Global standard	Range in countries	
Integrated programme	Four known but could be more	Midwifery content is integrated into a nursing curriculum. Graduates qualify with more than one discipline (SANC 2017)	None	12	None	36–48	It is difficult to ensure that all competencies for each discipline have been acquired at the end of the programme
Other (shorter courses)	Several LICs	Abbreviated content for nursing, midwifery and other areas is delivered in a shortened programme. Products are usually auxiliary workers of different titles, e.g. nurse midwife technician in Malawi and Zimbabwe; lady health visitor in Pakistan; family welfare volunteers in Bangladesh and maternal and child health aids in Sierra Leone	None	Varied	None	3–24	These programmes do not meet global standards. The content of the programme varies per country. The products in some countries are also called midwives. This leads to confusion in the community

Source: International Confederation of Midwives website www.internationalmidwives.org accessed August 2019

Annex 4.2: Education Models, Technological Advances and Innovations Instructional Technologies in Midwifery Education

Model/innovation	Brief description	Major benefits	Constraints	Comments
Synchronous systems Face to face onsite learning	Real-time learning face-to-face with the teacher. Usually teacher and students are in the same place	• Support is there and immediate • Students and teachers can form personal relationships • There is peer support • Teachers can identify students who have problems through direct observation and personal interactions	• The student has to be away from home and work • Can be expensive in time and money • Schools can be inaccessible for some, especially if they are only in cities	Modern technological advances are making this approach less necessary
Asynchronous modular systems	Teacher and student are not in the same place. Teacher can post a lesson at one time and students complete it later at a convenient time	• Students can take up the course from anywhere as long as there is connectivity • Student does not have to be away from the family for prolonged periods of time • Student does not have to be away from work for blocks of time	• Some asynchronous systems may need electricity and internet connections which may not be available everywhere in some countries • Requires personal motivation and self-discipline from students	The constraints can be offset by blended approaches where there is fixed schedule of some face-to-face time and some distance learning time

Model/innovation	Brief description	Major benefits	Constraints	Comments
Distance learning And e-learning or web-based learning	Distance learning is also called online learning. Students from one part of the world can take a programme run in another part of the world and become international student without needing to travel e-learning typically refers to the online interaction between a student and the teacher. Basically, the student receives the training through an online medium, even though the teacher may be in the same building. e-learning can be used in a classroom or an online setting. Additionally, it can be used to simulate and intensify work-based learning situations	• Increased access to midwifery education and degree programmes • Lectures, assignments, tests are all enabled by virtual platforms. A fully online university degree means the student does not have to travel at all for studies	• Requires a computer and connectivity which may not be available in those areas where the need for midwifery education is greatest • Very sensitive to civil and other types of population unrest	As the world gets more connected, there is expansion of the availability of electricity, computers and internet Discussion forums via email, videoconferencing, and live lectures (video streaming) are all possible through the web. Web-based courses may also provide static pages such as printed course materials
Some learner-centred instructional technologies				
Competency-based education methodologies	Focus is on the acquisition of pre-determined set of competencies and combines with mastery learning	Acknowledges that individuals learn at different paces and therefore does not focus on the time it takes for the student to be declared competent. Assessment is ongoing and frequent to determine competence. Useful in all learning domains and most observable results are in clinical skills	Low-dose, high-frequency practice where students learn one or two competencies by practising over short periods of time frequently	Some critics are challenging the approach stating that it breaks learning down to too small elements for gestalt (big picture) learning
Problem-based education methodologies	Students learn about a subject through the experience of solving an open-ended problem	It is student centred. Fosters better understanding and retention of knowledge and develops problem-solving skills and critical thinking, self-directed learning and upholds life-long learning	Depending on utilisation of resources which might not be available in most schools of midwifery and tutor facilitation in some settings, the teachers are not familiar with the approach. It is time consuming Very challenging to students who would have learnt in the previous years that the teacher is the main disseminator of knowledge. Students might therefore spend a lot of time unfocused trying to get to grips with the approach	The problems must be well defined for it to produce the desired effect

Model/innovation	Brief description	Major benefits	Constraints	Comments
Enquiry-based learning	Enquiry-based learning is a form of active learning that starts by posing questions, problems or scenarios. It contrasts with traditional education, which generally relies on the teacher presenting facts and his or her knowledge about the subject Includes three steps: Question, investigate and communicate results	• There is evidence that inquiry-based learning can motivate students to learn and advance their problem-solving and critical thinking skills • Students develop stronger relationships with their classmates, improve their communication skills and increase their confidence in their own ideas	The effectiveness of inquiry-based learning depends on the guidance provided by teachers The teachers have to be conversant with the approach to provide effective guidance to students	In many low-income countries, very few teachers learn using this approach, and it may be difficult for them to guide students to use it. The situation was progressively improving at the time of writing
Simulation learning using a variety of simulators Low-fidelity models • Basic low-tech models • High-tech models designed to look and feel human • High-fidelity patient simulators	Simple effective and sometimes made by the students in the school. Low cost and therefore affordable and easy to maintain Look and feel human, thus providing a more realistic experience to the student Sometimes expensive and difficult to maintain. Some are even difficult to operate Computerised manikins that simulate real-life scenarios. Long used in medical schools, now quickly becoming essential for many midwifery schools	Simulation provides students with opportunities to practice their clinical and decision-making skills through various real-life situational experiences	With low-fidelity simulators, there is no direct interaction with the model, but interaction can be integrated by having a fellow student acting as the woman. The Mama Natali set, produced by Laerdal Global Health is one effective low-fidelity but highly effective range of such models High-fidelity simulators may be expensive and difficult to maintain, requiring technicians to maintain them	Not all education institutions in the areas where midwifery education is needed most can afford or have access to models of any level of fidelity

Model/innovation	Brief description	Major benefits	Constraints	Comments
Online platforms, e.g. • Virtual classroom • Unfolding case study • Online return demonstration of clinical skills	An online classroom that allows participants to communicate with one another, view presentations or videos, interact with other participants and engage with resources in workgroups Uses innovative evidence-based teaching and learning strategies Available on mobile devices anywhere, thus providing greater flexibility of when and where to learn	Collaborative, interactive and flexible. Attractive to the generation used to gaming as it gamifies learning Can be omni-synchronous, i.e. at times there can be real-time teacher–student interaction and real-time group session as well as private tutoring Encourages creativity for teachers to develop more inspiring, engrossing and effective learning content and allow learners to interact with lessons in a new way Potential to involve more artificial intelligence and virtual reality Enhances students' experiences More students including those in rural and underserved regions who might otherwise have been unable to attend the traditional onsite campus have access to midwifery education at their desired level (certificate, diploma, degree and masters)	Might take time to reach the poorest of the poor	Educators should stay alert to the advent of these new technologies. Not every innovation is successful. It is important to find the right solutions for each course and for the learners sometimes by trial and error. Educators have to be continuing learners too Students treat them like their messaging apps, and audio lessons are consumed like podcasts and mini quizzes as micro games that can be played during lunch break, given the proliferation of mobile devices in the twenty-first century
Virtual and augmented reality Augmented reality	A technology that allows the student to immerse her/himself in an artificial world using a virtual reality head set (*Journal of Education Technology* 2019). The world can be purely imaginary or a reproduction of the real world. Can be visual, auditory Augmented reality refers to a virtual interface, in 2D or 3D, that enhances (or augments) what we see by overlaying additional information (digital content) onto the real world. Immersion in the virtual world is not total, because we can always see the real world around us	• Allows the student to manipulate and interact with the object through the use of controllers enabling practice and learning. Allows the doing of tests and experiments without taking physical risks • Can improve and facilitate learning, increase memory capacity and making • Enables better decisions whilst working in a stimulating and entertaining environment. Students can 'see' internal organs and processes, thus enhancing understanding • The learner feels more engaged, more motivated and more receptive and ready to learn and communicate with others	• Implementation not yet generalised but it is taking root. Integration of these technologies requires radical changes and new teaching and learning models and a close collaboration between educators and education engineers	Having physical access to all what we learn is not possible, hence the importance of VR, which allows access to everything virtually. This allows a better understanding of things and phenomena with less cognitive efforts on the part of the learner, and less cost for the institute that deals with learning. Virtual reality-based learning has been proven to increase learners' level of attention by 100% and improve test results by 30%. VR will not only transform the way we entertain ourselves, but it will also completely change the way students learn

Annex 4.3: Resources Available for the Strengthening of Midwifery Education Globally

Resource	Source Comments
Global Strategic Directions for Nursing and Midwifery, 2016–2020	https://www.who.int/hrh/nursing_midwifery/en/
Nurse Educator Competencies, 2014	
Strengthening Quality Midwifery Education: WHO Meeting Report, 25–26 July 2016	
Strengthening Midwifery Education Action Plan, 2016–2030	
The global midwifery advocacy strategy	
The midwifery services framework	https://www.internationalmidwives.org/our-work/education/
Global Standards for Midwifery Education, 2013	
Global Standards for Midwifery Regulation, 2013	
Essential Competencies for Basic Midwifery Practice, 2011, reviewed 2017	
Model Curriculum Outlines for Midwifery Education, 2013	
Midwifery Services Gap Analysis Tools, 2013	
Manual on Competency-Based Education Methodologies, 2015	
Philosophy and model of midwifery care	

Other source organisations:
    United National Population Fund (UNFPA)
    Jhpiego
    Global Health workforce Alliance
Midwifery organisations which have a global outreach section:
    1. Canadian Association of Midwives
    2. Japanese midwives association
    3. American College of Nurse Midwives
    4. Royal College of Midwives (United Kingdom)
    5. Royal Dutch Organization of midwives (KNOV)
	https://www.unfpa.org/search/site/Midwifery%20education
	http://resources.jhpiego.org/search?text=Midwifery+education&sort_bef_combine=search_api_relevance_1+DESC

Additional Resources for Reflection and Further Study

Global Health Workforce Alliance (2011) Outcome statement of the second global forum on human resources for health, Bangkok, 27–29 January 2011: http://www.who.int/workforcealliance

The 'midwifery map' ICM website. https://www.internationalmidwives.org/icm-publications/map.html compares the available data on midwifery education in several countries. Consider how these interrelate with maternal and newborn mortality statistics in those countries

What is the difference between e-learning and blended learning? https://www.distancelearningportal.com/articles/269/whats-the-difference-between-blended-learning-e-learning-and-online-learning.html

World Health Organisation (2014) Nurse educator competencies. WHO, Geneva

Videos

Source: International Journal of Emerging Technologies in learning—ISSN:1863-0383, vol 14, no. 03, 2019.

Augmented reality and virtual reality in education. Myth or Reality? Noureddine Elmqaddem. https://doi.org/10.3991/ijet.v14i03.9289. Accessed Aug 2019

XENODU. Virtual environments for personal and social development. Tag Archives: nursing and midwifery training: how virtual reality is transforming nursing and midwifery learning (incl. video). March 8, 2018. Learning, Virtual Environments medical education, nursing and midwifery training, technology enhanced learning, virtual reality training simulation

https://www.youtube.com/watch?time_continue=86&v=IJT1K8Vjtmk

Some Examples of Mobile Applications and Some Videos

Giftedmom. http://www.giftedmom.org/. Accessed 10 Oct 2019. A mobile health provider based in Africa works with NGOs to provide free mobile services to expectant mothers and women with newborn children. A combination of apps and informational text messages, GiftedMom provides a wide range of health services through mobile devices, some of which are donated to women in need of the service. The app was first launched in Cameroon, where more than 7000 women die per year in pregnancy-related complications. To help curb maternal mortality rates in the country, GiftedMom subscribes pregnant women and new mothers to free text messages to educate them on prenatal care, vaccines and reproductive health. The messages also remind mothers of important pregnancy milestones and health services their newborns should be receiving. More than 6700 mothers currently use the app in Cameroon and Nigeria

Zero Mothers Die. https://www.youtube.com/watch?time_continue=15&v=8gdZl8Ac3uY. Accessed Oct 2019. This application provides small mobile phones to women in Africa—specifically Ghana, Gabon, Mali, Nigeria and Zambia—at no cost, with the goal of curbing maternal health care inaccessibility. The phones use SMS text messaging to provide women living in isolated areas with essential information for having a healthy pregnancy and birth. The short, digestible messages help empower women to be active in their own health care, whilst also giving them information they can pass along to women in their communities. The phones come preloaded with calling minutes at no additional cost, which women can use to call local healthcare providers in the event of an emergency. Zero Mothers Die also uses mobile connectivity to help educate healthcare workers through a partner app, increasing their knowledge as well as improving their role in the care of pregnant women

Maymay. http://pulse.psi.org/spring-2015/#maternal. Accessed Oct. Maternal and infant mortality rates in Myanmar are significantly higher than those in neighbouring nations—and the app maymay is helping address it. The free app sends out three tailored health alerts every week to pregnant women, providing tips on having a successful, healthy pregnancy. The app, created by Population Services International, provides a wide array of tips—such as nutritional advice, explanations of early signs and symptoms of pregnancy, and recommendations for safe baby items—catered to a user's stage in pregnancy. The app also allows pregnant women to find doctors in their area, sorting by specialty and medical institution

Safe Delivery. https://www.maternity.dk/. Accessed Oct 2019. https://www.youtube.com/watch?time_continue=6&v=qI5PMSYa_BM. Developed by the Maternity Foundation, the Safe Delivery app provides simple instructions to health workers in remote areas on how to assist with non-routine births. The app hopes to strengthen the quality of care and reduce maternal and newborn mortality rates by increasing a birthing attendant's knowledge in times of crisis. First launched in Ethiopia and Ghana, Safe Delivery uses animated videos to provide instruction to health workers, focusing on what to do when faced with birthing complications, like a newborn who is not breathing or a prolonged labour. The app also has flashcards, so an attendant can self-assess their knowledge outside of emergency situations. Safe Delivery is available in English and regional languages, breaking access barriers with tailored narration

Mama. https://unfoundation.org/. Accessed Oct 2019. The Mobile Alliance for Maternal Action (MAMA) created an app of the same name that delivers free health messages to new and expectant mothers in Bangladesh, South Africa, India and Nigeria. Women receive stage-based, culturally sensitive messages two to three times per week, which helps empower mothers with the health knowledge they are often denied. The messages address three main areas important to women throughout their experience with motherhood: warning signs, reminders and encouragement. That last point is especially notable: Along with health-based tips and information, users receive affirmation that they are succeeding as mothers—and that can be just as important as hard facts

Mobile Midwife. https://www.youtube.com/watch?time_continue=56&v=USRvTsPwihg. MOTECH Suite: Ghana Mobile Midwife. Accessed Oct 2019. To provide increased healthcare access to women in Ghana, the Mobile Midwife app utilises text messages and pre-recorded voice messages to help spread information to pregnant women, new mothers and their families. The app's messages are time-specific, providing information relevant to women that hinges on their stage in motherhood. Mobile Midwife is also used in conjunction with a Nurses' Application, which medical providers use to collect patient data and upload records to a centralised database. Through the application, providers can track patient care and identify those who are due for medical services

Safe Pregnancy and Birth. https://hesperian.org/books-and-resources/safe-pregnancy-and-birth-mobile-app/. Accessed Oct 2019. An award-winning app for expectant mothers in developing countries, Safe Pregnancy and Birth provides maternal health knowledge to both expectant mothers and healthcare providers. The app focuses on four major points: data collection, patient monitoring, health education or appointment reminders. Available in both English and Spanish, the Safe Pregnancy and Birth app relays information to pregnant women on how to stay healthy during pregnancy, how to recognise prenatal health concerns and what to do in an emergency situation. It also has step-by-step instructions for community health workers, explaining how to perform procedures such as taking blood pressure, treating someone in shock and stopping bleeding post-birth

References

AbouZahr C (2003) Safe motherhood: a brief history of the global movement 1947–2002. Br Med Bull 67(1):13–25. https://doi.org/10.1093/bmb/ldg014. Accessed 15 July 2019

Adegoke AA, Utz B, Msuya S et al (2012) Skilled birth attendants. Who is Who? A descriptive study of definitions and roles from nine Sub Saharan African countries. Plos One. 7(7)e40220

American College of Nurse Midwives (2017) Comparison of certified nurse midwives, certified midwives, certified professional midwives, clarifying the distinctions among professional midwifery credentials in the US. https://www.midwife.org/acnm/files/ccLibraryFiles/FILENAME/000000006807/FINAL-ComparisonChart-Oct2017.pdf

Apay SE, Kanbur A, Ozdemir F et al (2012) Midwifery education in Turkey. Coll Antropol 36(4): 1453–1456

Beran D et al (2019) High-quality health systems: time for a revolution in research and research funding. Lancet Glob Health 7(3):e303–e3e4

Bharj KK, Luyben A, Avery MD et al (2016) An agenda for midwifery education: advancing the State of the World's Midwifery. Midwifery 33:3–6

Burst HV (2005) The history of nurse-midwifery/midwifery education. J Midwifery Womens Health 50(2):129–137

Buttler MM (2018) Competence for basic midwifery practice: updating the ICM essential competencies. Midwifery 66(16875):137

Campbel OM, Graham W, Althabe F et al (2016) Maternal health. Every woman, every newborn, everywhere has the right to good quality care. Executive summary of the Lancet Series

Cassells J (2000) The Manhattan Midwifery School. (Master Thesis) New Haven: Yale University School of Nursing.

Castro-Lopes S, Nove AA, Ten Hoope-Bender P et al (2016) A descriptive analysis of midwifery education, regulation and association in 73 countries: the baseline for a post-2015 pathway. Hum Resour Health 14:37. https://doi.org/10.1186/s12960-016-0134-7

Ceschia A, Horton R (2016) Maternal health: time for a radical reappraisal. Lancet 388(10056):2064–2066

Chipeta E (2016) Working relationships between obstetric care staff and their managers: a critical incident analysis. BMC Health Serv Res 16(1):441

Chou D (2015) Ending preventable maternal and newborn mortality and stillbirths. BMJ 351:h4255

Deller B, Tripathi V, Stender S et al (2015) Task shifting in maternal and newborn health care: key components from policy to implementation. International Journal of Obstetrics and Gynecology. https://doi.org/10.1016/j.ijgo.2015.03.05

Evans CL, Maine B, McCloskey L et al. (2009) Where there is no obstetrician: increasing capacity for emergency obstetric care in rural India: an evaluation of a pilot program to train general doctors. International Journal of Obstetrics and Gynaecology. 107(3):277–282

Filby A, McConville F, and Portella A (2016) What prevents quality midwifery care? A systematic mapping of barriers in Low and Middle Income countries from the provider perspective. https://doi.org/10.1371/journal.pone.153391

Finerty G, Bosanque A, Aubrey D (2013) Charting the history of midwifery education. Pract Midwife 16(8):23–25

Ford S (ed) (2010) Tackling discrimination requires urgent change. Direct entry means no exit from the midwifery profession. Practice comment. Nursing Times, 7 June 2010

Fullerton JT, Johnson P, Thompson JB et al (2011) Quality considerations in midwifery pre-service education: exemplars from Africa. Midwifery 27(3) 308–315

Fulton BD, Scheffler RM, Sparkes SP et al. (2011) Health workforce skill mix and task shifting in low income countries: a review of recent evidence. Human Resources for Health. 9(1):1

Global Health Workforce Alliance (2010) Mid-level health providers a promising resource to achieve the health Millennium Development Goals. Geneva: WHO

Grady K, Ameh C, Adegoke AA et al (2011) Improving essential obstetric and newborn care in resource poor countries. Journal of Obstetrics and Gynecology. 31(1):18–23

Gherrisi A, Tinsa F, Soussi S et al (2016) Teaching research methodology to student midwives through a socio-constructivist educational model: the experience of the high school for science and health techniques of Tunis. Midwifery 33:46–48

Gilkison A, Pairman S, McAra-Couper J et al (2016) Midwifery education in New Zealand: education, practice and autonomy. Midwifery 33:31–33

Hagtvedt ML (2008) Jordmorutdanning - den første formelle udanningen for kvinner i Norge. Tidsskrift for Jordmødre. 114(6):36–40.

Harvey S (2007) Are skilled birth attendants really skilled? A measurement method, some disturbing results and potential way forward. Bulleting of the World Health Organisation 85(10):783–790

Harvey SA, Blandon YC, McCaw-Binns A et al (2007) Are skilled attendants really skilled? A measurement method, some disturbing results and a potential way forward. Bulletin of the World Health Organisation 85(10):783–790

Hellman LM (1971) Nurse Midwifery: Fifteen years. Bulleting of the American College of Nurse Midwifery. 16(3):1542–2011

Hobbs AJ (2019) Scoping review to identify and map the health personnel considered skilled birth attendants in low-and-middle income countries from 2000–2015. PLoS One 14(2):e0211576

Högberg U (2004) The Decline in Maternal Mortality in Sweden: the role of community midwifery. Am J Public Health 94(8):1312–1320. https://doi.org/10.2105/AJPH.94.8.1312

Homer CSE, Frieberg IK, Bastos Dias MA et al (2014) The projected effect of scaling up midwifery. Lancet 384(9948):1146–1157

Hughes AJ and Fraser DM (2011) 'SINK or SWIM': the experiences of newly qualified midwives in England. Midwifery 27(3):382–386

International Confederation of Midwives (2011) Young midwifery leaders curriculum for latin america and the caribbean. www.internationalmidwives.org

International Confederation of Midwives (2013a) Essential competencies for basic midwifery practice

(2010) revised in 2013 and 2019. www.internation-almidwives.org. Accessed 15 May 2019

International Confederation of Midwives (2013b) Global standards for midwifery education (2010) amended in 2013. www.internationalmidwives.org. Accessed 14 May 2019

International Confederation of Midwives (2014) A manual for competency based education methodologies for midwifery educators. https://www.internation-almidwives.org/documents

International Confederation of Midwives (2017) Definition of the midwife. International Confederation of Midwives. https://www.internationalmidwives.org/our-work/policy-and-practice/icm-definitions.html. Accessed 01 Oct 2019

Jhpiego (2019) Gender analysis toolkit for health systems [Internet] 2019 [cited 2019 Apr 1]. https://gender.jhpiego.org/analysistoolkit/gender-analysis/

Limura B (2015) History of Midwifery in Japan. Midwifery Today. midwiferytoday.com/summer

Lukasse M, Lilleengen AM, Fylkesnes AM et al (2017) Norwegian midwives opinion of their midwifery education – a mixed methods study. BMC Med Educ 17:80

Luyben A, Barger M, Avery M et al (2017) Exploring global recognition of quality midwifery education: vision or fiction? Women Birth 30:184–192

Magge H (2015) Mentoring and quality improvement strengthen integrated management of childhood illness implementation in rural Rwanda. Arch Dis Childhood 100(6):565–570

Magobe DK, Ncube E (2006) Evolution of formal midwifery education in Botswana, 1926 – 2005. Botswana Notes Rec 38:89–98. Published by: Botswana Society. https://www.jstor.org/stable/41235989. Accessed 15 July 2019

Making Pregnancy Safer (2014) The critical role of the skilled attendant. A joint statement by WHO, ICM and FIGO. World Health Organisation

Manzi A (2014) Clinical mentorship to improve pediatric quality of care at the health centers in rural Rwanda: a qualitative study of perceptions and acceptability of health care workers. BMC Health Serv Res 14(1):275

March C (2019) A guide to gender analysis frameworks. Oxfam GB, Oxford, p 145

McPake B, and Mensah K (2008) Task shifting in health care in resource poor countries. Lancet 372(9642):870–871

MEASURE (2016) Evaluation Bangladesh maternal mortality and health care survey 2016: summary [Internet]. 2018. [cited 2018 January 30]. https://www.measure-evaluation.org/resources/publications/fs-17-245-en/

Mivsec P, Baskova M, Wilhelmova R (2016) Midwifery education in Central-Eastern Europe. Midwifery 33:43–45. https://doi.org/10.1016/j.midw.2015.10.016

National Midwifery Institute Incorporated. Direct Entry Midwifery. https://www.nationalmidwiferyinstitute.com/. Accessed Oct 2019

Newman C (2016) Integration of gender-transformative interventions into health professional education

reform for the 21st century: implications of an expert review. Hum Resour Health 14(1):14

Nove A (2018) La qualité de la formation des sages-femmes dans six pays francophones d'Afrique sub-saharienne. Sante Publique, Paris. https://www.cairn.info/revue-sante-publique-2018-HS-page-45.html#

Lekasses M, Lillengen AM et al (2017) Norwegian midwives' opinion of their midwifery education - a mixed methods study. BMC Medical Education

O'Connell R, Bradshaw C (2016) Midwifery education in Ireland- the quest for modernity. Midwifery 33:34–36

Peabody JW, Taguiwalo MM, Robalino DA et al. (2006) Improving the quality of care in developing countries. In: Jamison DT, Breman JG, Measham AR, et al. (eds) Disease control priorities in developing countries (2nd edn), chap 70. Co-published by Oxford University Press, New York. https://www.ncbi.nlm.nih.gov/books/NBK11790/

Rosskam E (2011) A 21st century approach to assessing the protection of workers' health. Work: A Journal of Prevention, Assessment & Rehabilitation, 38(3):265–278

Renfrew M, McFadden A, Bastos MH et al (2014) Midwifery and quality care : findings from a new evidence -informed framework for maternal and newborn care. Lancet. 384(9948):1129–1145

Rumsey M (2017) Building nursing and midwifery leadership capacity in the Pacific. Int Nurs Rev 64(1):50–58

Schytt E, and Waldenstrom U (2013) How well does midwifery education prepare for clinical practice? Exploring views of Swedish students, midwives and obstetricians. Midwifery 29(2):102–109

Scottish Government (2017) The best start maternity and neonatal care plan executive summary. The Scottish Government. ISBN: 978-1-78652-764-6. www.gov.scot

South African Nursing Council (2017) Analysis of persons on the register. https://www.sanc.co.za/stats/stat2017/Age%20stats%202017.pdf

Speirs J (1985) Midwifery education in Malawi. Midwifery. 1(3):146–149 September 1985

Stones W, Arulkumaran S (2014) Health-care professionals in midwifery care. Lancet 384(9949):1169–1170

Ten Hoope-Bender P, de Bernis L, Campbell J et al (2014) Improvement of maternal and newborn health through midwifery. Lancet 384(9949):1226–1235

The Partnership for Maternal Newborn & Child Health (2011) A global review of the key interventions related to Reproductive, Maternal, Newborn and Child Health (RMNCH). PMNCH, Geneva

Turrittin (2002) Colonial midwives and modernising midwifery in West Africa. In: Berger I (ed) Women in twentieth-century Africa. Cambridge University Press, Cambridge

United Nations Population Fund (2011). The State of the World's Midwifery Report. Delivering health. Savng lives. UNFPA New York

United Nations Population Fund (2014) The state of the world's midwifery. A universal pathway. A woman's right to health. New York, United Nations Population Fund

Van Lerberghe W, Matthews Z, Achadi E et al (2014) Country experience with strengthening of health systems and deployment of midwives in countries with high maternal mortality. Lancet 384:1215–1210

Varney et al. (2004) Varney's midwifery, 4th Edition, Jones and Bartlett, Sudbury, MA

Vitale TR (2018) Nurse leader mentorship. Nurs Manage 49(2):8–10

Wagner M (2007) Global midwifery – traditional and official – humanisation of birth. Midwifery Today 2007:55–57

Way S (2016) Consistent, quality midwifery care: how midwifery education and the role of the midwife teacher are important contributions to the Lancet Series. Midwifery 33:1–2

Welcome Trust (2005) Midwifery in Colonial India. The role of traditional birth attendants in colonial India. White Rose Research online. White Rose University Consortium. Universities of Leeds Sheffield and York

World Health Assembly (2013) Transforming health workforce education in support of universal health coverage. In: Sixty sixth World Health Assembly, 2013. WHA, vol 66, p 23

World Health Organization (2008) Task shifting: global recommendations and guidelines. World Health Organization, Geneva. https://www.who.int/health-systems/TTR-TaskShifting.pdf?ua=1. Accessed 02 Oct 2019

World Health Organization (2013) Midwife educator core competencies. www.who.int. Accessed 13 May 2019

World Health Organization (2016) Global strategy for human resources for health: workforce 2030. World Health Organization. ISBN 978-92-4-151113-1

World Health Organization (2017) Strengthening quality midwifery education. WHO Meeting report July 25–26, 2016. In support of Global Strategy for Women's, Children's and Adolescents' Health 2016–30. World Health Organization

World Health Organization (2018) Definition of skilled health personnel providing care during childbirth. The 2018 joint statement by WHO, UNFPA, UNICEF, ICM, ICN, FIGO, IPA. https://www.who.int/reproductivehealth/publications/statement-competent-mnh-professionals/en/. Accessed 29 April 2020

World Health Organization (2019) Strengthening quality midwifery education for universal health coverage 2030: framework for action. ISBN: 978-92-4-151584-9

Midwifery Regulation

5

Expected Learning Outcomes
By the end of the chapter, the reader should be able to:

1. Define midwifery regulation
2. Present the purpose of midwifery regulation
3. Outline the key elements of regulation
4. Outline the principles of good regulation
5. Discuss approaches to midwifery regulation
6. Map out midwifery regulation across the globe
7. Describe the role of midwifery regulation in strengthening the profession
8. Access existing resources on developing midwifery regulation

nisms beyond the midwife's own personal compassion and care. Midwives also need to feel safe from litigation by the presence of documented parameters within which they are designated to function. Midwifery regulation fills this role for women, their families and midwives.

A strong health workforce is the backbone of a well-functioning health system (Renfrew et al. 2014; UNFPA 2011, 2014; WHO AFRO 2016; WHO 2016, 2017, 2019). In order to achieve the objectives of some of the global health initiatives, the education, recruitment, deployment and retention of health workers including midwives are imperative (Renfrew et al. 2014; WHO 2017, WHO AFRO 2016), and yet these remain major challenges in many low- and middle-income countries' health systems especially in Africa (WHO AFRO 2016). Systems are required to be in place to ensure maintenance of standards for the education and practice of health workers and to protect the health of the public (WHO EMRO 2002).

5.1 The Work of Midwives

The midwife works with women and families during some of the most emotionally intense and vulnerable periods of their lives. Sometimes the events of childbirth are so intense that women and families are vulnerable and completely dependent on the healthcare providers. It is during such moments that the public need to feel safe and protected by appropriate official mecha-

5.2 What Is Midwifery Regulation?

The International Confederation of Midwives (ICM) defines midwifery regulation as the set of criteria and processes arising from the legislation that identifies who is a midwife and who is not and describes the scope of midwifery practice (ICM

© Springer Nature Switzerland AG 2021
J. Kemp et al., *Global Midwifery: Principles, Policy and Practice*,
https://doi.org/10.1007/978-3-030-46765-4_5

2019). The ICM Regulation Toolkit (2016:2) describes midwifery regulation as the mechanism by which the social contract between the midwifery profession and society is expressed. Society grants the profession authority and autonomy to regulate itself and expects the profession to act responsibly, ensure high standards of care and maintain public trust (ICM 2016). Regulation is a dynamic framework within which professional standards can be enforced for the protection of the public.

5.3 Characteristics of Midwifery Regulation

Midwifery regulation is a part of a nation's laws relating to midwifery education and practice. Effective regulation is resilient, flexible, adaptive and responsive to the environment. It must be fit for context and fit for purpose (WHO EMRO 2002; ICM 2016). Regulation should be broad and flexible enough to allow the profession to respond to emerging health needs and demands as well as professional growth. When not properly written, regulation can limit services to women and their families. For example, the ability of midwives to provide contraception can be restricted by limits in midwives' prescriptive authority (Osborne 2015; Kennedy et al. 2018). Additionally, the regulation process should be transparent, fair and robust and should be reviewed regularly.

Regulation must be properly focused to make it enforceable. It must be clear, visible and comprehensive on who is responsible to whom and for what and provide an appeal process when these stipulations are breached. Regulation must be consistent with other existing health laws and regulations (ICM 2016). Any inconsistencies are likely to cause confusion to the midwives, the population and the government.

5.4 The Purpose of Midwifery Regulation

5.4.1 Maintenance of Standards

Political, social and economic changes taking place globally impact on the delivery and organisation of midwifery care. Midwifery regulation supports midwives to work autonomously within their full scope of practice (ICM 2011; Kennedy et al. 2018) and ensures maintenance of standards in education and practice. It ensures quality of services and the safety of women and their families in all settings (WHO AFRO 2016). Globalisation has led to an inevitable increase in world trade, with health care being considered as a transferable commodity (WHO EMRO 2002). The changing political and structural boundaries, increasing disparity of access to health care amongst different population sectors, climate, environmental and demographic changes, natural and humanitarian disasters and rapid technological developments all impact on care provision and the way in which and by whom services are provided (WHO EMRO 2002). Midwifery regulation enforces the maintenance of quality, guides policymakers and politicians on how to ensure quality and protects the title 'midwife' especially in an era where consumer expectations are increasing.

5.4.2 Protection of the Public, the Care Provider and Quality Assurance

Regulation exists to protect both the public and the care provider and provides mechanisms for gate keeping in relation to who is allowed to provide care, what institutions are allowed to provide education and training and what facilities are deemed suitable for providing health services. All these are mechanisms of quality assurance (Borgren and Berg 2012). Regulation enables the government to demand quality from the profession in all aspects of the healthcare and service provision wherever the profession functions through processes such as accreditation, registration, licensure and re-licensure,[1] enforcement of codes of conduct and ethics as well as addressing complaints and disciplinary processes (ten Hoope-Bender et al. 2014). Without regulation, complaints would be settled in criminal courts rather than constructive administrative processes. Regulation provides a mechanism for consumers and stakeholders to register concerns or complaints and clear processes for

---

[1]These terms are defined in Annex 5.1.

receipt, investigation, determination and resolution of complaints. It ensures transparency, fair treatment without bias and a fair hearing, separating the powers of investigation, hearing and judgement (Camacho et al. 2015).

5.4.3   Professional Self-Regulation

Effective regulation raises the profile of midwifery by allowing the profession to govern itself (WHO AFRO 2016; ICM 2016). It enables autonomous care leading to the improvement of the health of women and newborns and the status of women (ICM 2011). In cases of task shifting and multiskilling, regulation provides a framework within which midwives are supported and enabled to practise their full scope autonomously with neither professional- nor other attribute-based discrimination (Castro Lopes et al 2015). When midwives practise their full scope of practice autonomously, the health outcomes of women and newborns improve (Yang et al. 2016; Vedam et al. 2017).

5.5   The Values and Principles of Midwifery Regulation

The ICM Regulation Toolkit (ICM 2016) sets out five values and principles for midwifery regulation (ICM 2016). These are presented in Box 5.1.

Box 5.1. The five values and principles of midwifery regulation
Midwifery regulation recognises that…

1. Each woman has the right to receive care in childbirth from an educated and competent midwife authorised to practise midwifery.
2. Midwives are autonomous practitioners; that is, they practise in their own right and are responsible and accountable for their own clinical decision-making.
3. The midwife's scope of practice describes the circumstances in which

---

the midwife may make autonomous clinical decisions and in what circumstances the midwife must practise in collaboration with other health professionals such as doctors.
4. Midwifery is a profession that is autonomous, separate and distinct from nursing and medicine. What sets midwives apart from nurses and doctors is that only midwives can practise the full scope of midwifery practice and provide all the competencies within this scope.
5. Wherever a qualified registered midwife with a midwifery practising certificate works with pregnant women during the childbearing continuum, no matter what the setting, she is practising midwifery. Therefore, when a midwife holds dual registration/qualification as a nurse, she cannot practise simultaneously as a midwife and as a nurse. In a maternity setting a registered/qualified midwife always practises midwifery.

Source: ICM Regulation Toolkit (2016)

Both ICM and the International Council of Nurses (ICN) outline principles of professional regulation which provide a benchmark against which regulatory processes can be assessed. These are presented in Box 5.2.

Box 5.2. Principles of professional regulation
Necessity: Is the regulation necessary? Are current rules and structures that govern this area still valid? Is the legislation purposeful? A purposeful regulatory system should be designed to achieve that purpose with systems in place for continuous monitoring of all aspects of quality in relation to the purpose.
Effectiveness: Is regulation properly focused or targeted to enable unambiguous enforcement and monitoring? Is it achievable and is it flexible and enabling?

Flexibility: Is the regulation sufficiently flexible rather than too prescriptive? Effective regulation should be sufficiently broad and flexible to achieve the objectives at the same time permitting freedom of innovation, growth and change. Neither too general nor too specific. Instead, it should give broad but clear guidance to midwives and employers, enabling midwives to respond to changes in the practice environment whilst still working safely and effectively from an evidence base.

Proportionality: Do the advantages of having the regulation outweigh the disadvantages of having none? Can the same objectives be achieved in another way? There is a danger of regulation placing too much emphasis on the details of the system without paying adequate attention to the underpinning principles. The risk is for the regulation to be self-defeating since regulation and standards are slow to change, making it less and less relevant within a short period of time. Hence, regulation should provide and be limited to those controls and restrictions necessary to achieve their objectives.

Representational balance: Does the regulation and its design acknowledge and balance interdependent interests? No profession should be entirely free in managing its own regulation as there is a danger of indulgent self-interest, lack of accountability and catastrophic loss of public confidence. All those parties with legitimate interests should have explicit and visible roles and responsibilities (the public, the profession and its members, government, employers and other professions) with no one profession dominating another.

Transparency: Is the regulation clear and accessible to all? Have stakeholders been involved in the development? Similar to representational balance, the involvement of other parties, particularly and increasingly those who are the users of midwifery services, is vital for public protection policies.

Accountability: Is it clear who is responsible to whom and for what? Is there an effective appeal process?

Consistency: Will the regulation give rise to anomalies and or discordance in relation to another regulation that is already in place for the area? Are best practice principles being applied? There should be coherence and coordination in relation to other existing laws and regulation.

Source: ICM Regulation Toolkit 2016. ICN Regulation and Governance Toolkit (2013)

5.6 The Functions of Midwifery Regulation

5.6.1 Defining the Midwife and Midwifery

Regulation provides a clear definition of the midwife and the type of practice called midwifery, enabling individual midwives to honour their personal and professional accountability. Titles or roles should not be confusing (WHO 2002). This demands that regulation be clear on what competencies bestow the title 'midwife' and what additional insignia identify those who have acquired additional competencies.

Regulation defines midwifery practice and the midwife's role, recognising that professions and their practice are evolving over time, making professional boundaries increasingly fluid. These definitions need to be communicated to the public. According to the WHO (2016), there is a public misunderstanding of what a midwife is and what a midwife does. This misunderstanding means that important dimensions of midwifery are misunderstood and undervalued.

5.6.2 Setting the Scope of Practice

Regulation delineates or circumscribes the professional parameters within which midwives can practise, enabling midwives to ensure that they have the competencies required to deliver effective care at all times (Elwood 2013). Midwives are the only care providers able to provide the full scope of midwifery practice (Renfrew et al. 2014). Regulation therefore facilitates and encourages the fullest development of the midwife in relation to the anticipated or potential social contribution.

5.6.3 Stipulating Pre-registration Education and Qualifications

Regulation guides the education processes and programmes to provide individuals with the relevant competencies to earn the title 'midwife'. Specific, clear, transparent standards relating to the student body, the physical structures needed, the financial and human resources required for effective programme implementation, the curriculum, the teaching and learning methods, evaluation techniques and the quality of educators must be adhered to. Regulation enforces these through accreditation of programmes and institutions, registration and licensure of the professionals and provides processes and criteria for the assessment of equivalence of applicants who do not meet the requirements set for the country's midwifery education.

5.7 Foundation Documents and Tools

Foundation documents (Box 5.3) provide midwifery regulation with measurable benchmarks on which midwifery programmes can be developed. These documents form the basis for quality assurance tools including the status of midwifery regulation in a country. Regulation facilitates the education of midwives such that midwifery has a common set of basic competencies for effective practice in all settings (WHO 2002). These are summarised in Box 5.3.

Box 5.3. Bases for regulation and tools to measure status of regulation in a country

- *Definition of the midwife* (ICM 2014). Regulation uses this definition as the basis of determining who is allowed to use the title 'midwife'.
- *Global standards for basic midwifery education* (ICM 2013a). Regulation will accredit only those midwifery education programmes which meet the global standards.
- *Global standards for midwifery regulation* (ICM 2016). Countries use these standards to assess or develop their own regulation.
- *Essential competencies for basic midwifery practice* (ICM 2019). Regulation ensures that all programmes cover and enable students to acquire all these competencies.
- *Midwifery philosophy and model of care* (ICM 2011). Competency includes the ability to offer care that demonstrates recognition of the value of women. Midwife-led care epitomises this philosophy.
- *Model curriculum outlines for midwifery education* (ICM 2015). Used by countries to decide what type of curriculum to develop or what to modify in their existing curricula.
- *Nurse educator competencies*. Help countries to determine the quality of the midwifery educators required for quality products.

Tools:
- *Midwifery Education Accreditation Tool (MEAP)* (ICM 2019). Assesses midwifery education programmes.
- *ICM Regulation Gap Analysis Tool* (ICM 2011). Assesses the status of midwifery regulation in a country.

- *Member Association Capacity Assessment Tool* (ICM 2013b). Measures the association's perception of midwifery regulation in a country.
- *The ICM Curriculum Concordance* (ICM 2013c). Measures the extent to which a curriculum covers the essential competencies.

Excellent tools are also available in other organisations which regulate midwifery.

5.8   Registration, Licensure and Re-licensure

Regulation confirms the quality of an education programme by entering successful candidates onto a midwifery register, thus acknowledging the programme as academically sound and enabling the acquisition of competencies for individuals to earn the title 'midwife'. Licensure gives the midwife permission to practise midwifery. Regulation demands demonstrations of continuing competency for renewal of license (re-licensure) and also provides criteria for assessing midwives educated in other countries prior to licensure and criteria for assessing readiness to return to practise of midwives who have been out of practice for a defined period. Thus, regulation encourages midwives to regularly engage in continuing professional development and highlights the role of the employer and the regulatory bodies in enabling this to happen.

5.9   Mechanisms for Addressing Complaints and Issues of Discipline

Regulation stipulates the procedures for addressing issues of discipline and fair pathways for resolving conflict whilst ensuring that the midwife feels safe and anticipates fair non-discriminatory investigation, hearing and treatment.

5.10   Mechanisms for Enforcing Codes of Conduct and Ethics

Regulation engenders a feeling of security in a midwife even in times of distress through codes of conduct and of ethics. A code of ethics outlines what is accepted as professionally ethical behaviour whilst a code of conduct stipulates what constitutes acceptable professional behaviour. Whilst a code of conduct protects the public from disrespectful care, a code of ethics goes further to protect the public against professional malpractice.

5.11   The Midwifery Regulatory Body

The creation of a midwifery regulatory body is a national undertaking involving multiple stakeholders.

Ideally, the majority of its members should be midwives representing all the types of midwives in the country. The body should be led by midwives and the government and chaired by a midwife. The public, other stakeholders including other professions should be represented to ensure that midwifery is not only addressing its own interests at the expense of the interests of the public and others.

The regulatory body hires manpower for the implementation of the regulation. It keeps the register of midwives and different types of licensure statuses, i.e. temporary, full licensure, provisional, conditional and suspended. These registers are available to the public. The body defines expected standards of conduct, what constitutes unprofessional conduct or misconduct and imposes reviews and penalties, sanctions and conditions of practice. It collects information on midwives and their practices, creates databases and contributes to workforce planning and research. The body commissions experts to deal with different aspects including investigating and hearing cases of complaints and misconduct. It develops assessment tools for education and practice. Where midwifery is regulated through other means, there should be a specific committee or subcommittee to attend to and retain the final authority over the affairs of midwifery.

5.12   Models of Midwifery Regulation

5.12.1 Through Legislation

Midwifery can be regulated through state laws which enable the creation of the profession and of the regulatory body. In some countries, the laws which are intended to protect the public can end up restricting care. For example, in the United States of America, half of the US states have laws that prohibit Certified Nurse-Midwives and Certified Midwives from full-practice authority. Six require physician supervision, although the American College of Nurse Midwives and the American College of Obstetricians and Gynaecologists, in a joint statement, state that Obstetrician-Gynaecologists and Certified Nurse-Midwives and Certified Midwives are experts in their respective fields of practice. They are educated, trained and licensed independent providers who may collaborate with each other based on the needs of their patients. This demonstrates that the ability of a profession to practise its full scope is directly affected by the laws of the country (Kennedy et al. 2018).

5.12.2 Through the Government

In many countries, midwives are regulated through a part of the Ministry of Health that takes on the role of regulating midwifery practice and education through an umbrella regulation for all healthcare providers, a Health Professions Act and/or a Health Professions Council.

5.12.3 By the Professional Association

In quite a few countries, regulation of the profession is by the professional association. One example is in Lebanon. The midwives' associa-

tion was transitioned to the Order of Midwifery, so that it could take on the role of a regulatory body (ICM Membership Report 2016). The regulation is specific to midwifery and is overseen by midwives.

5.12.4 Through a Government-Approved Organisation

Another model is regulation by an autonomous or a semi-autonomous body which regulates all healthcare professions. For example, Zimbabwe, up until 2010, had a Health Professions Council before the development of the Nurses Council in 2013. The Health Professions Council was a semi-autonomous organisation with a separate section for each profession.

5.12.5 Regulation by Another Profession

In some instances, midwifery is regulated by another profession's council like a nurses' council or a medical council. Midwifery regulation is a section or part of that other profession's regulation especially in countries where midwifery is perceived as a specialisation of nursing, is not clearly understood or has a very low profile. The worst-case scenario is where midwifery is subsumed in nursing giving the understanding that nursing regulation applies equally to midwifery. For example, the Eastern Mediterranean and the European regions of the World Health Organization (EMRO and EURO respectively), whilst developing a regional regulatory framework for nursing and midwifery stated, '("Nursing" in this instance and throughout the document *also includes midwifery*) has long been influenced by a range of people' (WHO EMRO 2002:9, italics mine). Throughout, they discuss nursing regulation to govern and improve the quality of nursing *and midwifery*. An Australian study demonstrated that regulation that subsumes midwifery into nursing lacked consistency and had discrepancies in the standards of midwifery education and practice. The authors argue for '…a need for change in the view and legal positioning of the Australian Nursing Council and all Nurses' Boards regarding the identification of midwifery as distinct from nursing' (Brodie and Barclay 2001:9).

5.12.6 Through a Regulatory Collaborative

Midwifery can also be regulated through a regulatory collaborative which spans across multiple countries. Examples include the African Health Collaborative developed in 2011 to regulate midwifery in 17 African countries (Gross et al. 2018) in response to the high burden of HIV infections in the face of severe staff shortages. The same situation was experienced in East Central and Southern Africa (ECSA) and led to the review and development of the ECSA nursing and midwifery regulatory reform across 13 countries (McCarthy et al. 2013a) and in the United States of America and led to the publication of the statement of commitment to health equity in maternal and newborn health and diversity (US MERA 2015a) and a set or principles for the development and implementation of midwifery regulation across all 50 United States of America states (US MERA 2015b).

5.12.7 Through a Nurses and Midwives Council

In this model, the council regulates nursing and midwifery with distinct sections for each profession and a specific midwifery committee representing midwifery (Royal College of Midwives 2019). The committee has the responsibility of conducting a 'sense check' on the impact of planned change and advising the council on the wisdom of doing so. In such a setting, the midwifery committee must retain the final authority over midwifery regulation (Kennedy et al. 2018).

5.12.8 Through a Midwives' Council

This model is the ideal. Midwives and midwifery are governed by an independent midwifery-specific regulatory body—a midwives' council.

The regulation is specific to midwifery, presenting a true picture of the profession regulating itself. However, not many countries have this in place. In 2017, only 15 out of 113 countries with ICM members had regulation specific to midwifery (ICM 2017).

5.13   Midwifery Regulation Across the World

Regulation has been identified as the weakest pillar of the midwifery profession. Less than half of the 73 Count Down countries (Annex 5.1) said they had legislation recognising midwifery as an autonomous, regulated profession. None of the six Western Pacific Region[2] countries had such legislation, and only one in the South East Asian Region had. Seventy eight percent of these 73 countries reported having a recognised definition of a professional midwife and in 92% midwifery regulation was by a government department or government-approved organisation which, in some countries, was reported as not fully functional or needing support. All the seven EMRO[3] countries amongst the 73 Count Down countries reported that they had no midwifery legislation (WHO 2002). In 2011, two countries in EMRO had legislation for midwifery; however, in 2014 this figure had reduced to one as the second country had retracted its previous legislation (UNFPA 2011, 2014). In the Americas, the United States Midwifery Education Regulation and Association (US MERA) consisting of seven midwifery organisations[4] produced a consensus document for the regulation of midwifery in the United States as there was confusion amongst policymakers and consumers (Camacho et al. 2015; Kennedy et al. 2018). Because of this widespread

---

[2]Cambodia, China, Lao People's Democratic Republic, Papua New Guinea, Solomon Islands, Viet Nam.

[3]Afghanistan, Djibouti, Morocco, Pakistan, Somalia, Sudan, Yemen.

[4]American College of Nurse-Midwives, American Midwifery Certification Board, Midwives Alliance of North America, Midwifery Education Accreditation Council, National Association of Certified Professional Midwives, North American Registry of Midwives, Accreditation Commission for Midwifery Education.

lack or weakness of midwifery regulation, midwifery is not an autonomous profession and therefore not involved in policy planning and decision-making. Decisions are made for and about the profession without midwives (Castro Lopes et al. 2015). The 'reinforcement of regulation through the development of legislation for midwifery…would benefit the profession generally' (Castro Lopes et al. 2016:10).

Widespread midwifery regulatory inconsistencies exist despite guidelines provided by the WHO, ICM and the Framework by Renfrew et al. 2014 (Bharj et al. 2016). The definition of a midwife is not used consistently across countries, and the competencies of midwives are varied because of weak regulation and legislation (WHO 2016). The States of the World's Midwifery reports in 2011 and 2014 found some reported improvements in midwifery regulation over the three period between each report. Whereas, in 2011, 39 out of 54 countries reported existing legislation, by 2014 that number had increased by 7 (Castro Lopes et al. 2016; UNFPA 2011, 2014). The Pan American Health Organisation (PAHO) reported the highest proportion of countries with legislation compared to the Western Pacific Region (WPRO) where legislation was non-existent. In 113 ICM Member countries, 85 reported having some form of midwifery regulation (ICM 2017). Despite this promising improvement, regulation remains the pillar where most variability lies.

The formation of regulatory collaboratives has led to improvement in Southern Africa and the ECSA region. Though the US MERA is not strictly speaking a collaborative, the function is the same, as the consensus document adopted in 2015 facilitates similar understanding of regulation across all 50 states (Kennedy et al. 2018). EMRO and EURO came together as early as 2002. This gives hope that with time, midwifery regulation will become the norm in an increasing number of countries.

Most efforts for introducing midwifery regulation in a country or region are driven by midwives' associations. Where they exist, midwives' associations, with strong support from ICM, advocate for the introduction of midwifery regulation.

5.14 Barriers to Midwifery Regulation

There is a lack of investment in midwifery regulation (WHO 2016; Renfrew et al. 2014; UNFPA 2014). Many governments perceive the cost of supporting a relatively small group of professionals too high to warrant significant investment (Kennedy et al. 2018). Other long-standing barriers to midwifery regulation include restrictive state laws, which fail to recognise midwifery as an autonomous profession, and resistance from other professionals and government departments who perceive midwifery to be a part of nursing. Economic and political restrictions for midwives to provide the full scope of practice, and social and cultural norms which do not uphold women's rights to education and employment are also barriers to effective midwifery regulation (Kennedy et al. 2018). Bharj et al. (2016) also cite economic and political restrictions for midwives to provide the full scope of practice. Also, social and cultural norms which mitigate against women's rights, education and employment are perceived as barriers against effective midwifery regulation.

5.15 Building a Case for Midwifery Regulation

Midwifery regulation is important for the achievement of the SDGs. Well-educated, regulated and supported midwives can contribute to the reduction of up to 80% of maternal deaths plus 50 additional positive health outcomes for women and newborns (WHO 2016, 2017, 2019). Midwifery education is only effective when standards are met through the enforcement of regulation. Quality of care depends on the effective regulation of practice and regulatory processes like accreditation, registration, licensure and relicensure of practitioners. The 2016 WHO meeting acknowledged that strengthening midwifery education globally requires strong and effective midwifery regulation, just as the Global Midwifery Advocacy Strategies (WHO 2019) highlighted the lack of investment in midwifery regulation and autonomy as a barrier to the advocacy process. Of the 12 indicators on education listed in the Global Strategic Directions for Strengthening Nursing and Midwifery 2016–2020, eight are regulatory processes (Box 5.4).

Box 5.4. The 12 'regulation-related' indicators focused on education: 2020

Global strategic Directions for Strengthening Nursing and Midwifery 2016–2020:

1. # countries' accreditation
2. # countries' curricula endorsed by regulatory body or institution
3. #countries' data on educational institutions, regulatory bodies and regulatory information on licensing, registration and scopes of practice
4. #countries' competency-based curricula
5. # partners supporting regulatory bodies to monitor and evaluate training
6. #countries' implemented national standards for education and practice and nursing and midwifery services
7. # countries' reviewed and revised professional regulation
8. # availability and status of information systems (e.g. for education, workforce, regulation)

Source: Reference to Global strategic Directions for Strengthening Nursing and Midwifery 2016–2020

The value of regulation lies in its enabling ability to implement and enforce rules in order to get the desired outcome. Regulation makes it possible for women to claim their right to quality care. Without regulation, women would not know what is due to them. Regulation implies implementation of agreed benchmarks or standards—the minimum acceptable level. Hence, regulation is required to enforce the right type of education to produce the right type of practitioner who will provide the right type of care and produce the right type of health outcomes. Studies have shown that when regulation is specific to midwifery, health outcomes for women and their newborn are better. Yang et al. (2016) argued that allowing midwives autonomous practice impacts positively on women's health outcomes with less caesarean sections and other invasive procedures. A study by Vedam et al. (2017) demonstrated that favourable midwifery regulation led to higher rates of spontaneous vaginal births, higher numbers of vaginal births after caesarean rates, and lower caesarean rates. For babies, there were lower rates of preterm birth and low birth weight. Although the reasons for these outcomes are multifactorial, this critical study highlights the potential impact of midwifery legislation on birth outcomes.

5.16   Why Midwifery Regulation and Strengthening Midwifery?

Effective midwifery regulation raises the profile of midwifery, making it recognised as an autonomous profession. Once autonomous, the profession is able to practise to its full scope and thus increase access of care to women and their families. Regulation also strengthens the profession by providing governments and policy- and decision-makers with clear guidelines and benchmarks on whom to call a midwife. It is also clear what can be expected from the appropriately qualified midwife. This is because effective regulation ensures quality midwifery education which enhances competence and instils the desire for continuing professional development and life-long learning. Thus, regulation promotes the profession, identifies and excludes imposters, contributes to addressing crises and ensures that institutions providing services are fit to do so. It guides the midwife in ways of behaviour and enforces the philosophy of woman- and family-centred care, providing women with choices during childbirth. These matters increase the possibility of equity, informed choice, safety and seamless access to quality midwifery care as a right to every birthing family (Kennedy et al. 2018). All these factors contribute to the strengthening of the profession and to increasing public trust and confidence in midwives and midwifery. When there is no legislation to support midwifery regulation activities, the recognition and scope of midwifery practice can be limited even if the government is the main regulator (McCarthy et al. 2013b).

5.17 Developing and Strengthening Midwifery Regulation

Strong and persistent advocacy for midwifery regulation is required despite the barriers. There is lack of clarity in many countries around the role and scope of practice of the midwife. This flows into uncertainties in education and practice (Castro Lopes et al. 2016). Midwives in every country need to advocate for such clarity through legislation. Midwives must work with women's groups and indigenous populations to advocate for midwifery regulation. Castro Lopes et al. (2016), the Lancet (Renfrew et al. 2014) and the SoWMy reports (UNFPA 2011, 2014) all state that the reinforcement of regulation through the development of legislation would benefit the development of the other two pillars. If education, regulation and association (ERA) are key components for the development of an effective midwifery workforce, simultaneous and holistic improvements to all three elements are required as strengthening one in isolation is unlikely to address the overall quality. Assuring the development or strengthening of legislation that recognises midwifery would support education and association. Midwives should advocate for the integration of all ERA elements in national planning and strategies for SRMNH and health workforce plans, involve stakeholders and provide evidence of the value of midwifery regulation.

5.18 Conclusion

Midwifery regulation is a complex dynamic issue. There is much work ahead to work closely with legislators and policymakers, educating and advising them about midwives and midwifery and the importance of regulating midwifery in the interest of public health. This…

> …will require a unified commitment to an ongoing exploration of the issues as they arise. Just as some labours are long and hard, pushing both woman and midwife to their own private edges of discouragement and exhaustion, there is sometimes no better answer than support, advocacy, and patient passage of time to bring about the birth. (Kennedy et al. 2018:9)

As more and more countries recognise and license midwives, the world can look forward to a future in which equity, informed choice, safety, and seamless access to quality midwifery care will be available to every birthing family leading to the anticipated 80% reduction of maternal and newborn mortality globally.

5.18.1 Principles

The principle of midwifery being an autonomous profession which provides skilled practitioners for whole populations is unquestionable. In order to achieve this, regulation is required in order to ensure that the midwifery profession is educated and practises to approved standards.

5.18.2 Policy

Midwifery regulation should be an integral part of healthcare policy in all countries. This should complement the regulation of other healthcare professions with which midwives may need to liaise but to remain separate rather than being subsumed by them.

5.18.3 Practice

In order to address the unacceptably high global maternal and perinatal mortality and morbidity rates, the practice of midwifery must be controlled and directed by a recognised regulatory framework. Within such a framework, midwives should be enabled to provide skilled, respectful care.

Questions for Reflection or Review

1. Examine midwifery regulation in your country in relation to the models described in this chapter and reflect on the following:
   - What are the strengths and challenges in the model in your country?
   - How can the challenges be addressed?
2. In your opinion, what would be the steps to be followed in the process of harmonising midwifery regulation globally?

   What would be the advantages of harmonising midwifery regulation globally?

Annex 5.1: Definition of Terms

Accreditation: A voluntary self-regulatory process by which non-governmental associations recognise educational institutions or programmes that have been found to meet or exceed standards and criteria in the quality of education. Accreditation also assists in the further improvement of the institutions or programmes as related to resources invested, processes followed and results achieved. This process also ensures professional development opportunity and validation of faculty (WHO AFRO 2016).

Regulation: All the legitimate and appropriate means and rules (governmental, professional, private and individual) through which order, identity, consistency and control are brought to the profession (governance). Regulation defines the professional, the profession, the scope of practice and the type of education one has to undergo, including what constitutes ethical and competent practice. Regulation also stipulates systems of accountability.

It is the set of criteria and processes arising from the legislation and prescribed by the regulatory authority that controls the practice of midwifery in a jurisdiction, including identifying who can hold the title 'midwife' and practise midwifery. Regulation includes registration, licensure, accreditation of education programmes, setting standards of practice and conduct and processes of holding midwives accountable to professional standards (ICM Regulation standards 2011).

Regulatory body: A formal organisation designated by law or an authorised governmental agency to implement the regulatory processes, procedures and reform in a manner which maintains order, consistency and control to the profession.

Registration: The process of providing authority to use an exclusive title to those persons entered onto a register after successful completion of a prescribed midwifery programme in an accredited institution of that country. Registration acknowledges qualification but is not synonymous with it. Qualification is a pre-requisite for registration. The possession of a midwifery qualification does not automatically entitle an individual to registration. Just as registration does not permit an individual to practise. Licensure does. In other words, qualification is a pre-requisite of registration provided the registering authority is convinced that the qualification is from a programme that meets certain standards (accredited). Being on a professional register is a pre-requisite to licensure as long as the licensing agency is convinced that the individual is competent in the skills, knowledge and attitudes that enable the individual to practise safely and competently (proof of competence).

Register: A documentation of persons and their qualifications in a particular field of practice. Individuals may be registered in more than one part of the register, for example, midwives who are also nurses can be on the nurses' and the midwives' registers. The register is maintained and updated by an authorised regulatory body.

Licensure: This is a process sanctioned by law that grants exclusive power or privilege to persons who meet established standards which allow them to engage in a given occupation or profession and to use the specific title as designated by law. Licensure confers on an individual the right to practise their profession according to the dictates of the law. Licensure confirms fitness to practise one's profession safely and the required standard.

Re-licensure: A process that confirms that a practitioner is still fit to practise. This is usually after a break in service or after practising for a designated period of time.

Legislation: A law or act of parliament which sanctions the existence of the profession, the titles used, the scope of practice and criteria for the education process of the professionals. It provides protection for all categories of midwives and midwifery practice. Only people who meet certain criteria can use the title 'midwife'. Legislation forms the basis for regulation. Legislation should be informed by policy and linked to overall policy for development of human resources for health.

Source: Derived from McCarthy et al. (2013a, b); Africa Health Professional Regulation Collaborative for Nurses and Midwives (ARC), International Council of Nurses (2013) and International Confederation of Midwives (2016).

Annex 5.2: The 73 Countdown Countries

AFRO ($n = 41$)	SAERO ($N = 6$)	WPRO ($N = 6$)	PAHO ($N = 6$)	EMRO ($N = 9$)	EURO ($N = 5$)
Angola, Benin, Botswana, Burkina Faso, Burundi, Cameroon, Central African Republic, Chad, Comoros, Congo Democratic Republic, Ivory Coast, Eritrea, Ethiopia, Gabon, Gambia, Ghana, Guinea, Guinea Bissau, Kenya, Lesotho, Liberia, Madagascar, Malawi, Mali, Mauritania, Mozambique, Niger, Nigeria, Rwanda, Sao Tome and Principe, Senegal, Sierra Leone, South Africa, South Sudan, Swaziland, Tanzania, Togo, Uganda, Zambia, Zimbabwe	Bangladesh, India, Indonesia, Korea Democratic Republic, Myanmar, Nepal	Cambodia, China, Lao People's Democratic Republic, Papua New Guinea, Solomon Islands, Viet Nam	Bolivia, Brazil, Guatemala, Haiti, Mexico, Peru	Afghanistan, Djibouti, Egypt, Iraq, Morocco, Pakistan, Somalia, Sudan, Yemen	Azerbaijan, Kyrgyzstan, Tajikistan, Turkmenistan, Oezbekistan

Source: A descriptive analysis of midwifery education, regulation and association in 73 countries: the baseline for a post-2015 pathway (Castro Lopes et al. 2016)

Key Messages

Midwifery regulation is the anchor of midwifery education and association as it provides benchmarks for quality and professional identity.

Midwifery regulation, when well developed and implemented enhances the autonomy of the profession.

Without effective midwifery regulation, it is difficult to establish a true niche for midwives in the provision of maternal and newborn health care.

Additional Resources for Reflection and Further Study

Foundation documents are found at https://www.internationalmidwives.org/regulation

Principles for Model U.S. Midwifery Legislation and Regulation. https://www.usmera.org/wp-content/uploads/2015/11/US-MERALegislativeStatement2015.pdf

The Midwifery Education Accreditation Programme. https://www.internationalmidwives.org/what-we-do/

WHO Nurse Educator Core Competencies. https://apps.who.int/iris/handle/10665/258713

References

Africa Health Professional Regulation Collaborative for Nurses and Midwives (ARC) (2013). https://www.google.com/search?sxsrf=ACYBGNQcc9ra9M5GFfNVFmT57kB7HnXZLA%3A1573485008258&source=hp&ei=0HnJXenjDY-LlwSM6aDYCw&q=african+health+professional+regulatory+collaborative+for+nurses+and+midwives

Bharj KK, Luyben A, Avery MD et al (2016) An agenda for midwifery education: Advancing the state of the world's midwifery. Midwifery 33:3–6

Borgren MU, Berg M (2012) Midwifery education, regulation and association in six South Asian Countries – a descriptive report. Swedish Assoc Midwives 3(2):67–72

Brodie P, Barclay L (2001) Contemporary issues in Australian midwifery regulation. Aust Health Rev 24(4):103–118

Camacho CK, Collins-Fulea C, Krulewitch C et al (2015) The United States midwifery, education, regulation, and association work group: what is it and what does it hope to accomplish? J Midwifery Womens Health 60(2):125–127

Castro Lopes S, Titulaer P, Bokosi M et al (2015) The involvement of midwives' association in policy planning bout the midwifery workforce: a global survey. Midwifery 31:1096–1103

Castro Lopes S, Nove A, ten Hoope-Bender P et al (2016) A descriptive analysis of midwifery education, regulation and association in 73 countries: the baseline for a post-2015 pathway. Hum Resour Health 14(37):0134–0137

Elwood TW (2013) Patchwork of scope-of-practice regulations prevent allied health professionals from fully participating in patient care. Health Aff 32(11):1985–1989. https://www.healthaffairs.org/doi/full/10.1377/hlthaff.2013.0530. Accessed 30 April 2020

Gross MJ, McCarthy CM, Verani AR et al (2018) Evaluation of the impact of the ARC program on national nursing and midwifery regulations, leadership, and organisational capacity in East Central and Southern Africa. BMC Health Serv Res 18:406. https://bmchealthservres.biomedcentral.com/articles/10.1186/s12913-018-3233-4. Accessed 30 April 2020

ten Hoope-Bender P, de Bernis L, Campbell J et al (2014) Improving maternal and newborn health through midwifery. Lancet 384:1226–1235. http://linkinghub.elsevier.com. Accessed November 2019

International Confederation of Midwives (2011) Philosophy and model of midwifery care. https://www.internationalmidwives.org/documents

International Confederation of Midwives (2013a) Global standards for midwifery education. https://www.internationalmidwives.org. Accessed 30 March 2020

International Confederation of Midwives (2013b) Member Association Capacity Assessment Tool (MACAT). https://www.internationalmidwives.org/what-we-do/association-coredocuments/macat.html. Accessed November 2019

International Confederation of Midwives (2013c) Global standards for Midwifery regulation. www.internationalmidwifery.org/regulation-resources/. Accessed 30 March 2020

International Confederation of Midwives (2014) Definition of the midwife. https://www.internationalmidwives.org/documents

International Confederation of Midwives (2015) Model curriculum for midwifery education. https://www.internationalmidwives.org/education

International Confederation of Midwives (2016) The regulation toolkit. www.inertnationalmidwives.org/regulation-resources. Accessed 30 March 2020

International Confederation of Midwives (2017) The ICM Midwives map. https://www.internationalmidwives.org/midwives_map. Accessed 30 March 2020

International Confederation of Midwives (2019) Essential competencies for basic midwifery practice. https://www.internationalmidwives.org/competencies. Accessed 30 March 2020

International Council of Nurses (2013) Regulatory and Governance Toolkit. https://www.icn.ch/sites/default/files/inline-files/2014_Regulatory_Board_Governance_Toolkit.pdf. Accessed 30 March 2020

Kennedy HP, Myers-Ciecko JA, Camacho Carr K et al (2018) United States model of Midwifery Legislation and regulation: development of consensus document. J Midwifery Womens Health 63:652–659

McCarthy FC, Voss J, Salmon M et al (2013a) Nursing and Midwifery regulatory reform in East Central and Southern Africa: a survey of key stakeholders. Hum Resour Health 2013:11–29

McCarthy FC, Voss J, Verani AR et al (2013b) Nursing and Midwifery regulation and HIV scale up: establishing a baseline in east, central and southern Africa. J Int AIDS Soc 16(1):18051

Osborne K (2015) Regulation of prescriptive authority for certified nurse-midwives and certified midwives: national overview. J Midwifery Womens Health 60(5):519–533

Renfrew MJ, MacFadden A, Bastos MH et al (2014) Midwifery and quality care: findings from a new evidence-informed framework for maternal and newborn care. Lancet 384(9948):1129–1145

Royal College of Midwives (2019) Review of midwifery regulation by the Nursing and Midwifery Council (NMC) - a briefing paper. www.rcm.uk. Accessed October 2019

UNFPA (2011) State of the World's Midwifery. Delivering health, saving lives. United Nations Population Fund, New York

UNFPA (2014) State of the World's Midwifery. A universal pathway. A woman's right to health. United Nations Population Fund, New York

US Midwifery Education, Regulation, and Association (2015a) US MERA statement of Commitment to Health equity in maternal and new-born health and to greater diversity in Midwifery, 15 Sept 2015. US Midwifery Education, Regulation, and Association: http://www.usmera.org/index.php/2015/09/15/us-mera-. Accessed Nov 2019

US Midwifery Education, Regulation, and Association (2015b) Principles for model US Midwifery legislation and regulation, 12 Oct 2015. US Midwifery, Education, Regulation, and Association. http://www.usmera.org/index.php/2015/11/20/principles-for-model-u-s-midwifery-legislation-regulation/. Accessed Nov 2019

Vedam S, MacDorman M, Declercq E et al (2017) Collaboration Across Birth Settings in the United States. Obstetrics & Gynecology 129:183S

World Health Organisation (2002) Strategic directions for strengthening nursing and midwifery. WHO Geneva 2002

World Health Organization (2016) Strengthening quality midwifery education. WHO meeting report, 25– 6 July 2016. www.who.int/maternal_child_adolescent/en. Accessed 10 Oct 2019

World Health Organisation (2017) Strengthening quality midwifery education: meeting report July 25–26 2016. WHO Geneva 2017

World Healht Organisation (2019) Strengthening quality midwifery education for universal health coverage 2030: framework for action. WHO Geneva 2019

World Health Organization Regional Office for Africa (2016) The regional professional regulatory framework for Nursing and Midwifery: creating a common approach to regulation, educational preparation and practice: future directions for nursing and midwifery development in the African Region. https://apps.who.int/iris/handle/10665/331472. Accessed 30 March 2020

World Health Organization Regional Office of the Eastern Mediterranean; Regional Office for Europe Cairo (2002) Nursing and Midwifery: a guide to professional regulation. WHO technical publication series: 27. https://apps.who.int/bookorders/anglais/detart1.jsp?codlan=1&codcol=45&codcch=27. Accessed 30 March 2020

Yang TY, Attanasio LB, Kozhimannil KB (2016) State of scope of practice laws, nurse-midwifery workforce, and childbirth procedures and outcomes. Womens Health Issues 26(3):262–267

Midwives' Associations

6

Expected Learning Outcomes

By the end of the chapter, readers should be able to:

1. Describe a midwives' association
2. Outline the types and distribution of midwives' associations across the globe
3. Provide a brief description of the International Confederation of Midwives including its purpose and function
4. Describe the role of midwives' associations in promoting the profession, education, regulation and service provision
5. Examine resources, as recommended reading, for strengthening midwives' associations as organisations able to fulfil their own objectives.
6. Access recommended materials on creating, nurturing and maintaining a healthy midwives' association

6.1 What Is a Midwives' Association?

A midwives' association is defined by ICM as 'a platform for developing strong, supportive, positive relationships among midwives and between the profession of midwifery and other stakehold-

ers such as women, governments and other health care providers' (ICM 2014a, b). It consists of an organised body of persons engaged in a common professional practice, sharing information, career advancement objectives, in-service training, advocacy and other activities (Castro Lopes et al. 2016). Ideally, the midwives forming the associations would be those who have acquired all the essential competencies for basic midwifery practice as described by the International Confederation of Midwives (2019a, b). However, it is acknowledged that it is not all countries who educate midwives to global standard (Renfrew et al. 2014; UNFPA 2014). Hence, even those associations created by individuals who do not possess all the essential competencies (ICM 2019a, b) but are recognised as midwives in their countries are included in the discussion. Midwives' associations are professional bodies organisations or health professional associations. The Empire State Association Society of Association Executive (2019:1) define a professional association as, 'an organisation of individuals who come together to expand their own knowledge of their profession and the guidelines under which they operate'. They go on to state that associations are created to establish strength and unity in working towards common goals and are intended to be continuing organisations with rules and by-laws, membership requirements and other aspects of an organisation. Midwives' associations fit this description. They are non-profit,

© Springer Nature Switzerland AG 2021
J. Kemp et al., *Global Midwifery: Principles, Policy and Practice*,
https://doi.org/10.1007/978-3-030-46765-4_6

non-governmental organisations which exist to further the interests of midwives, women and their families and the public at large.

6.2   The Purpose of Midwives' Associations

The key reason for the creation of midwives' associations is to facilitate strengthening midwives and midwifery, promoting the profession, advocating for women and newborns and contributing to the provision of quality midwifery services (ICM 2019a, b). They inform the public and the government on midwifery issues and guide and support their members (Bogren 2016; Bogren et al. 2012). According to the International Federation of Gynaecology and Obstetrics (FIGO) (2012), health professional associations have vital roles to play to ensure that the health professionals are well prepared for their roles in healthcare provision and in contributing to the achievement of the objectives of the global health agenda. ESSAE (2019) adds that professional associations assist in establishing government relations and other partnerships, in standardisation of practice including professional competency assessment, research, promotion of the profession, business ethics and public relations and may fulfil their mission through research, government certification, conferences, seminars and publications of books and journals.

6.3   Types of Midwives' Associations

Some midwives' associations are purely professional organisations, i.e. represent their members and ensure that their members provide the services expected of them by the government and partners (FIGO 2012). Some are both professional organisations and unions, i.e. they do not only attend to the interests of their members and the profession but also represent their members during labour discussions (conditions of service

and remuneration issues) (Castro Lopes et al. 2016). Some are purely unions, i.e. they represent their members during labour discussions. In some countries, midwives have formed associations as professional bodies and joined other professions for union issues. In Zambia and Uganda, there are both midwives' associations and nurses and midwives' unions with the unions taking on the labour responsibilities. Others also take on the roles of regulation, for example the Dutch Organisation of Midwives (KNOV) and the Lebanese Order of Midwifery.

6.3.1   The International Confederation of Midwives

The International Confederation of Midwives (ICM) is an accredited, global, non-governmental organisation that represents midwives' associations, midwives and midwifery to achieve common goals in the care of mothers and newborns (ICM 2019a, b). It is the sole representative of midwives globally, made up of 140 midwives associations (at the time of writing), representing 1,000,000 midwives in 121 countries (ICM 2019a, b). It is an association of midwives' associations. The number of associations in ICM membership continues to grow and so does the number of midwives represented. The member associations are spread out across the globe in six ICM regions (Box 6.1).

Box 6.1. Regions of the International Confederation of Midwives
Africa: Francophone and Anglophone
   Americas: North America and the Caribbean and South America
      Western Pacific
      Eastern Mediterranean
      South East Asia
      Europe: Northern, Central and Southern
      Source https://www.internationalmidwives. org [last accessed October 2019]

6.3.2 The Purpose of the International Confederation of Midwives

The ICM exists to support, represent and work to strengthen professional associations of midwives throughout the world. It works closely with other global bodies including United Nations (UN) Agencies (World Health Organization (WHO), United Nations Population Fund (UNFPA) and other UN agencies), other global professional bodies—International Federation of Gynaecology and Obstetrics (FIGO), International Paediatric Association (IPA), International Council of Nurses (ICN) and other global non-governmental organisations, bilateral and civil society groups (ICM 2019a, b). ICM is an advocate for midwives, midwifery, women and the newborn during global discussions on the world health agenda in general and specifically during global discussions and technical consultations impacting on sexual, reproductive, maternal, newborn, child and adolescent health (SRMNCAH) (ICM 2020).

Because of its vantage position on the global health arena and its access to the global decision-making bodies including the UN and global technical consultative meetings of the WHO, the ICM contributes to the development of global practice protocols on maternal, newborn and child health (MNCH) and uses its knowledge and expertise to produce reference and guidance documents on the production, management and regulation of midwives and midwifery services in countries worldwide including quality assurance in care provision. The ICM provides professional identity to midwives globally and contributes to the reduction of maternal and newborn morbidity and mortality through strengthening midwifery. It creates, nurtures and supports midwives' associations and provides quality management and workforce development. It provides service provision planning tools and evidence. The evidence enables governments to get full return on their investment in midwifery. It also enables them to effectively utilise midwives and the rest of the midwifery workforce. The ICM also sensitises governments on best practice developments and approaches in MNCH at any one time.

Because of its global reach, the ICM has access to experts in different fields not only of midwifery but also of other areas pertinent to maternal and newborn health service provision. These include researchers, health system specialists, expert evaluators and facilitators. Amongst midwives, the ICM has created and supported specialist networks and standing committees of experts across the globe. At the time of writing, there were three committees: The Education Standing Committee, the Research Standing Committee and the Regulation Standing Committee. The Standing Committees provide ICM's Midwives Associations with up-to-date information on all aspects of midwifery practice, education and service (ICM 2019a, b). The ICM Research Network brings together expert researchers and those midwives interested in research to share ideas, expertise and knowledge as well as to answer questions from students embarking on research. The standing committees support countries in strengthening their education, regulation and research programmes. They develop guidelines and respond to global queries on midwifery in their respective fields as well as contributing to the production of new knowledge specific to midwifery and maternal and newborn health (MNH). Education is discussed in detail in Chapter 4 and research in Chapter 12. At the time of writing, ICM did not as yet have a standing committee for midwifery practice. In several countries, there are no midwifery practice specialists; hence, such a committee could not be truly representative. However, with more universities now offering higher degrees in midwifery, formation of such a committee may be a possibility for the future.

Taking advantage of this wide reach of experts, the ICM has developed a consultancy service, including online training of consultants to ensure an understanding of ICM's core documents, resources and tools. The consultants will drive forward best practice and provide organisations, governments and programme implementers with a pool of accredited midwife consultants. This is one way of better utilising the skills and knowledge vested in individuals, partners, stakeholders and midwifery associations to identify and respond to needs and capitalise on opportunities (ICM 2019a, b). Issues relating to cross-cultural midwifery consultancy are discussed in Chapter 15.

6.3.3 Regional Midwives' Associations

ICM defines regional midwives' associations as those associations whose membership comprises midwives' associations from different countries within the same geographical region. Regional midwives' associations may include members and/or non-members of ICM and bodies that have the authority to regulate midwifery (ICM 2017). Regional midwives' associations exist in each of the six ICM regions. These associations represent and advocate for midwives and midwifery at regional level. They facilitate the adoption and adaptation of best practices in their regions and sensitise the ICM and other decision-making organisations of any region-specific issues requiring global policy attention. Examples of regional midwives' associations in existence at the time of writing include European Midwives Associations (EMA), South Asia Midwives Associations (SAMA), Confederation of African Midwives Associations (CONAMA), the Federation of French Speaking African Midwives Associations (FASFAF), the Caribbean Regional Midwives Associations (CRMA), Midwives Associations of North America (MANA) and Latin America Federation of Midwives (FLO).

Some regional associations represent special interests. One such body is the Lugina African Midwives Research Network (LAMRN) which is dedicated to improving maternal health outcomes in Africa through increasing evidence-based practice in midwifery. The network supports midwifery research, information sharing, networking and training activities in Kenya, Malawi, Zambia, Zimbabwe, Uganda and Tanzania. Further details about the African research net-

works are explored in Chapter 12. Similar bodies exist in other regions.

6.3.4 National Midwives' Associations

Midwives in many countries formed or have been assisted by partners to form a midwives' association. Many international organisations, specifically, ICM, in some countries, in collaboration with UNFPA and WHO, support midwives to form and to strengthen midwives' associations as one of the ways of promoting the profession and making it visible.

In some countries, only midwives are members. In some, other care providers in MNH can be members. A 2016 analysis across 73 low- and middle-income countries (LMICs) confirmed that, though professional associations open to midwives were widely available in all regions, they were not all exclusive to midwives (Castro Lopes et al. 2016). For example, in Mongolia, Feldshers (health workers limited to providing emergency treatment) are members of the midwives' association. In Turkey and Georgia, obstetricians could join a midwives' association whilst in Sierra Leone Maternal and Child Health Aids (MCH Aids) could be members. In some countries, the midwives' association is an umbrella body encompassing special interest groups within midwifery such as education, regulation and practice. Midwife educators, midwife researchers and midwife managers can form subgroups within the midwives' association. In some countries midwives of a certain ideology come together to form a separate association so that there are two or more midwives' associations in the same country, e.g. in the United Kingdom, Japan, Spain, Ghana and the United States of America (ICM 2017). In other countries like Canada, each province or state has its own midwives' association. The ICM encourages midwives to form one united body in a country whenever possible (ICM 2015).

6.4 Midwives' Associations Across the World

Midwives' associations vary in size, type and rate of progress (Castro Lopes et al. 2016). Additionally, there is a progressive increase of countries which are creating midwives' associations. In 2011, 51 out of the 73 Count Down Countries (Box 6.2), had a midwives' association. By 2014, 54 countries had a midwives' association (Castro Lopes et al. 2016).

Box 6.2. 73 Count Down countries included in an analysis of midwives' associations

AFRO (*n* = 41)	SAERO (*N* = 6)	WPRO (*N* = 6)	PAHO (*N* = 6)	EMRO (*N* = 9)	EURO (*N* = 5)
Angola, Benin, Botswana, Burkina Faso, Burundi, Cameroon, Central African Republic, Chad, Comoros, Congo Democratic Republic, Ivory Coast, Eritrea, Ethiopia, Gabon, Gambia, Ghana, Guinea, Guinea Bissau, Kenya, Lesotho, Liberia, Madagascar, Malawi, Mali, Mauritania, Mozambique, Niger, Nigeria, Rwanda, Sao Tome and Principe, Senegal, Sierra Leone, South Africa, South Sudan, Swaziland, Tanzania, Togo, Uganda, Zambia, Zimbabwe	Bangladesh, India, Indonesia, Korea Democratic Republic, Myanmar, Nepal	Cambodia, China, Lao People's Democratic Republic, Papua New Guinea, Solomon Islands, Vietnam	Bolivia, Brazil, Guatemala, Haiti, Mexico, Peru	Afghanistan, Djibouti, Egypt, Iraq, Morocco, Pakistan, Somalia, Sudan, Yemen	Azerbaijan, Kyrgyzstan, Tajikistan, Turkmenistan, Oezbekistan

Source: A descriptive analysis of midwifery education, regulation and association in 73 countries: the baseline for a post-2015 pathway (Castro Lopes et al. 2016)

The ICM was the only organisation at the time of writing which had a list of midwives' associations across the world. Some are huge organisations with a large membership, employees and several departments including global departments. Examples include Canadian Midwives Association (CAM), United Kingdom Royal College of Midwives (RCM), Japanese Midwives Association (JAMA), American College of Nurse Midwives (ACNM) and Royal Dutch Organisation of Midwives (KNOV) just to mention a few. Such midwives' associations contribute to the creation and strengthening of midwives' associations and midwifery in other countries through their global departments. They mobilise resources and carry out projects to reinforce midwifery. All four examples have carried out twinning and mentorship projects with associations in other countries (ICM 2013; Dawson et al. 2014; Kemp et al. 2018a, b; Sandwell et al. 2018; Ireland et al. 2015; Cadee et al. 2016). Some are not so big but are strong, stable organisations visibly achieving objectives. For example, the Zimbabwe Confederation of Midwives (ZICOM) was instrumental in lobbying the government to increase the period of midwifery education from 12 months to the global standard of 18 months (see Box 6.3).

Box 6.3. Role of Midwives Associations in education through advocacy

Government increases midwives training period

The government has increased the training period for midwives from 12 to 18 months beginning 2019 in order to cater for curriculum changes which are meant to improve service delivery. This was revealed by the President of Zimbabwe Confederation of Midwives (ZICOM), Dr Lillian Dodzo during an annual general meeting for midwives held in Nyanga. 'There is an increasing recognition that … Attaining universal health care is when a country has midwives with sound knowledge and skills for managing obstetrics and neonatal emergencies', said Dr Dodzo. She appealed for the creation of separate establishments of midwives in healthcare institutions.The Vice Chairperson of the Health Services Board, Professor Auxillia Chideme Munodawafa, the guest of honour, urged the midwives to get into research and come up with scientific solutions and recommendations for midwifery challenges and dilemmas. 'Midwives should work hard in reducing the current mortality rate which is at 651/1000', she said. The conference under the theme 'midwives respond to the global agenda on sustainable development and universal health care' was attended by midwives from across the ten provinces.

Article in a 2 December 2018 Zimbabwean newspaper: [Accessed October 2019 on https://bulawayo24.com/index-id-news-sc-national-byo-150841.html]

Other associations are very small with no employee, no office and a handful of members. Experience has shown that, in most cases, the smaller and weaker associations exist where midwifery is not yet well known and only beginning to be appreciated and where the midwifery identity is still vague. Such situations were observed in Kyrgyzstan and China (ICM 2013 and 2016). In both the countries, midwifery was not yet well understood and the associations were particularly small and weak (ICM 2013 and 2016).

6.5 Strengthening Midwifery Globally

Strengthening midwifery implies the process of developing and implementing interventions that lead to midwives in a country progressing towards better and greater ability in contributing effectively towards the provision of quality care and the resultant reduction in maternal newborn and child morbidity and mortality. The process should lead to countries reaping the rewards of their investment into the education of midwives and regulation of midwifery as the midwifery profession progressively moves towards providing care and services at global standard. The importance of regulation and various approaches to this are discussed in Chapter 5.

6.5.1 Why Midwives' Associations and Strengthening Midwifery?

Midwives' associations are more and more recognised as an important mechanism for strengthening midwifery (UNFPA 2011, 2014; ICM 2014a, b. Evidence shows the importance of an enabling work environment for midwives (Renfrew et al. 2014), and professional associations can contribute to this by optimising the value of midwives and providing a link between policy and implementation (ICM 2014a, b). According to the ICM Twinning Operational Manual (ICM 2014a, b), strengthening a midwives' association empowers the association with the capacity to identify challenges, develop context appropriate solutions for problems and enable the association to initiate interventions targeted at resolving identified MNCH care provision problems. When midwives in each country are supported to take their position as critical care providers especially for women, newborns, children and families, midwifery services will be of quality and maternal and newborn disability and deaths would be reduced (Renfrew et al. 2014; FIGO 2012; ICM 2014a, b). Strong professional associations provide leadership and can work together with governments and other stakeholders in setting and implementing health policies to improve the health of women, newborns, children and adolescents (FIGO 2012). There is increasing recognition of the role of midwives in improving SRMNH outcomes and of the environment enablers that improve the quality of midwifery practice (Atkinson 2012). Recent evidence positions midwives as being pivotal to effective SRMNH services (Ten Hoope-Bender et al. 2014; Renfrew et al. 2014). Hence, midwives' associations make it possible for midwives to optimise their value, take their position in care provision and contribute to policymaking and effective policy implementation.

However, it is a known fact that midwifery and midwives are often of a very low status in countries with a high rate of maternal and newborn morbidity and mortality because the status of midwives tends to match the status of women in a country (Ten Hoope-Bender 2014; Castro Lopes et al. 2015; ICM 2014a, b). Midwives' associations provide a nucleus from which the profession progressively grows. With this insight, global development partners and UN agencies including WHO and UNFPA work together with the ICM to create and strengthen midwives' associations as a means of strengthening midwifery and improving midwifery services. An improved status of midwives has the potential to lead to improving the status of women in a country (Renfrew et al. 2014).

6.6   The Roles of Midwives' Associations

6.6.1   Unifying the Profession

Midwives' associations unify midwives and the profession through giving a common vision and goal to members. They aggregate the efforts, thoughts and ideas of midwives, give a voice to the profession as well as power and credibility to the activities that are led by the profession. Midwives' associations provide structure and governance to the profession. When well-led and managed, midwives' associations provide a unified front through which midwives can work together to produce results and to achieve their individual and collective professional objectives (ICM 2011; FIGO 2012). According to Survive and Thrive (2016), professional associations harness resources, expertise, innovation and experience of the profession and contribute to its visibility. They are the powerhouse of midwifery expertise and the go-to organisations for midwifery information for the public, the media and other key stakeholders and partners (ESSAE 2019). They look after the welfare of their members and ensure that as many midwives in the country as possible become members through membership drives and creation of member benefits.

6.6.2   Legal Roles

To be credible to government, organisations have to be legal entities. The midwives' associations, as registered non-governmental organisations, constitute a legal representation of the midwifery profession and thus make midwives members of a legal organisation with which government and partners can enter into agreements. Registration gives the midwives' associations legal capacity to assume obligations, enter into contracts and create relevant partnerships and collaborations and gives legitimacy for the association to represent, defend and act on behalf of its members (Survive and Thrive 2018) and advocate for the welfare and rights of the population they serve. The associations can make demands on the government and partners on behalf of the profession, handle any legal issues impacting on midwives and ensure that midwives and midwifery practice are well regulated and supported for the benefit of the public. According to Module 4 of the Survive and Thrive package,

> …the legal name, logo, and graphic design contribute to profiling the profession. The strong visual identity and an attractive, informative website are tools that will help the population recognise the professional association. (Survive and Thrive 2018: Module 4:4)

In some countries, midwives' associations also participate in and help enforce the certification and licensing of members, as well as contribute to developing regulation that governs the profession (Survive and Thrive 2018). They are also a useful support in times of members' distress as they advise and/or represent members accused of misconduct or incompetence as well as negotiate work and/or salary issues with the government (Castro Lopes et al. 2016).

6.6.3 Education, Training and Keeping Members Up to Date

Midwives' associations ensure the effective education of their members spanning from pre-service to in-service education and continuing professional development (see Box 6.1). They take on the responsibility of keeping their members up to date. According to the 2016 survey of 73 countries (Castro Lopes et al. 2016), the associations are responsible for the continuing professional development (CPD) of their members and advising members on quality standards. They assist in establishing collaborative relationships with other healthcare professions associations, global bodies and development partners. They learn from these what are best practices at any given time and share that with their members through CPD activities, with midwifery education institutions and with the Ministry of Health. Midwives' associations also help enforce the relicensing of members as a way of ensuring that members remain up to date, thus assisting with quality assurance (Survive and Thrive 2018; Castro Lopes et al. 2016).

6.6.4 Service Provision and Health System Strengthening

Midwives know their country's context best and are therefore able to contribute to the adoption and adaptation of any best practices generated on the global health arena. They provide leadership and guide government in implementation processes (Castro Lopes et al. 2016) for the improvement of maternal health outcomes. Where they have capacity and are functioning well, mid-wives' associations provide a context-specific gateway for introducing evidence-based approaches for strengthening midwifery services and health systems. Midwifery services are so closely intertwined with the state of a country's health system that health system specialists can access the country's health system as well as policymakers and government officials through working with midwives' associations. As midwifery services are strengthened, so is the health system. Conversely, working with midwives' associations exposes some weaknesses in the health system and thus alert policymakers to the need for change and improvement (ICM 2015). However, the reality is that midwives' associations are often not so functional and do not always engage effectively with the health system.

Midwives' associations strategically position midwives and midwifery in the health system (ten Hoope-Bender et al. 2014). Hence, they provide an effective conduit for introducing innovative MNCH services planning approaches. One example was the introduction of the Midwifery Services Framework (MSF) (2014) developed by the ICM in 2015 to support midwifery services planning processes in six countries, viz. Afghanistan, Bangladesh, Ghana, Kyrgyzstan, Lesotho and Togo (Nove et al. 2018). Working with and through the midwives' associations, ICM was able to harness resources from donor agency (Bill and Melinda Gates Foundation), to introduce, implement and evaluate the impact of the MSF and to refine the tool prior to its introduction to a second set of countries (ICM 2018). The evaluation of the MSF's impact in these countries demonstrated varied levels of success but obvious impact on sensitisation of the countries to the value of midwives and midwifery (ICM 2019a, b). When it works well, the MSF facilitates the improvement of the quality of midwifery services and the reduction of preventable maternal morbidity and mortality (ICM 2015).

The variety in sizes and expertise amongst midwives' associations creates a rich field for collaborative mutually beneficial relationships: twinning. The twinning approach has been used by other agencies including WHO, universities, cities and even countries (WHO 2001). Other health professions associations, specifically FIGO, have also used the twinning approach to strengthen their societies for effective care provision. Twinning is described in detail in Chapter 16.

The ICM Midwifery Services Framework

The Midwifery Services Framework (MSF) (2014) for developing Sexual, Reproductive, Maternal and Newborn Health (SRMNH) Services by midwives is a tool developed by International Confederation of Midwives (ICM) and partners to support the development and strengthening of midwifery services across all countries focusing on a quality midwifery workforce.

The ICM supports a midwifery strengthening approach using the MSF: The framework provides health system developers and planners, maternal and newborn health experts, policymakers and other stakeholders such as midwives, educators, regulators and professional associations with an evidence-based tool from which to develop new or strengthen existing effective and efficient midwifery services. The MSF supports the implementation of the midwife-led model of care, which has proven to be an effective and desirable model of care provision for women and their families.

The framework is available on: https://www.internationalmidwives.org/assets/uploads/documents/MSF%20Documents/The%20ICM%20MSF.pdf. Accessed from the International Confederation of Midwives website https://www.internationalmidwives.org. Accessed 10 October 2019

6.6.5   Communication and Advocacy

Other key roles of the associations are communication and advocacy. Associations function as a conduit of communication between government, development partners and other stakeholders, including the population they service and the media. By becoming the mouthpiece of the profession, associations allow midwives to advocate for themselves, for women, their newborn and their families. They advocate for and contribute to the enforcement of human rights, including in times of crisis such as natural disasters and civil unrest. This advocacy role spans across representing midwives on policymaking bodies in relation to service provision, conditions of service and management of the quality care (UNFPA 2017). Advocating for quality of care includes the associations making demands for sufficient resources (equipment, infrastructure, human resources and finances) to enable the provision of optimum, respectful and culturally sensitive care for women and their families. Those which act as unions ensure fair treatment and remuneration of its members but with a major focus on improving the plight of women and newborn during the time they need care and support.

6.6.6   Gate Keeping in Midwifery Practice

The association is the gate keeper in midwifery practice, ensuring that, together with the regulatory body, only those individuals who qualify to provide care and service are doing so. They take on the responsibility for quality assurance as well as horizon scanning for and introduction of new approaches and technologies which improve quality in close communication with the Ministry of Health and the midwifery education institutions. In some countries, educators have expressed that when government and partners are introducing new technologies and approaches, the midwifery schools are often left out. The association has a responsibility to ensure that all midwives feel well represented irrespective of their area of function. The midwives' associations have a role to play in issues of recruitment and deployment of fit-for-practice staff, that the staff are well looked after and respected in order for them to provide respectful care to women and their families. As gate keepers and closely related to their advocacy role, associations are involved in service management issues, workforce management and development including requesting adequate staffing levels, availability of mentors, preceptors and support systems that enhance effective professional clinical practice.

6.6.7   Contributing to Implementation of Global Strategies

Midwives' associations advocate for and contribute to the implementation of activities emanating from agreed global strategies. For example, during the consultation phase of the Global Strategy for Women's Children's and Adolescents' Health 2016–2030 (WHO 2015) and the Global Strategy for Human Resources for Health: Workforce 2030 (WHO 2016), it was agreed that midwives' associations could be responsible for ensuring that midwifery education had sufficient emphasis in the new WRA-WHO-ICM Global Midwifery Advocacy Strategy (WHO 2017). Midwives' associations could also link advocacy for midwifery education to other ongoing advocacy platforms (WHO 2017). WHO has suggested that the Sustainable Development Goals (SDGs) provided an opportunity for midwives to position themselves as the main providers of MNH and take hold of power over that 15-year period (WHO 2016). They could do this through the midwives' associations. The global strategies present an unprecedented opportunity to increase the professional role and socio-economic status of midwives in the implementation of the strategies. This is the responsibility of the midwives' associations to take up this opportunity and raise the profile of midwives and midwifery. 'Midwives need to be at the table, they need to be at Ministries of Health meetings, midwives need to be present and represented' (WHO 2016:9). The face and voice of midwives is the midwives' association.

6.7   Creating, Nurturing and Sustaining a Midwives' Association

Survive and Thrive (2016) developed a nine-module package for strengthening professional associations. This package is practical, evidence based, easy to follow guidance on how to create, nurture and sustain a professional association. This package is available online. Each of the nine modules describes in detail an aspect of strengthening a professional association starting from creating one through its growth and development to how a healthy association can carry out its responsibilities such as developing a vision, strategic planning, managing membership and quality management. The characteristics of a healthy and unhealthy professional association are clearly described (Table 6.1). The package also contains 'how to' content to guide new associations in carrying out their responsibilities.

Table 6.1 Characteristics of an association's state of health

Characteristics of a healthy professional association	Characteristics of an unhealthy professional association
• Ability to maintain the visibility of the profession • Ability to fulfil objectives; the PA is creative and represents its members well • Serves as the go-to organisation for information related to the professional field • Goal-driven, well-led and managed, and produces results that are recognised by the target population and policy makers • Establishes a niche that can only be filled by itself and the members of the profession • Establishes professional unity, identity, and a sense of belonging amongst members • Produces evidence and contributes to the provision of quality care • Is considered a worthwhile partner and is sought out by other organisations, including other healthcare professional associations • Is invited to contribute to decision and policymaking circles and its opinion is valued • Contributes to the achievement of national health care provision strategies • Serves as a gatekeeper for quality of care	A professional association that is not functioning well is characterised by • Lack of a sense of identity and belonging amongst members • Bickering and fighting for leadership positions • No results that can be attributed to the profession • No representation of the profession in decision-making circles • Weak leadership • No common goal for the members • No sense of commitment or ownership of the association or its activities. Individuals are concerned about themselves rather than the greater professional good because they do not identify with the profession • Membership is low and sometimes those who are members are disgruntled. There is no visible benefit to be a member of the PA • Policymakers, the community and the population served are not aware of the contributions of the association or its members

Source: Strengthening Professional Associations. Survive and Thrive. Module 9 (revised 2018)

6.7.1   The Role of Leadership in Midwives' Associations

One key to the success of a midwives' association is effective leadership (ICM 2004, 2013). Effective leadership ensures that the association is a goal-driven, well-led and well-managed organisation that produces results, and the results are recognised by the population served (Survive and Thrive 2016). With effective leadership, the association has the ability to fulfil its objectives, represent its members well and maintain the visibility of the profession by 'establishing a niche that can only be filled by itself and members of the profession' (ICM Twinning Manual 2014). Because of the importance of leadership to the strength, development and survival of midwives' associations, ICM, UNFPA and other global organisations have invested time and resources in developing midwifery leadership across a number of countries. For example, since 2004, ICM developed, and has progressively refined and conducted, a global programme to develop leadership in young midwives—the Young Midwifery Leaders Programme (ICM 2019a, b) (Box 6.5).

The issue of leadership is discussed in some detail in Chapter 11.

Box 6.5. The ICM Young Midwifery Leaders (YML) programme

The ICM Young Midwifery Leaders (YML) programme is a 2-year programme which provides young midwives with a unique opportunity to learn how to develop as leaders in their professional lives and the communities they work in. The programme challenges young midwives to broaden their knowledge of key policy areas in maternal and newborn health and create innovative projects to address some of the biggest global health challenges of today. The YML programme consists of online, interactive learning on leadership and the role and function of International Confederation of Midwives, a combination of group and individual projects, atten-

---

dance in the ICM regional conferences (2019). ICM will support a chosen mentor for each YML to develop their mentoring skills. The programme aims to identify young midwives with the potential to become leaders within their national midwifery communities and to build their capacity to become the global and regional midwifery leaders of tomorrow.

Source: https://www.internationalmidwives.org/assets/files/project-files/2019/02/final-yml-advert%2D%2D-selection-c-and-process-document.pdf

---

6.7.2   Some Causes of Association Failure

Some associations fail because of personality differences. Organisations such as Professional associations, like any other organisation, are as good as the individuals who constitute them. It needs to be recognised that members of an association come from different backgrounds and have different ideas and preferences. These differences need to be factored in whilst creating, nurturing and supporting a midwives' association. In some instances, the members just do not have capacity to lead and manage an organisation. Hence, the need for the development partners and other organisations to strengthen leadership in midwives' associations.

6.8   Conclusion

Evidence abounds showing that midwifery services make a difference (WHO 2019; ten Hoope-Bender et al. 2014) and that midwives are key service providers in MNCH (Renfrew et al. 2014). When midwives are brought together in a well-led and well-managed association, midwifery becomes strong and more able to contribute to the reduction of maternal and newborn morbidity and mortality. The association ensures the integrity of the organisation and the profession it represents (Hovekamp 1997). This provides members with a sense of identity, inspires and motivates them to work towards a common goal in care provision. Thus, the association institutionalises thought processes, codes of conduct, change and change management within the profession (Galaskiewis 1985). When there is no association, there is no focal point for the profession. It is difficult for members to contribute to policy and decision-making, and it is difficult for the profession to be consulted in its own right.

6.8.1 Principles

Availability of midwives' associations is invaluable to the strengthening of midwifery services. Countries should ensure that their midwifery workforce is organised into a strong association.

6.8.2 Policy

Governments, development partners and key stakeholders should support the strengthening of midwives' associations as a means of enhancing quality midwifery services for women, newborns and their families.

6.8.3 Practice

Studies are required to determine the value of effective midwives' associations and the difference they make to the quality of care.

Key Messages

Midwives' associations are the entities that bring midwives together to represent the profession.

Midwives' associations provide the mechanism by which Ministroies of Health and other organisations can interact with midwifery on a professional basis.

Midwives' associations are the focal point through which the profession of midwifery can be strengthened and acquire an identity.

Questions for Reflection

1. This chapter posits that strengthening midwives' associations has a positive impact on midwifery services in a country. Discuss this thought highlighting key contributions which would otherwise be difficult when there is no or a weak association.

2. In many countries, midwives are not obliged to be members of the midwives' association. Discuss the benefits of membership to the association for
   (a) Individual midwives
   (b) The government
   (c) Key stakeholders

3. Examine the factors impacting on the development of a midwives' association and how challenges can be addressed.

Additional Resources for Reflection and Further Study

Alexander L, Igumbor EU, Sanders D (2009) Building capacity without disrupting health services: public health education for Africa through distance learning. Human Resour Health 7:28

Hailey J, James R, Wrigley R (2005) Rising to the challenges: assessing the impacts of organisational capacity building. Praxis Paper No. 2. The International NGO Training and Research Centre, Feb 2005

Howard GL (2016) Creating and nurturing an organisation. Survive and Thrive Global Development Alliance. Professional Association Strengthening Module 2. American College of Nurse-Midwives

International Confederation of Midwives (2011a) Member Association Capacity Assessment Tool (MACAT)

International Confederation of Midwives (2011b) Member Association Capacity Assessment Tool (MACAT). Guidelines

International Confederation of Midwives (2014) Why and how to create a midwives' association. https://www.internationalmidwives.org/who-we-are-/midwives-associations/create-a-nationa-association.html. Accesses 10 Feb 2020

International Confederation of Midwives (2019) The ICM Young Midwifery Leaders Programme. https://www.internationalmidwives.org/assets/files/project-files/2019/02/final-yml-advert%2D%2D-selection-c-and-process-document.pdf. Accessed 1 Feb 2020

Quimby CH, Mantz ML (2007) Expanding access to reproductive health through midwives: lessons learnt from the SEATS Project. MAPS Initiative. JSL,

SEATS Project 2000, Arlington. Quoted in Capacity Project Knowledge Sharing February 2007. www.who.int/workforce alliance/knowledge /toolkit/27_1.pdf. Accessed 2 March 2018

Robert K, Merton R (1958) The functions of a Professional Association. Am J Nurs 58(1):50–54. www.jstor.org/stable/pdf/3461366.pdf. Accessed 2 March 2018

Weiner B (2009) A theory of organisational readiness for change. Implement Sci 4:67

References

Atkinson R (2012) The value of professional associations. https://www.thinkhdi.com/library/supportworld/2012/professional-associations.aspx. Accessed 9 October 2019

Bogren MU (2016) Building a profession of Midwifery in South Asia. PhD Thesis, Institute of Health Care Sciences at Sahlgrenska Academy at the University of Gothenburg

Bogren M, Wiseman A, Berg M (2012) Midwifery education, regulation and association in six South Asian countries - A descriptive report. Sexual Reprod Healthcare 3:67–72. https://doi.org/10.1016/j.srhc.2012.03.004

Cadee F, Nieuwenhuijze MJ, Lagro-Janssen AL et al (2016) The state of the art of twinning, a concept analysis of twinning in healthcare. Global Health 12:66

Castro Lopes S, Titulaer P, Bokosi M et al (2015) The involvement of midwives' associations in policy planning about the midwifery workforce: a global survey. Midwifery 31(2015):1096–1103

Castro Lopes S, Nove A, ten Hoope-Bender P et al (2016) A descriptive analysis of midwifery education, regulation and association in 73 countries: the baseline for a post-2015 pathway. Hum Resour Health 14:37

Dawson A, Brodie P, Copeland F et al (2014) Collaborative approaches towards building midwifery capacity in low income countries: a review of experiences. Midwifery. 30(4):391–402. https://doi.org/10.1016/j.midw.2013.05.009

Empire State Association Society of Association Executive (2019) Value of associations. https://www.essae.org/advocacy. Accessed 10 Oct 2019

Hovekamp TM (1997) Professional associations or unions? A comparative look. Library Trends 46(2):232–244

International Confederation of Midwives (2004) The Young Midwifery Leaders Programme. https://www.internationalmidwives.org/projects

International Confederation of Midwives (2011) The Young Midwifery Leaders Programme for Latin America and the Caribbean. https://www.internationalmidwives.org/projects

International Confederation of Midwives (2013) Strengthening Midwifery services in China:helping mothers survive bleeding after birth. https://www.internationalmidwives.org/projects/china2013

International Confederation of Midwives (2014a) Twinning as a tool for strengthening midwives associations. Operational manual. The Hague International Confederation of Midwives

International Confederation of Midwives (2014b) Twinning programmes. https://www.internationalmidwives.org/projects-programmes/twinning-twinning-projects-programmes.html. Accessed 10 March 2020

International Confederation of Midwives (2016) Strengthening midwifery services in Kyrgyzstan: midwifery services framework country assessment workshop report. https://www.interntionalmidwives.org/projects

International Confederation of Midwives (2019a) (Web document) The International Confederation of Midwives Consultancy service. https://www.internationalmidwives.org/icm-publications/icm-consultancy-service.html. Accessed 10 Oct 2019

International Confederation of Midwives (2019b) (Web document) The ICM Regions. https://www.internationalmidwives.org/about-us/international-confederation-of-midwives/. Accessed 10 Oct 2019

International Confederation of Midwives. Vision, mission and purpose (www document). https://www.internationalmidwives.org/home. Accessed 10 March 2020

International Federation of Gynaecology and Obstetrics (2012) Strengthening organisational capacity of health professional associations. The FIGO LOGIC Toolkit. International Federation of Gynecology and Obstetrics, London, vol 122, no 3, pp 190–191

Ireland J, van Teijlingen E, Kemp J (2015) Twinning in Nepal: The Royal College of Midwives UK and the Midwifery Society of Nepal working in partnership. J Asian Midwives 2(1):26–33

Kemp J, Bannon E M, Muwema Mwanja M et al. (2018a) Developing a national standard for midwifery mentorship in Uganda. Int J Health Governance. ISSN: 2059-4631

Kemp J, Shawe E, Musoke MG et al (2018b) Developing a model of midwifery mentorship for Uganda: The MOMENTUM project 2015–2017. Midwifery 59:127–129

Nove A, Moyo NT, Bokosi MA et al (2018) The Midwifery Services Framework: the process of implementation. Midwifery 58:96–101

Renfrew MJ, McFadden A, Bastos MH et al (2014) Midwifery and quality care. Findings from a new evidence informed framework for maternal and newborn care. Lancet 384:1129–1145

Sandwell R, Bonser D, Hebert E et al (2018) Stronger together: midwifery twinning between Tanzania and Canada. Globalization Health 14:123

Survive and Thrive (2016) Introduction to the professional association strengthening manual. American College of Nurse Midwives. http://www.strongprofassoc.org/wp-content/uploads/2016/07/PAS-Introduction-060316.pdf. Accessed 5 Aug 2020

Survive and Thrive (2018) Professional Association Strengthening: a series of modules to strengthen health professional associations. American College of Nurse Midwives (2016) revised 2018. www.strongprofassoc.org. Accessed October 2019

Ten Hoope-Bender P, de Bernis L, Campbell J et al (2014) Improvement of maternal and newborn health through midwifery. Lancet 384:1226–1235

The Midwifery Services Framework (2014) For strengthening sexual reproductive maternal and newborn health. https://www.internationalmidwives.org/documents/msf

United Nations Population Fund (2011) State of the World's Midwifery report 2011: delivering health, saving lives. United Nations Population Fund, New York

United Nations Population Fund (2014) The State of the World's Midwifery report: a universal pathway. A woman's right to health. United Nations Population Fund, New York

United Nations Population Fund (2017) UNFPA Strategic Plan 2018 – 2021: working together to support implementation of the 2030 Agenda. https://www.sdgfund.org/publication/working-together-support-implementation-2030-agenda-sustainable-development-joint-annex. Accessed 11 Jan 2020

World Health Organisation (2001) Guideines for city twinning. WHO Regional Office of Europe. Copenhagen

World Health Organisation (2015) Global strategy for women's, children's and adolescents' health 2016–2030

World Health Organization (2016) Strengthening quality midwifery education. WHO meeting report, 25–26 July. In support of Global strategy for women's, children's and adolescents' health 2016-30. World Health Organization, Geneva

World Health Organisation (2017) Midwifery education and the Global Midwifery Advocacy Strategy. WHO, ICM and White Ribbon Alliance. WHO Geneva

World Health Organisation (2019) Strengthening quality midwifery education for Universal Health Coverage 2030. WHO Geneva

Part III

Midwifery Practice

Models of Midwifery Practice

7

Expected Learning Outcomes

By the end of the chapter, the reader should be able to:

1. Identify the different models of midwifery practice that are in use
2. Examine the differences in the medical and midwifery models of care
3. Discuss the differing perceptions of birth and how these influence the philosophy and practicality in care provision
4. Present examples of the uses and benefits of various models of midwifery practice that have been shown to provide safe and satisfying care in a range of countries
5. Discuss the need for respectful maternity care, providing examples of disrespect and abuse and efforts being made to address human rights issues in this context
6. Identify documents and resources that support the promotion of respectful maternity care

7.1 Models of Care

Models of midwifery practice vary within countries and across the world. These largely focus on either a medical/obstetric/nursing model or a midwifery model. How birth is perceived (Box 7.1) and the philosophies of care vary considerably between these models.

Box 7.1. Differing perceptions of birth

Midwifery perception

- Birth is usually a normal, physiological process.
- Birth is a social event, a normal part of a woman's life.
- Birth is the work of the woman and her family.
- The woman is a person experiencing a life-transforming event.

Medical Perception

- Childbirth is a potentially pathological process.
- Childbirth is a 'risk state'.
- Birth is the work of doctors, nurses, midwives and other experts.
- The woman is a patient.

Source: Berg (2005), ICM (2014), Birthlink (2019)

© Springer Nature Switzerland AG 2021
J. Kemp et al., *Global Midwifery: Principles, Policy and Practice*,
https://doi.org/10.1007/978-3-030-46765-4_7

Emerging from the perceptions of birth, the philosophies and practice surrounding birthing are very different when the medical and midwifery models are compared. Whilst practitioners in both professions inevitably vary and there can be no dogmatic classification of their individual approaches, the models in use tend to offer dissimilar types of care. It needs to be remembered that both midwives and obstetricians have different but complementary roles in order to meet the needs of pregnant and birthing women. During normal childbirth women do not need medical attention, but sometimes midwives opt for the medical approach rather than using a midwiferymodel in providing essential care. A comparison of these approaches is presented in Table 7.1.

Table 7.1 Different approaches used by midwives using different models

Midwives using a midwifery model	Midwives (or doctors) using a medical model
See birth as a holistic process	Necessarily focus on the medical aspects
Consider that there is no class distinction between birthing women and those providing their care	Approach can be more 'paternalistic', an authoritarian attitude existing between obstetricians or midwives and their clients
Expect decisions to be shared between them in this equal relationship	Refer to women as their patients
Information is shared using familiar language and imagery	Tendency to use medical terminology
Efforts are made to provide information sensitively, and there is often strong emotional support	In a traditional approach, information may not always be shared adequately
Often provide longer and more in-depth antenatal care sessions	Inclined to use brief and less-personalised care with little emotional support
Believes that the female body is designed for birth with no harm to either mother or baby	Assumes that the female body is prone to fail, and so childbirth is considered very risky
Believes in the integrity of birth and use technology only when needed	Doctors who are consulted when problems are suspected tend to value technology and use it more readily

Derived from Birthlink (2019)

In both the professions, modern educational methods increasingly emphasise the importance of interpersonal communication skills and the use of empathic approaches in providing sensitive as well as safe standards of care. The medicalisation of childbirth has been justified by several arguments. These surround the concern for safety, the need for defensive medical practice and the concept of women's choice (OU 2005).

It is because the medical model assumes that the female body is prone to fail, childbirth is considered very risky. In this context, hospital birth has been advocated as it is considered the safest in spite of some research evidence demonstrating that, for a healthy woman with a normal pregnancy, out of hospital settings such as midwifery-led units (MLUs) or a planned home birth is as safe as a hospital birth though more research is advocated on this subject (MacDonald 2009). Clearly the emphasis is placed on the woman selecting the right place in her individual circumstances (Birthchoice UK 2019) though it has been recommended that a woman at 'low risk' in the UK may choose any birth setting (UKMidSS 2017). What is considered safe in one country may not be so in another, and the home and health facility circumstances need to be taken into consideration as well as the country infrastructure and support system that is available for home births (Olsen 2012). Koblinsky et al. (2016:2308) emphasise that '…despite the diversity in models of providing care, the starting point is the same for all countries: to ensure that every woman, everywhere, delivers in a safe environment'. They maintain that every country needs to make its own unambiguous statement detailing the care that should be provided for pregnant women, identifying the care that needs to exist for uncomplicated births; in addition the systems required to make a timely response when complications arise and the essential referral linkages need to be in place.

However, because the safety and well-being of the woman and her newborn are of primary concern, midwives are expected to work in collaboration with other health professionals (ICM 2014) and as indicated above, in considering models of midwifery practice, the issue of the place of birth inevitably surfaces. It has been established that 10–15% of women will need some obstetric intervention in order to facilitate a safe birth (WHO 2015a), and therefore, cooperation and mutual respect between medical staff and midwives is crucial.

In order to promote safer childbirth, the importance of skilled attendance during childbirth has become a dominant issue in reducing the global statistics of maternal and perinatal mortality and morbidity (WHO 2018), and this is discussed in Chapter 2. However, although the place of birth may influence the model of care used, it does not necessarily dictate it. In the UK, it has been concluded that for women having their second or subsequent baby, births in a midwifery unit or at home appear to be safe for the baby and certainly offer the mother some benefits (NPEU 2017). This resonates with the findings in the Netherlands cited above (MacDonald 2009), both countries providing a skilled and supported community midwifery service.

In the midst of a multitude of approaches, perhaps a Canadian study offers wisdom in stating that a variety of intrapartum care models need to be available because no single model proposes to meet the needs of all maternity care providers. It is stressed that attention must be given to eliminating barriers to collaborative inter-professional practice, along with enhancing factors that facilitate the delivery of intrapartum care (Smith et al. 2009).

7.2   The Transition of Philosophies of Care

In a rapidly changing world, philosophies of midwifery care have changed somewhat more slowly. The philosophies of obstetric/medical/nursing models of care are gradually evolving into woman-centred care provided by skilled midwives as efforts to 'humanise' birth gain momentum. It has been claimed that birth is one of the most powerful of all human experiences. Although in some circumstances it can be disem-

powering, there is evidence across the globe that there are societies that respect the desires of women and honour the normal physiological process of labour. Birthing models with a philosophy that offers women true choice and where interventions are minimal have been shown to be more acceptable. In the best models of care, women are respected and trusted (Davis-Floyd et al. 2009:1). There is clearly a continued need for a transition of the philosophy of care to focus on women rather than risk, but a holistic and comprehensive approach must always ensure that safety is a priority whilst maintaining a woman-centred approach. Drawing from three qualitative studies considering midwifery models of care for women at high risk, Berg (2005) identifies three components of what is termed 'ideal midwifery'. Primarily 'a dignity-protective action' is described. This incorporates the caring relationship of the midwife with a childbearing woman who is at high risk. It comprises 'mutuality, trust, ongoing dialogue, enduring presence, and shared responsibility'. Secondly, she identifies the midwife's embodied knowledge which consists of 'theoretical, practical, intuitive, and reflective knowledge'. Lastly, Berg stresses that midwives hold a singular responsibility in balancing 'the natural and medical perspectives in the care of childbearing women at high risk'. This recognises a woman's 'inborn capacity to be a mother and to give birth in a natural manner'. The author stresses the uniqueness of every woman which needs to be respected in organising her care. It is therefore purported that the philosophy identified here in caring for women at high risk is no less relevant to all childbearing women (Berg 2005:9). Renfrew et al. (2014:1132) in developing an evidence-informed framework consider that:

> Optimising biological, psychological, social, and cultural processes; strengthening woman's capabilities' is an important philosophy and that there should be expectant management, using interventions only when indicated.

The International Confederation of Midwives (ICM) has considered and repeatedly revised its midwifery philosophy of care, and this is specified in Box 7.2.

Box 7.2. The ICM philosophy of midwifery care

- Pregnancy and childbearing are usually normal physiological processes.
- Pregnancy and childbearing are a profound experience, which carry a significant meaning to the woman, her family, and the community.
- Midwives are the most appropriate care providers to attend childbearing women.
- Midwifery care promotes, protects and supports women's human, reproductive and sexual health and rights, and respects ethnic and cultural diversity. It is based on the ethical principles of justice, equity and respect for human dignity.
- Midwifery care is holistic and continuous in nature, grounded in an understanding of the social, emotional, cultural, spiritual, psychological and physical experiences of women.
- Midwifery care is emancipatory as it protects and enhances the health and social status of women and builds women's self-confidence in their ability to cope with childbirth.
- Midwifery care takes place in partnership with women, recognising the right to self-determination, and is respectful, personalised, continuous and non-authoritarian.
- Ethical and competent midwifery care is informed and guided by formal and continuous education, scientific research and application of evidence.

Source: ICM (2014)

In considering what makes midwifery models of care safe, Fahi (2012:1) acknowledges that inconsistent definitions of these models cause claims of safety to be a challenge. However, she makes it plain that such a definition must include skilled midwives who are knowledgeable in midwifery philosophy, who work in partnership with women and provide care which focuses on facili-

tating the natural process of birth whenever possible. This concurs with Berg's philosophy described above. Fahy compares midwifery models of care with 'midwife provided-care models' which are dominated by obstetric philosophy and practice; the latter concentrate on risk rather than on women. However, Berg (2005) stresses that for the woman's sake, it is crucial that medical and midwifery care exist on equal terms.

7.3 The Emergence of Midwife-Led Care

In an extensive review of the available evidence (Cochrane 2016), it was recommended that the majority of women should be offered 'midwife-led continuity of care'. This is because it has been shown to provide benefits for women and their babies, with no adverse effects being identified. The evidence reviewed did not include women with pre-existing serious pregnancy or health complications. Nevertheless, the review suggested that women who received midwife-led continuity models of care by comparison with women who received other models of care were less likely to experience adverse outcomes or interventions when giving birth. They were also more inclined to express satisfaction with their maternity care. In considering the options, Fahi (2012:1) contends that 'skilled, well-supported midwives are needed to attend women who refuse hospital care' and suggests that there is overwhelming evidence anyway for supporting a midwifery model of care because it is a safe option.

Concerning antenatal care, WHO (2016) recommends using a model with a minimum of eight contacts between woman and care provider if perinatal mortality is to be reduced and the woman's experience of care improved. The midwifery model of care can be provided in a number of different ways and examples are offered in Box 7.3. The model may be used in the community, hospital, health facility or birthing centre, and the key issue usually focuses on the centrality of the woman and meeting her needs holistically whether this is met through partnership, team midwifery or other model in use.

Box 7.3. Examples of midwifery models of care

- Group antenatal care or 'CenteringPregnancy'
- Caseloading
- Midwife-led care including birthing centres, alongside midwifery units, freestanding midwifery units
- Continuity of care/carer
- Partnership
- Team midwifery

Sources: Mackenzie Bryers and van Teijlingen (2010), Clow (2010), Oosthuizen et al. (2019), Page (2003), Sandall (1997)

Midwifery units in the UK may be in the form of a 'Freestanding Maternity Unit' (FMU), an Alongside Maternity Unit (AMU) or an obstetric unit (OU). An evaluation of these three models demonstrated that FMUs had slightly better outcomes than AMUs. The reasons for this were considered complex with medical respondents, suggesting that AMUs tended to attract more affluent, white women and cater less well for those from different ethnic and social groups. It was thought that the difference could also relate to staffing and management of the units and whether women 'opted in' to give birth there or 'opted out' preferring to go to an OU or stay at home. Obstetricians were generally in favour of AMUs because they gave them more time to focus on women at higher risk. It was acknowledged that more research is needed on this topic, that there should be clear criteria set for admission to AMUs allowing women to make a truly informed choice. Since it was observed that women often get sent home from various maternity units in early labour, it was proposed that there should be more midwifery support available for women in early labour at home regardless of where they planned to give birth (Nove 2015).

Models of care can and have been adapted in various ways to meet specific needs. Experience from Australia describes the importance of identifying vulnerabilities and offering care specifi-

cally designed to meet these needs, for example the very young and those who are culturally or linguistically diverse (Everitt 2016).

Group antenatal care has emerged as an innovative model comprising all aspects of antenatal care, some focusing particularly on education (Abrams et al. 2018; Shimpuku et al. 2019; Oguntunde et al. 2019). Groups are established, and professional healthcare providers act as facilitators. Sometimes referred to as 'CenteringPregnancy', this has become popular within the context of the healthcare system of the United States of America (USA) where it has been acclaimed as safe and effective. But until more recently, less has been known about the experience of adapting this model of care in settings outside the USA. However, the CenteringPregnancy model has been adapted for use in Mexico and has demonstrated both opportunities and challenges. From this experience, emphasis has been placed on the need to understand the health system context when such an approach is used in diverse settings across the globe (Heredia-Pi et al. 2018).

Sayinzoga et al. (2018) modified the CenteringPregnancy model for use in providing both antenatal and postnatal care in Rwanda. The authors suggest that the group process is an effective method of providing care and is a key to local ownership and therefore uptake of healthcare provision. A later study in Rwanda revealed that although concerns about privacy were initially expressed, lack of financial resources and lack of male partner support were cited as the major concerns. It was proposed that additional human resources at health centres, intensive efforts to provide 'reminder communications' and large-scale community outreach were required in order to benefit the largest number of pregnant and postnatal women. It was concluded that these additional resources were required if a group care model were to be scaled up successfully (Musabyimana et al. 2019).

Similarly for Spanish-speaking women within the USA, Trudnak et al. (2013) discovered that although group antenatal care appeared to make no difference to the perinatal outcomes, it did improve the uptake of care which concurs with the findings of Robertson et al. (2009) who indicate that by comparison with traditional care provided for Hispanic women, group care met with a high level of satisfaction. Whilst adapting models of care from one country to another inevitably presents its challenges, from their experience in Haiti Abrams et al. (2018) offer insights into modifying the group approach to meet the needs of low resourced countries. The challenges identified include language, literacy, cultural issues, socio-political climate and available space. The authors suggest numerous approaches designed to assist in addressing these issues across the world in low-resourced countries (Box 7.4).

Space
- Consider space and location in order to build capacity and partnerships within a community
- Consider that group arrangement can promote or inhibit group dynamics and communication
- Arrange meetings in easily accessible sites that can comfortably accommodate the group and be reasonably private

Derived from Abrams et al. (2018)

It is worthy of note that a family-oriented antenatal group education programme in rural Tanzania, designed to promote birth preparedness and complication readiness, showed that participants were better prepared with better outcomes. Consequently, women attended antenatal clinic more than four times and were aware of a health facility in case of emergency. The place of birth was selected with or by the pregnant women who arranged for a companion to accompany them to a health facility. The intervention group had less bleeding and seizures during labour and birth, fewer Caesarean sections and less neonatal complications (Shimpuku et al. 2019). Educating men about danger signs of pregnancy, labour, birth, newborn and child health was found to be crucial in improving maternal and newborn health outcomes in the northern Nigeria. Here the establishment of male support groups included interpersonal skills and household decision-making. These efforts were effective in educating men and motivating some to become advocates, so influencing the community and improving health-service utilisation, promoting decision-making for women when the need arose to seek professional help (Oguntunde et al. 2019). This may indeed be the key to improving effectiveness of antenatal education and care in other areas, especially where men continue to be the main decision-makers.

Box 7.4. Adapting CenteringPregnancy approaches in low-resourced countries: lessons from Haiti

Language
- Conduct group-level interventions in participants' native language
- Learn key phrases in the language
- If necessary, train bilingual nationals to co-facilitate

Literacy
- Consider alternative methods of evaluation for low-literacy participants

Culture
- Ensure materials and approaches are culturally tailored
- Use national advisers to balance any foreign advisers not allowing the latter to outnumber the former

The socio-political climate
- Raise awareness that the presence of foreigners in previously colonised countries will influence group dynamics
- Conduct transparent discussions on identities prior to initiating programmes

7.4 The Concept of Continuity

Continuity of care and more recently continuity of *carer* have long been associated with improved clinical outcomes and greater satisfaction, though what women value about these approaches has been less well defined (Perriman et al. 2018). Continuity of carer has been shown to result in lower pre-term births, fewer inductions of labour and interventions, more spontaneous vaginal births and an increased incidence of breastfeeding (Homer et al. 2017, Sandall et al. 2016). It has been claimed that the ideology of continuity of carer overlaps with that of team midwifery or midwife-led care and birth centre care which confer similar benefits. However, it is not easy to disentangle the components of these approaches. Whereas models that promote continuity of care can make the continuity of carer more likely, midwife caseloads are considered the 'gold standard' in ensuring continuity of carer (Warren 2003). There is evidence that this approach offers midwives more job satisfaction, and they experience less burnout (Dixon et al. 2017; Fenwick et al. 2017; Jepson et al. 2017; Foster et al. 2011). However, McInnes (2018) maintains that in order to implement continuity of carer, midwives' roles need to be changed and maternity services require restructuring.

A meta-synthesis undertaken to examine qualitative research papers in Australia, New Zealand, Denmark, the United Kingdom (UK) and the USA sought to obtain a deeper understanding of woman's perspectives in receiving continuity of maternity care. The study concluded that the midwife–woman relationship is the vehicle through which personalised care, trust and empowerment are achieved in this model (Perriman et al. 2018).

It has been acknowledged above that achieving continuity is likely to need reorganisation of midwives' roles and the maternity services in high income countries. However, examining the issue in the context of low- and middle-income countries is bound to present extra challenges given the inevitability of limited resources both human and fiscal. Considering the findings from a systematic review and examining whether continuity of care improved the quality of care and the maternal and neonatal outcomes, Sandall et al. (2016) conclude that the applicability of this model in low-income countries requires consideration of several issues where midwives may provide the majority of care but may not lead it or have clear referral systems. They recommend that the availability and training of midwives, the midwives' workload, accessibility for childbearing women and the baseline risk for the anticipated outcomes should be carefully examined. However, WHO (2019a, b) urges the use of this model stating that no adverse outcomes but rather substantial benefits are associated with midwife-led care. WHO therefore recommends midwife-led continuity of care, adding that case-loading midwifery is both safe and cost-effective.

In a study evaluating a midwife-led continuity model in rural areas of the Palestinian West Bank, given the better uptake of care and improved outcomes, it was concluded that this could be a useful approach in other low- and middle-income countries but that more research was needed (Mortensen et al. 2018:9).

An Australian study comparing 'standard midwifery care' with caseload midwifery concluded that the latter is a safe and cost-effective approach to care for women experiencing any level of risk (Tracy et al. 2013).

A study conducted following a natural disaster in the Queensland area, showed that the benefits of continuity of midwifery carer during pregnancy extended beyond a more positive birth experience, resulting in enhanced birthing and infant outcomes. It also alleviated the effects of high stress levels experienced by women in this context and promoted better postnatal mental health (Kildea et al. 2018). This concurs with the experience of the continuity of carer provided in the wake of a hurricane in the United States (Giarratano et al. 2015).

In the context of the Sustainable Development Goal 3, WHO commends the concept of continuity of care (Box 7.5).

7.5   Disrespect and Abuse: A Pandemic to be Tackled!

Disrespect and abuse are a matter of concern across centuries, across generations and across continents. This has been referred to as 'a global epidemic' (Miller and Lalonde 2015:S49). There is increasing evidence of this scourge affecting not only women, but other vulnerable adults and children too (WHO 2017, 2019a, b). Abuse of adults has been defined as 'a single or repeated act or lack of appropriate actions, occurring within any relationship where there is an expectation of trust, which causes harm or distress to a vulnerable person' (Tidy 2016). Sometimes referred to as 'obstetric violence' when this occurs to the childbearing woman, it is defined as '…the appropriation of the body and reproductive processes of women by health personnel during pregnancy, childbirth and post-partum' (WHO 2015b).

The legal term 'obstetric violence' was first described in Latin America (Perez 2010), but there is evidence of concern about this issue in Europe and North America (Reader and Gillespie 2013, Rivaldi et al. 2018) and of widespread abuse of adults, across many other parts of the world (WHO 2017). WHO defines child maltreatment as abuse or neglect which can take many forms; this may be physical, sexual, emotional or constitute neglect and states that 1 in 4 adults have been physically abused as children. Many of these incidents go unreported but the consequences can last a lifetime or result in early

death (WHO 2019b). In the context of maternity care, abuse of neonates includes undertaking treatment without parental consent and refusing treatment because a baby is 'too sick to save' (Sacks 2017). With almost half the global population exceeding one billion children experiencing violence in a given year, this has been aptly described as endemic and has accelerated over recent decades. Disrespect and abuse have been acknowledged as a public health, human rights and social problem, but at the same time the fact that this is largely preventable has emerged (Hillis 2016) and constitutes part of the 2030 agenda (United Nations 2015). Violence against women and girls has been recognised as a global pandemic affecting one in three women during their lifetime (World Bank 2019). Inequity and abuse during pregnancy and birth have been shown to be more prevalent in women of colour and those challenged by social, economic or health issues (Vedam et al. 2019).

In the context of childbirth, the problem of women accessing safe and skilled care has been complicated by this lack of respect and physical and emotional abuse that is sometimes inflicted on them by those providing their care (Bowser and Hill 2010, Abuya et al. 2015). atfGherissi et al. (2016) and Brailey et al. (2017) have associated disrespectful care with the poor education of midwives. Disrespect and abuse have been classified into seven main categories (Box 7.6).

A qualitative study in Nigeria considered the social norms and acceptability of the abuse of women during childbirth and identified intimidation, shouting, threats of a poor outcome, physical restraint to a bed and slapping as common strategies. There was a difference of opinion as to whether these measures constituted abuse or whether they were acceptable in order to gain compliance. The authors conclude that these practices can reflect what is socially acceptable but that blaming women in these circumstances equates with much of the literature on intimate partner violence, so that the practices create a power gradient between midwives and women and perpetuate the low status of women and gender inequality (Bohren et al. 2016). Given the widespread abuse of and violence against children (Hillis 2016, WHO 2019b) and the discrimination against women and girls (World Bank 2019), there is little wonder that such behaviours entrenched within society reach unchallenged into the domain of childbirth. In a study of intrapartum care in India, Jha et al. (2016) claim that it is women in poor socio-economic circumstances who make use of the free government maternity care facilities provided. These women appreciated the provision of food, ambulance services and free care, but they experienced physical and verbal abuse. A medical model of care was in use with some evidence-based practices and some harmful practices, and women had no control over the process of their labour. In order to avoid abuse, the women in the Indian study were frequently subordinated and became submissive.

This evidence finds resonance with practices observed across sub-Saharan Africa. In a review of facility-based intrapartum care across this region, Bradley et al. (2016) propose that attitudes and approaches relate to the model of care that is in use. Both women and midwives are frequently caught between a medical model of birth, which dictates the way services are organised, and the social forces and traditional expectations which surround a 'social model of birth'. In such situations, women do not receive the compassion and care they need; neither the safety that they sought in an institutional setting. Women frequently lack the presence of a midwife and of any birthing companion. They conclude:

> …the harshness of their treatment, disproportionately meted out to more marginalised women, justifies their continued eschewal of facility-based delivery or a calculated, but risky, decision to arrive at the facility as close to delivery as possible. The false compartmentalisation of technical quality and safety from the interpersonal aspects of care has done women in resource-poor settings a considerable disservice. (Bradley et al. 2016:168)

Knowledge and skills are essential for all providing reproductive health care, but inappropriate attitudes all too often discourage women from seeking the recommended professional help at the time of birth (Bohren et al. 2014).

7.6   Respectful Maternity Care

Alongside the increasing recognition of the pandemic of disrespect and abuse, an initiative to advance 'Respectful Maternity Care' (RMC) has been actively and increasingly promoted in recent years (White Ribbon Alliance 2011). This will continue to be a matter for urgent action whilst there is considerable evidence that disrespectful care, the attitudes of staff and the quality of care can influence whether a woman and her family will seek the services of a skilled birth attendant (UNAIDS 2000, Filippi et al. 2006, Swahnberg et al. 2007, Uys et al. 2007, 2009, McMahon et al. 2014, Jha et al. 2016). WHO (2015b:1) states that: 'Every woman has the right to the highest attainable standard of health, which includes the right to dignified, respectful health care'.

RMC has therefore become a crucial issue in promoting safer childbirth and in seeking to lower the maternal and perinatal mortality and morbidity rates whilst women continue to bypass facilities that fail to offer quality care (Kruk 2009, WHO 2015b). Respect and dignity in the context of reproductive healthcare provision have gradually become part of the human rights agenda (Engender Health 2003, UNFPA 2014) though it has been acknowledged that

...the human rights lens failed to focus as rapidly on abuses during childbirth or links between adverse maternal outcomes and abusive practices and lack of quality of care. (Miller and Lalonde 2015:S50)

The issue of quality of care is discussed more fully in Chapter 8. Strategies to reduce disrespect and abuse include raising awareness, training, supportive supervision, clarification of values and criterion-based audits. In analysing audit data, it has been stressed that an objective and systematic approach is needed where the quality of care is measured against an identified set of criteria denoting best practice (van den Broek and Graham 2009).

The concept of RMC has markedly evolved and developed since an international conference on the humanisation of childbirth was held in Brazil in 2000. This was inspired as a response to the established trend of the medical model of childbirth which was epitomised in the global surge in births by caesarean section. In addition, the mounting disquiet about 'obstetric violence' led to the concept of a woman-centred approach (Maternal Health Task Force 2019).

The Global Respectful Maternity Care Council (GRMCC) was established in 2015. This is a multisectoral group of 22 organisations, representing over 200 members from across the globe. Members include clinicians, professional associations, advocates, researchers, United Nations agencies and donors who are committed to identifying, implementing and advocating for strategies to promote RMC. Through addressing the issue of disrespect and abuse during childbirth, the Council members aim to improve the quality of reproductive, maternal and newborn health care (Every Woman Every Child 2015).

Raising awareness of the issue is obviously the first but essential step in attempting to change staff attitudes and women's expectations. Evidence from Tanzania has demonstrated that workshops resulted in healthcare providers becoming aware of their negative attitudes but recommend further research to examine the impact of any interventions. It is stressed that research should focus on whether attitudinal changes of the providers are sustained and on the women's perceptions of the quality of the healthcare services (Webber et al. 2018). The importance of implementing behaviour change interventions focusing on the care providers has been identified as central to promoting RMC. This conclusion emanated from a study in Kenya where working relationships and environment were shown to impact the providers' emotional health. The latter causing burnout and influencing their interactions with women and the quality of care they provide (Ndwiga et al. 2017). Similarly, Burrowes et al. (2017) from a qualitative study in Ethiopia emphasise that addressing structural issues surrounding provider workload needs is key and should complement all interventions that aim to improve midwives' interpersonal interactions with women.

Key Messages

Principles

Models of midwifery practice should be developed within a philosophy of woman-centred, safe and satisfying care.

Policy

Strategies to afford continuity of care and carer need to be utilised within a country-specific context where safety and respectful care are never compromised. The infrastructure should support effective and timely referrals where needed.

Practice

Maternity care should be provided by skilled midwives who have been trained to international standards and work in collaboration with obstetricians, paediatricians and other professionals as necessary.

Questions for Reflection or Review

1. Consider the different perceptions of birth and how these influence the philosophy of care. Determine your own perception of birth and consider how this influences your personal philoso-

phy of midwifery care and your preferred model of care.

2. Consider the lessons learned in Haiti concerning adapting a model of care from a western model for use in low-resourced countries (Box 7.4). Since 'midwife-led continuity of care models' are recommended by WHO (Box 7.5), what criteria would be helpful in adapting such a model from a high-income to low- or middle-income country setting?

3. Disrespect and abuse during childbirth have been linked with various issues including human rights, the status of women and intimate partner violence. Identify approaches that are needed in order to promote Respectful Maternity Care within an identified community and in the provision of maternity services there.

Additional Resources for Reflection and Further Study

A short video entitled 'Understanding Respectful Maternity Care' produced by Medical Aid Films. https://www.medicalaidfilms.org/film/understanding-respectful-maternity-care/. Accessed 10 Oct 2019

The White Ribbon Alliance produces constantly updated information and resources on Respectful Maternity Care. https://www.whiteribbonalliance.org/resources. Accessed 10 Oct 2019

Davis-Floyd R, Barclay L, Tritten J et al (eds) (2009) Birth models that work. University of California Press, San Diego

Mortensen B, Lukasse M, Diep L et al (2018) Can a midwife-led continuity model improve maternal services in a low-resource setting? A non-randomised cluster intervention study in Palestine. BMJ. https://bmjopen.bmj.com/content/8/3/e019568. Accessed 05 Oct 2019

World Health Organization (2019) The case for midwifery. World Health Organization, Geneva. https://www.who.int/maternal_child_adolescent/topics/quality-of-care/midwifery/case-for-midwifery/en/. Accessed 05 Oct 2018

References

Abrams J, Forte J, Bettler C et al (2018) Considerations for implementing group-level prenatal health interventions in low-resource communities: lessons learned from Haiti. J Midwifery Womens Health 63(1):121–126

Abuya T, Warren C, Miller N et al (2015) Exploring the prevalence of disrespect and abuse during childbirth in Kenya. PLoS One 10(4):e0123606. https://doi.org/10.1371/journal.pone.0123606. Accessed 10 July 2019

AtfGherissi CM, Tinsa F, Soussi S et al (2016) Teaching research methodology to student midwives through a socio-constructivist educational model: The experience of the high school for science and health techniques of Tunis. Midwifery 33:46–48. https://doi.org/10.1016/j.midw.2015.10.015

Berg M (2005) A midwifery model of care for women at high risk: genuine caring in caring for the genuine. J Perinat Educ 14(1):9–21. https://www.ncbi.nlm.nih.gov/pmc/articles/PMC1595225/. Accessed 06 July 2019

BirthchoiceUK (2019) Where is the safest place to give birth? https://www.which.co.uk/birth-choice/faqs#where-is-the-safest-place-to-give-birth. Accessed 03 July 2019

Birthlink (2019) Midwife vs medical models of care. https://birthlink.com/midwife-vs-medical-models-of-care/. Accessed 03 July 2019

Bohren M, Hunter E, Munthe-Kaas H et al (2014) Facilitators and barriers to facility-based delivery in low and middle income countries: a qualitative evidence synthesis. Reprod Health 11(1):71. https://doi.org/10.1186/1742-4755-11-71

Bohren M, Vogel J, Tuncalp O et al (2016) "By slapping their laps, the patient will know that you truly care for her": a qualitative study on social norms and acceptability of the mistreatment of women during childbirth in Abuja, Nigeria. Popul Health 2:640–655

Bowser D, Hill K (2010) Exploring evidence for disrespect and abuse in facility-based childbirth: report of a landscape analysis. USAID-TRAction Project, University Research Corporation, LLC, and Harvard School of PublicHealth, Bethesda. http://www.tractionproject.org/sites/default/files/Respectful_Care_at_Birth_9-20-101_Final.pdf

Bradley S, McCourt C, Rayment J et al (2016) Disrespectful intrapartum care during facility-based delivery in sub-Saharan Africa: a qualitative systematic review and thematic synthesis of women's perceptions and experiences. Soc Sci Med 169:157–170

Brailey S, Luybens A, van Teijlingen E et al (2017) Women, Midwives, and a Medical Model of Maternity Care in Switzerland, International Journal of Childbirth 7(3). https://doi.org/10.1891/2156-5287.7.3.117

van den Broek N, Graham W (2009) Quality of care for maternal and newborn health: the neglected agenda. BJOG 116(suppl 1):18–21. https://doi.org/10.1111/j.1471-0528.2009.02333.x

Burrowes S, Holcombe S, Jara D et al (2017) Midwives' and patients' perspectives on disrespect and abuse during labor and delivery care in Ethiopia: a qualitative study. BMC Pregnancy Childbirth 17:263. https://bmcpregnancychildbirth.biomedcentral.com/articles/10.1186/s12884-017-1442-1. Accessed 08 Oct 2019

Clow S (2010) Out-of-hospital midwife obstetric units in the Cape Peninsula, South Africa. Paper prepared as a background document for the State of the World's Midwifery 2011. http://citeseerx.ist.psu.edu/viewdoc/download?doi=10.1.1.636.5192&rep=rep1&type=pdf. Accessed 22 May 2020

Cochrane (2016) Midwife-led continuity models of care compared with other models of care for women during pregnancy, birth and early parenting. https://www.cochrane.org/CD004667/PREG_midwife-led-continuity-models-care-compared-other-models-care-women-during-pregnancy-birth-and-early. Accessed 28 June 2019

Davis-Floyd R, Barclay L, Tritten J et al (eds) (2009) Birth models that work. University of California Press, Berkeley

Dixon L, Guilliland K, Pallant J et al (2017) The emotional wellbeing of New Zealand midwives: comparing responses for midwives in caseloading and shift work settings. N Z Coll Midwives J 53:5–14

EngenderHealth (2003) COPE handbook: a process for improved quality in health services (revised edn). http://www.engenderhealth.org/pubs/quality/cope-handbook.php. Accessed 28 June 2019

Everitt L (2016) Flexible models of care for vulnerable women. Aust Midwifery News 16(1):22–23

Every Woman Every Child (2015) Global Respectful Maternity Care Council. Every Woman Every Child. https://www.everywomaneverychild.org/commitment/global-respectful-maternity-care-council-grmcc/. Accessed 29 June 2019

Fahi K (2012) What makes a midwifery model of care safe? Women Birth Midwives 25(1):1–3

Fenwick J, Sidebotham M, Gamble J et al (2017) The emotional and professional wellbeing of Australian midwives: a comparison between those providing continuity of midwifery care and those not providing continuity. Women Birth 31(1):38–43. https://doi.org/10.1016/j.wombi.2017.06.013. Accessed 30 Aug 2019

Filippi V, Ronsmans C, Campbell O et al (2006) Maternal health in poor countries: the broader context and a call for action. Lancet 368(9546):1535–1541

Foster D, Newton M, McLachaln H et al (2011) Exploring implementation and sustainability of models of care: can theory help? BMC Public Health. 11(S5):S8

Giarratano G, Harville E, de Mendoza B et al (2015) Healthy start: description of a safety net for perinatal support during disaster recovery. Matern Child Health J 19(4):819–827. https://doi.org/10.1007/s10995-014-1579-8. Accessed 30 Aug 2019

Heredia-Pi I, Fuentes-Rivera E, Andrade Z et al (2018) The Mexican experience adapting CenteringPregnancy: lessons learned in a publicly funded health care system serving vulnerable women. J Midwifery Womens Health 63:602–610

Hillis S (2016) Global prevalence of past year violence against children: a systematic review and minimum estimates. Pediatrics 137(3):1–14. https://pediatrics.aappublications.org/content/137/3/e20154079. Accessed 29 June 2019

Homer C, Leap N, Edwards N et al (2017) Midwifery continuity of carer in an area of high socio-economic disadvantage in London: a retrospective analysis of Albany midwifery practice outcomes using routine data (1997–2009). Midwifery 48:1–10

International Confederation of Midwives (2014) Philosophy and model of midwifery care. Core document. International Confederation of Midwives, The Hague. https://www.internationalmidwives.org/assets/files/definitions-files/2018/06/eng-philosophy-and-model-of-midwifery-care.pdf. Accessed 06 July 2019

Jepson I, Mark E, Foureur M et al (2017) A qualitative study of how caseload midwifery is experienced by couples in Denmark. Women and Birth 30(1):e61–e69 https://doi.org/10.1016/j.wombi.2016.09.003 [last accessed 08/11/2020]

Jha P, Christensson K, Svanberg A et al (2016) Cashless childbirth but at a cost : a grounded theory study on quality of intrapartum care in public health facilities in India. Midwifery 39:79–86

Kildea S, Simcock G, Liu A et al (2018) Continuity of midwifery carer moderates the effects of prenatal maternal stress on postnatal maternal wellbeing: the Queensland flood study. Arch Womens Ment Health 21(2):203–214

Koblinsky M, Moyer C, Calvert C et al (2016) Quality maternity care for every woman, everywhere: a call to action. Lancet 388:2307–2320

Kruk ME (2009) Bypassing primary care facilities for childbirth: a population-based study in rural Tanzania. Health Policy Plan 24(4):279–288

MacDonald H (2009) Home birth as safe as in hospital for low risk women, study shows. BMJ. https://www.bmj.com/content/338/bmj.b1616. Accessed 11 Oct 2019

MacKenzie Bryers H, van Teijlingen E (2010) Risk, theory, social and medical models: a critical analysis of the concept of risk in maternity care. Midwifery 26(5):488–496. https://doi.org/10.1016/j.midw.2010.07.003. Epub 2010 Aug 17. PMID: 20719418.

Maternal Health Task Force (2019) Respectful maternity care. Maternal Health Task Force. Harvard Chan School Center of Excellence in Maternal and Child Health, Boston. https://www.mhtf.org/topics/respectful-maternity-care/. Accessed 29 June 2019

McInnes RJ (2018) Midwifery continuity of carer: developing a realist evaluation framework to evaluate the implementation of strategic change in Scotland. Midwifery 66:103–110

McMahon S, George A, Chebet J et al (2014) Experiences of and responses to disrespectful maternity care and abuse during childbirth; a qualitative study with women and men in Morogoro region, Tanzania. BMC Pregnancy Childbirth 14:268. https://doi.org/10.1186/1471-2393-14-268

Miller S, Lalonde A (2015) The global epidemic of disrespect and abuse during childbirth: history, evidence, interventions and FIGO's mother-baby friendly birthing facilities initiative. Int J Gynaecol Obstet 131(S1):S49–S52

Mortensen B, Lukasse M, Diep L et al (2018) Can a midwife-led continuity model improve maternal services in a low-resource setting? A non-randomised cluster intervention study in Palestine. BMJ Open. https://bmjopen.bmj.com/content/8/3/e019568. Accessed 05 Oct 2019

Musabyimana A, Lundeen T, Butrick E et al (2019) Before and after implementation of group antenatal care in Rwanda: a qualitative study of women's experiences. Reprod Health 16:90. https://doi.org/10.1186/s12978-019-0750-5. Accessed 01 Aug 2019

National Perinatal Epidemiology Unit (2017) Birthplace in England research programme. Nuffield Department of Population Health, University of Oxford. https://www.npeu.ox.ac.uk/birthplace. Accessed 03 July 2019

Ndwiga C, Warren C, Ritter J et al (2017) Exploring provider perspectives on respectful maternity care in Kenya: "work with what you have". Reprod Health 14:99. https://doi.org/10.1186/s12978-017-0364-8. https://reproductive-health-journal.biomedcentral.com/track/pdf/10.1186/s12978-017-0364-8?site=reproductive-health-journal.biomedcentral.com. Accessed 08 Oct 2019

Nove A (2015) Alongside midwifery units. AIMS J 27:4. https://www.aims.org.uk/journal/item/alongside-midwifery-units. Accessed 19 Oct 2019

Oguntunde O, Nyenwa J, Yusuf F et al (2019) The experience of men who participated in interventions to improve demand for and utilization of maternal and child health services in northern Nigeria: a qualitative comparative study. Reprod Health 16:104. https://doi.org/10.1186/s12978-019-0761-2. Accessed 01 Aug 2019

Olsen (2012) Benefits and harms of planned hospital birth compared with planned home birth for low-risk pregnant women. Cochrane database. https://www.cochrane.org/CD000352/PREG_benefits-and-harms-of-planned-hospital-birth-compared-with-planned-home-birth-for-low-risk-pregnant-women. Accessed 11 Oct 2019

Oosthuizen SJ, Bergh AM, Grimbeek J et al. (2019) Midwife-led obstetric units working 'CLEVER': Improving perinatal outcome indicators in a South African health district January 2019 South African medical journal = Suid-Afrikaanse tydskrif vir geneeskunde 109(2):95

Open University (2005) Why is childbirth a medicalised procedure? Open Learning from the Open University. https://www.open.edu/openlearn/body-mind/health/nursing/why-childbirth-medical-procedure. Accessed 03 July 2019

Page L (2003) One-to-one midwifery: restoring the "with woman" relationship in midwifery. Journal of Midwifery and Women's health. 2003;48:119–125

Perez R (2010) Obstetric violence: a new legal term introduced in Venezuela. Gynecol Obstetr 111(3):201–202

Perriman N, Davis D, Ferguson S (2018) What women value in the midwifery continuity of care model: a systematic review with meta-synthesis. Midwifery 62:220–229

Reader TW, Gillespie A (2013) Patient neglect in healthcare institutions: a systematic review and conceptual model. BMC Health Serv Res 13:156. https://doi.org/10.1186/1472-6963-13-156

Renfrew M, Mcfadden A, Bastos M et al (2014) Midwifery and quality care: findings from a new evidence informed framework for maternal and newborn care. Lancet Midwifery Ser 384:1129–1145

Rivaldi C, Skoko E, Battisti A et al (2018) Abuse and disrespect in childbirth assistance in Italy, a community based survey. Eur J Obstet Gynecol Reprod Biol 224:208–209

Robertson B, Ayckock D, Darnell LA (2009) Comparison of centering pregnancy to traditional care in Hispanic mothers. Matern Child Health J 13(3):407–414

Sacks E (2017) Defining disrespect and abuse of newborns: a review of the evidence and an expanded typology of respectful maternity care. Reprod Health 14:66. https://doi.org/10.1186/s12978-017-0326-1

Sandall J (1997) Midwives' burnout and continuity of care. BJOM. Published Online:20 Feb 2014 https://doi.org/10.12968/bjom.1997.5.2.106

Sandall J, Devane D, Soltani H et al (2016) Midwife-led continuity models versus other models of care for childbearing women. Cochrane Database Syst Rev (4):CD004667

Sayinzoga F, Lundeen T, Gakwerere M et al (2018) Use of a facilitated group process to design and implement a group antenatal and postnatal care program in Rwanda. J Midwifery Womens Health 63:593–601

Shimpuku Y, Madeni FE, Horiuchi S et al (2019) A family-oriented antenatal education program to improve birth preparedness and maternal-infant birth outcomes: a cross sectional evaluation study. Reprod Health 16:107. https://doi.org/10.1186/s12978-019-0776-8. Accessed 01 Aug 2019

Smith C, Brown JB, Stewart M et al (2009) Ontario care providers' considerations regarding models of maternity care. J Obstet Gynaecol Can 31(5):401–408

Swahnberg K, Thapar-Björkert S, Berterö C (2007) Nullified: Women's perceptions of being abused in health care. J Psychosom Obstet Gynecol 28(3):161–167

Tidy C (2016) Safeguarding adults. Professional articles. https://patient.info/doctor/safeguarding-adults-pro#ref-1. Accessed 26 June 2019

Tracy SK, Welsh A, Hall B et al (2013) Caseload midwifery care versus standard maternity care for women of any risk: M@NGO, a randomised controlled trial. Lancet 382(9906):1723–1732

Trudnak TE, Arboleda E, Russell SK et al (2013) Outcomes of Latina women in CenteringPregnancy group prenatal care compared with individual prenatal care. J Midwifery Womens Health 58(4):396–403

United Kingdom Midwifery Study System (2017) UK Midwifery Study System. Nuffield Dept Population of Health, University of Oxford https://www.npeu.ox.ac.uk/research/ukmidss-320. Accessed 14 Oct 2019

United Nations (2015) Transforming our world: the 2030 agenda for sustainable development. United Nations general assembly; seventieth session, New York, 18 Sept

United Nations AIDS (2000) HIV and AIDS-related stigmatization, discrimination, and denial: forms, contexts, and determinants. Research studies from Uganda and India

United Nations Population Fund (2014) International conference on population and development. United Nations Population Fund. http://www.unfpa.org/icpd. Accessed 28 June 2019

Uys K, Thapar-Björkert S & Berterö,C (2007) Nullified: Women's perceptions of being abused in health care, Journal of Psychosomatic Obstetrics & Gynecology 28(3):161–167.

Uys L, Chirwa M, Kohi T et al (2009) Evaluation of a health setting-based stigma intervention in five African countries. AIDS Patient Care STDs 23(12):1059–1066

Vedam S, Stoll K, Taiwo TK et al (2019) The Giving Voice to Mothers study: inequity and mistreatment during pregnancy and childbirth in the United States. Reprod Health 16:77. https://reproductive-health-journal.biomedcentral.com/articles/10.1186/s12978-019-0729-2. Accessed 01 Aug 2019

Warren C (2003) Exploring the value of midwifery continuity of carer. Br J Midwifery 3(11):S34–S37

Webber G, Chirangi G, Magatti N (2018) Promoting respectful maternity care in rural Tanzania: nurses' experiences of the "health Workers for Change" program. BMC Health Serv Res 18:658. Accessed 08 Oct 2019

White Ribbon Alliance (2011) Respectful maternity care. White Ribbon Alliance. http://www.safemotherhood-forall.org.au/position-statements/respectful-maternity/. Accessed 28 June 2019

World Bank (2019) Gender based violence (violence against women and girls. https://www.worldbank.org/en/topic/socialdevelopment/brief/violence-against-women-and-girls. Accessed 29 June 2019

World Health Organization (2015a) WHO statement on caesarean section rates. WHO/RHR/15.02. https://www.who.int/reproductivehealth/publications/maternal_perinatal_health/cs-statement/en/. Accessed 06 July 2019

World Health Organization (2015b) The prevention and elimination of disrespect and abuse in facility based childbirth, World Health Organization Statement. https://apps.who.int/iris/bitstream/handle/10665/134588/WHO_RHR_14.23_eng.pdf;jsessionid=745EB6115879B05BE913341F4707C987?sequence=1. Accessed 27 June 2019

World Health Organization (2016) WHO recommendations on antenatal care for a positive pregnancy experience. World Health Organization, Geneva. https://apps.who.int/iris/bitstream/handle/10665/250800/WHO-RHR-16.12-eng.pdf;jsessionid=0D0744BF286494D60F9FC1EC4E3B92DB?sequence=1. Accessed 07 Oct 2019

World Health Organization (2017) Elder abuse: fact sheet: World Health Organization. https://www.who.int/news-room/fact-sheets/detail/elder-abuse. Accessed 26 June 2019

World Health Organization (2018) Definition of skilled health personnel providing care during childbirth: the 2018 joint statement by WHO, UNFPA, UNICEF, ICM, ICN, FIGO and IPA. Department of Reproductive Health, World Health Organization, Geneva

World Health Organization (2019a) The case for midwifery. World Health Organization, Geneva. https://www.who.int/maternal_child_adolescent/topics/quality-of-care/midwifery/case-for-midwifery/en/. Accessed 05 Oct 2018

World Health Organization (2019b) Child maltreatment (child abuse) violence and injury prevention. World Health Organization. https://www.who.int/violence_injury_prevention/violence/child/en/. Accessed 26 June 2019

Midwifery and Quality of Care in Different Settings

8

Expected Learning Outcomes

By the end of the chapter, the reader should be able to:

1. Discuss the importance of quality care and identify the barriers that impede its acquisition in midwifery practice
2. Consider the key factors that facilitate quality care
3. Discuss the relevance of evidence-based care in midwifery in aspiring towards quality care
4. Explore available resources and approaches for providing AAAQ (availability, accessibility, acceptability and quality)
5. Consider the differing nomenclature in use which describes midwifery care providers across countries and how these can impact on the quality of care
6. Examine quality as it is perceived by women and their families

8.1 Introduction

It has been recognised that 'Quality of care is essential for further progress in reducing maternal and newborn deaths'. Furthermore, it is accepted that 'The integration of educated, trained, regulated and licensed midwives into the health system is associated with improved quality of care and sustained decreases in maternal and newborn mortality' (Filby et al. 2016:1). Evidence-based care has become the expected norm in modern midwifery practice, and this is explored more extensively in Chapter 12 within the framework of midwifery research. However, in the context of providing quality care, reliance on constantly updated evidence needs to form the foundation of midwifery policy and practice. Only within such an environment can safe childbirth be promoted and death and disability become rarities across the world. Factors that facilitate quality care have been identified, but barriers to its provision also abound and both these are discussed below. The situation is further complicated by the various cadres of staff who provide maternity care. In addition to midwives, there are several categories of healthcare workers who inevitably vary in their level of education and skills. This issue has been discussed in Chapter 2, and the cadres are itemised in Fig. 2.4. This issue inevitably makes a significant impact on the matter of quality.

© Springer Nature Switzerland AG 2021
J. Kemp et al., *Global Midwifery: Principles, Policy and Practice*,
https://doi.org/10.1007/978-3-030-46765-4_8

8.2   The Barriers and Facilitators to Quality Care

In an extensive systematic analysis carried out on behalf of the World Health Organization (WHO) and cited above Filby et al. (2016), numerous barriers have been identified that impede the provision of quality care and a significant proportion of these relate to the status and situation of the midwife. In Bangladesh, a recent study has provided specific examples of these social, professional and economic barriers preventing the provision of quality midwifery care. It was established that in that country social barriers were shaped by beliefs associated with religion, society, and gender norms placing midwives in 'a vulnerable situation facing cultural prejudice' (Bogren and Erlandsson 2018:3). But professional barriers also existed including heavy workloads, staff shortages and staff not being utilised to their full capacity within the health system. Professional barriers stemmed from a lack of recognition in the medical hierarchy which resulted in midwives having low levels of autonomy. Economic barriers were evident in lack of supplies and shortage of hospital beds, midwives being on low and/or irregular salaries, and a deficiency in opportunities for recreation. Personal insecurity presented another issue and was associated with lack of housing and transportation. (Bogren and Erlandsson 2018). These barriers are by no means unique to Bangladesh as the WHO study has revealed, such barriers are evident in numerous low- and middle-income countries (LIMCs) across the world (Graham and Varghese 2012; Filby et al. 2016). Copious examples which have become evident in recent decades still exist across the globe. Lack of education and training has been identified as a major barrier to safe midwifery practice and quality care. In a study in a district hospital in Uganda, training in immediate care of the newborn and infection prevention was deemed deficient, just two-thirds of midwives had any training in essential obstetric care and only a third were able to document and interpret a partograph (Kaye 2000). Nurse-midwives in Malawi reported hesitance in resuscitating babies because of their lack of training and paediatric support (Bream et al. 2005). It was established that in Nepal none of the training programmes for skilled birth attendants incorporated the International Confederation of Midwives (ICM) essential competencies (Kc and Bajracharya 2013) and that in Pakistan it was possible to graduate from a midwifery programme having experienced only rote learning (Gibson 2000). More recently, in Pakistan, a midwifery coaching programme has proved helpful in enhancing clinical skills, and a community midwifery training extended to 18 months in 2008 was subsequently extended to 2 years by 2018 (UNFPA 2017).

Working conditions and staff shortages contribute to hazardous experiences in a number of countries. Although the number of births increased by 500% over a 6-year period in a Ghanaian hospital, no further midwifery staff were employed, so that four midwives were responsible for up to 1200 births a month and around 50 in 24-hour periods (Floyd 2013). In Malawian hospitals, midwives frequently worked long hours overtime and were rarely remunerated for this (Thorsen et al. 2011). Community-based midwives have also been discovered to carry unrealistic workloads. For example, midwives in Indonesia may need to serve up to five villages, often some considerable distances apart (D'Ambruoso et al. 2009), and a lone community midwife in the Philippines could be on call for a population of up to 30,000 whilst also taking responsibility for up to 40 Department of Health initiatives (de la Gente 2008). Examples of social barriers can be drawn from various corners of the globe. Evidence from Afghanistan and Zimbabwe describes assisting women in childbirth as low skilled and 'women's work' (Currie et al. 2007, Fauveau et al. 2008) whilst in Pakistan midwives were considered to be uneducated and of doubtful moral character (Gibson 2000). Promoting evidence-based care in some cultural settings obviously presents challenges, and 70% of Ghanaian women are reported to ignore professional advice in favour of traditional practices such as umbilical cord care (Moyer et al. 2012). Midwives in Mozambique had problems implementing early skin to skin care because of cultural attitudes towards body fluids (Pettersson et al. 2006, Pettersson 2007) and encouraging early feeding with colostrum presents problems across much of South Asia and in other continents too in spite of the research evidence emphasising the value of this (Blum et al. 2006).

Decades ago, the 'three delays model of care' was presented to illustrate some of the barriers that women faced in attempting to receive maternity care. The third level of delay focused on a lack of quality care even when women had overcome the first two hurdles of delay, namely in seeking care and then delay in reaching care (Thaddeus and Maine 1994). The world has been slow in grasping the significance of sub-standard care and the death sentence which the absence of quality maternity care spells for millions of women in many countries.

Different models of maternity care have been discussed in Chapter 7. In a global systematic analysis exploring factors that facilitated quality care, approaches that provided integrated care (Allen et al. 2009), continuity of care (Butler et al. 2011) and comprehensive care (Cohen et al. 2011) were, in general terms, found to impact positively on the health system goals (Nair et al. 2014). This metareview which studied 98 systematic reviews with 110 interventions designed to improve the quality of care identified key barriers and key facilitators in the context of quality care provision for maternal, newborn and child health (MNCH), and these are summarised in Boxes 8.1 and 8.2.

Box 8.1. Barriers to quality MNCH care

- Language barriers in information and communication
- Power difference between users and providers
- Health systems not accounting for user satisfaction
- Variable standards of implementation of standard guidelines
- Shortage of resources in health facilities
- Lack of studies assessing the role of leadership in improving QoC

Derived from Nair et al. (2014)

Box 8.2. Facilitators to quality MNCH care

- Active and regular interpersonal communication between users and providers
- Respect, confidentiality, comfort and support during care provision
- Engaging users in decision-making
- Continuity of care
- Effective audit and feedback mechanisms

Derived from Nair et al. (2014)

The issue of disrespect and abuse and the importance of respectful maternity care are discussed in some detail in Chapter 7, and the facilitating factors identified by Nair et al. (2014) and cited above serve to underline this as an indispensable component in promoting quality care.

Chapter 14 considers issues that will confront professionals and students in traversing international borders. In this context, a 'quality gap' has been identified (Maclean 1998, 2013), and the factors contributing to it are specified in Fig. 14.3. This gap which illustrates the enormous divide which exists between the health services and particularly the Sexual, Reproductive, Maternal and Neonatal Health (SRMNH) services between nations must be eliminated if the lives of women and babies are to be saved from every avoidable cause. WHO has emphasised that quality plays an important part in ensuring universal health coverage so that 'all people obtain the good-quality essential health services that they need without enduring financial hardship' (WHO 2017).

8.3   AAAQ: And All That!

WHO has stated that effective health services coverage should encompass four domains that have been specified as availability, accessibility, acceptability and quality of care (AAAQ) (WHO 2017). These have been defined and extensively explored by the international community in

AVAILABILITY	ACCESSIBILITY	ACCEPTABILITY	QUALITY
Need to have sufficient quantity of functioning public health and health-care facilities, goods and services, and programmes	Health facilities, goods, and services have to be accessible (physically accessible, affordable, and accessible information) to everyone within the jurisdiction of the State party without discrimination	The social and cultural distance between health systems and their users determine acceptability. All health facilities, goods, and services must be respectful of medical ethics and culturally appropriate, sensitive to gender and age. Also designed to respect confidentiality and improve the health status of those concerned	Health facilities, goods, and services must be scientifically and medically approved and of good quality

Fig. 8.1 The AAAQ Framework. (Derived from WHO 2016a)

examining midwifery across the globe (UNFPA 2014). The AAAQ Framework is displayed in Fig. 8.1.

Availability relates to both midwifery services and the midwifery workforce. This must be measured by full-time equivalents rather than a headcount, and numerous other issues need to be taken into account such as the proportion of time spent in providing SRMNH services, age, distribution of staff and attrition. In order to achieve the required workforce, it is stressed that this encompasses active management of midwifery education which 'involves ensuring that the number of training places available, in both the private and the public sectors, is sufficient and of high enough quality to meet future needs, taking into account student selection and attrition' (UNFPA 2014:16). Since 78% of midwifery and medical education programmes in the study perceived it a challenge to recruit candidates with a suitable educational background, this presents a continuing global dilemma. As discussed above, midwifery is not perceived as a respected and well-paid profession in many countries, and this matter needs addressing in any area aiming to meet the first dimension of the AAAQ framework. The other issue is a maldistribution of healthcare providers. In a workshop convened to

consider the implications of this framework and attended by participants from 36 LIMCs, it was considered that availability of care was hampered by having inadequate numbers of relevant workers in the workforce. This was partly attributed to insufficient numbers being educated, but in a number of countries, there was a lack of efficient and timely deployment of staff once they were trained. Three countries stated that workers refused to report to their appointed place of duty because of political or personal reasons including fears for their personal security (Homer et al. 2018).

In order to improve recruitment into midwifery, the White Ribbon Alliance for Safe Motherhood in Tanzania established a campaign entitled 'Increasing Women's Access to Healthcare through Promotion of Midwifery as a Career in Tanzania'. This has been aimed at secondary school students, their parents, politicians and the community (Windau-Melmer 2010). Progress has been made in some countries through media and advocacy, for instance by creating awards that recognise the work of midwives and the importance of maternal and newborn health. The African Union's Mama Afrika award is an example of this strategy (CARMMA/ African Union 2013). Cambodian midwives have been officially recognised as providing the key to reducing maternal and newborn deaths. Midwives have received a larger pay increase than other health personnel with a similar professional education, and as an incentive, they are financially rewarded for births conducted at public health facilities. Midwives receive priority when the Government of Cambodia recruits civil servants for the Ministry of Health (UNFPA 2014).

Accessibility is the second dimension referring to accessibility to health services and specifically to the midwifery workforce. However, even if 'there are enough health workers, adequately remunerated and with the competencies to provide the continuum of care that women and newborns need, accessing the care that they provide remains a problem in many countries' (UNFPA 2014:16). Furthermore, women need to be active decision-makers in choosing to access the midwifery workforce and services and be able to afford them. Gender discrimination can often deny them of this right with the crisis accentuated in case of emergency. Countries have been urged to develop a 'minimum guaranteed benefits package' for SRMNH. This is defined as 'a set of health services that the government has committed itself to making available to all, free at the point of access'. Further, it is emphasised that 'Equity-focused approaches will be required that target the poorest, if both aggregate and equity goals for SRMNH coverage are to be achieved in the future'. Although 70 of the 73 countries participating in the State of the World's Midwifery study possessed a minimum guaranteed benefits package, it is reckoned that there remain gaps in what are considered essential interventions and that 'many countries will face significant challenges to ensure universal coverage, especially for the poorest 40%' (UNFPA 2014:21).

Midwives' Associations have played an important part in addressing some of the issues relating to accessibility. For example, in Togo, the Midwives' Association coordinated national workshops. These activities generated data which helped to strengthen relationships between the Midwives' Association, the Ministry of Health, UNFPA and WHO. Another Midwives'

Association in Afghanistan organised two stakeholder workshops. They collected data, validating them and prompting policy discussion. From this exercise, plans emerged to disseminate vital information via the media and establish roundtable policy discussions (UNFPA 2014).

Acceptability is the third dimension in this context. It is evident that even if midwifery care is both available and accessible, effective coverage will be limited if the care offered or the midwifery workforce itself is unacceptable to women, their families and their communities. Acceptability of maternal and newborn health services has been strongly associated with discrimination against women. Although an increasing percentage of women have been giving birth in health facilities in recent years where there are professional healthcare workers, because of the absence of respectful care, this discourages women accessing the service (UNFPA 2014). The matter of respectful maternity care has been discussed in Chapter 7 and cannot be overestimated in its relevance to the uptake of care. Acceptable care demands that all health facilities, goods and services should be respectful. This includes medical ethics and culturally appropriate approaches respecting women whatever their age, culture or status (WHO 2010; UNFPA 2014). Efforts to improve respectful care worldwide are being encouraged by the White Ribbon Alliance (WRA) and partnerships established for this purpose. Cooperation between Zimbabwe and a maternity unit in Wales is believed to be having an impact, and there is hope that such a scheme can be extended across sub-Saharan Africa (WRA 2018a). From its global base, WRA followed the lead of WRA India in launching a multi-country 'What Women Want' campaign. This involved 356 partners and aimed to extend and reinforce the necessity to enable women's and girls' voices to be heard and help create global and national health agendas which are based on priorities specified by women and girls (WRA 2018b). In Bangladesh, a new partnership between the WRA and the Bangladesh Midwifery Society has been established in an effort to emphasise the need for respectful maternity care. The 'What Women Want' campaign has resulted in engaging other healthcare leaders in the efforts and influential media channels also (WRA 2018b).

Quality of care provides the fourth dimension in this context. If the midwifery workforce proves to be available, accessible and acceptable, poor-quality care can markedly limit the possibility of women receiving effective care. There is evidence that even where 100% institutional care is provided for birthing, maternal mortality levels sometimes remain high when the quality of care is deficient (WHO 2014). Quality of care is multifaceted and includes staffing levels, resources and the working environment. The quality of the health services refers to the 'Dimension of the right to health, which requires that health facilities, goods and services must be scientifically and medically appropriate and of good quality' (Ki-moon 2013).

The quality of the health workforce embraces 'The competencies, skills, knowledge and behaviour of the health worker assessed according to professional norms and as perceived by users' (WHO 2011). The WRA Global Secretariat has helped in embedding quality, equity and dignity in health services as one of six priority pillars of the 'Every Woman Every Child Global Strategy for Women's, Children's and Adolescents' Health' (UN 2015; WRA 2018b). The Quality Maternal and Newborn Care Framework is presented in Chapter 3: Annex 3.3. This clearly and succinctly presents the characteristics of care that comprise the essence of quality care for the woman and her newborn.

It has been stressed that high-quality education along with continuing professional development and clear career pathways are vital in addressing several challenges presented by the AAAQ framework. This particularly applies to the provision of quality care which is urgently needed to promote and ensure both accessibility and acceptability (WHO 2016b). WRA Indonesia gained the President's endorsement of the 'What Women Want' campaign. This has demonstrated the importance of linking the power of realising women's and girls' health demands with improved health outcomes. Whilst WRA Kenya has ensured that through its Ministry of Health, the country has become part of the Quality of Care Network and acquired the approval of quality of care standards (WRA 2018b).

8.4   Perceptions of Women and Families

Undoubtedly, the ultimate test of quality is how it is perceived by the consumers or clientele. The issues of respect as well as skilled care keep recurring in ascertaining the views of those who use the maternity services. Researchers evaluating the maternity care experiences of 701 women in both private and public facilities in the central hills district of Nepal conclude that the woman's assessment of quality is critical. They stress that emotional support, attention to cultural needs and respectful care are vital during labour and birth (Karkee et al. 2014).

In a National Health Service (NHS) study involving more than 18,000 women across England, their level of satisfaction showed some improvement from previous studies. In this context, the examination of women's perceptions of care was deemed important because 'The quality of the care women receive during this life-changing period will influence not only the health of mother and child, but also their interactions with health services throughout the rest of their lives' (NHS 2018:3). In 2016, the National Maternity Review presented a 5-year forward plan to promote 'better births'. This was designed in line with the guidelines set out by the National Institute for Clinical Excellence (NICE) (The National Maternity Review 2016). This review proposed 'a reform of the nature of maternity care provision, with an emphasis on the importance of achieving a series of "shared goals" that are central to quality care standards (NHS 2018:9).

In a cross-sectional national study involving 2400 women undertaken in the United States of America, it was emphasised that high-quality communication and a positive patient–provider relationship were considered to be aspects of patient-centred care. It was stressed that these are crucial elements in the provision of quality care. It is reported that more than 40% of women experienced communication problems in receiving antenatal care; furthermore, 24% perceived discrimination whilst they were in hospital giving birth. Women who suffered hypertension or diabetes were much more reluctant to ask questions.

Black and Hispanic women by comparison with white women perceived discrimination relating to their race or ethnicity (Attanasio and Kozhimannil 2015).

In an extensive study in India involving more than a thousand women, the respondents perceived the need for more sensitivity in care during childbirth as well as addressing the needs of those who provide the care. The incidence of Fear of Birth (FoB) as well as depressive symptoms were found to be associated with the quality of care received during childbirth. These issues also related to the type of facility where the birth took place; the primary care providers and the mode of delivery as well as the services received. Women considered that labour wards were functional. However, they thought that for women giving birth interpersonal processes comprising information-sharing along with sensitive treatment urgently needed improvement. It also emerged that women were anxious about operative procedures and for those who had undergone an emergency caesarean section, this was closely associated with FoB. The study recommended that in order to improve quality of care, future healthcare reforms should aim to improve interpersonal relationships and implement evidence-based care in labour rooms (Jha 2017). A correlational study in Swaziland with 383 women participants who had given birth in two regional hospitals showed that there was suboptimal satisfaction with the quality of intrapartum care practices. It is recommended that improvement should focus on woman-centred evidence-based intrapartum care that involves clients in decision-making. It was also proposed that there should be a comprehensive education programme for pregnant women (Gamedze-Mshayisa et al. 2018). Woman-centred care has long been recognised as an important approach in examining the satisfaction of women in England. In the context of examining team midwifery, it was noted that the midwife–woman relationship was an important aspect of satisfaction perceived by women and that this needs greater recognition (Tinker and Quinney 1998).

In Malawi, an extensive study was undertaken across six districts involving 58 women who had experienced maternity care at various facilities. The study indicated that the majority of women were satisfied with the quality of the maternity services that provided antenatal care. However, it was established that those who were accompanied by their spouses found that the quality of care they received was more acceptable than that experienced by others, for example those who were escorted by a female relative. Nevertheless, most of the respondents were not satisfied with the quality of services received during labour, birth and postnatally. There were reports of women being shouted at by healthcare providers and that they were not treated with the respect they had anticipated. The study also established that women delayed accessing and utilising maternal health services. Although this was related in part to cultural beliefs including the fear of being bewitched, it also related to the poor-quality maternity care that was available to them. It is suggested that in order to improve the uptake of care, it is necessary to promote and initiate partners' involvement. This is advocated if an effective quality of care is to be provided in most maternal health care facilities across the country. It is acknowledged that most women report not being treated with respect when they are seeking quality care. This factor encourages the use of high-risk care outside of the health facilities. It is recommended that service quality audit checks should be implemented periodically in order to monitor standards and assess quality. In addition, promoting community-based reproductive health education advocacy with male involvement in maternal healthcare services was advocated. It is considered that there is a need to promote understanding about some cultural beliefs; it is also considered important that health care providers receive continuing education. It is believed that this will offer a long-term 'positive perspective on the quality of maternal health care delivery and will subsequently promote use of the services' (Machira and Palamuleni 2018:34). The recurrent themes resulting in recommendations that emerge from the evidence and suggesting approaches to improving the quality of care from the woman's perspective are summarised in Fig. 8.2.

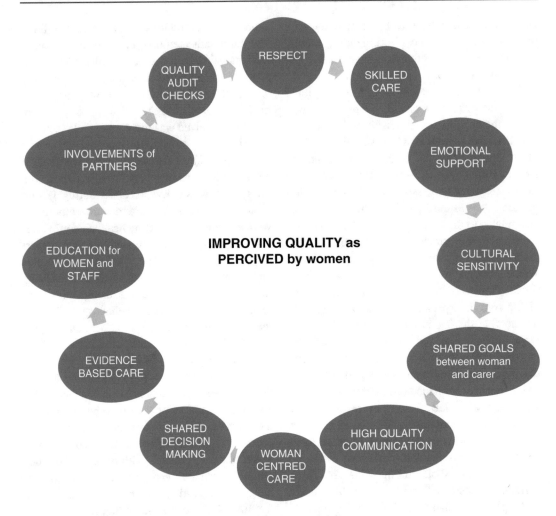

Fig. 8.2 Recommendations for improving quality: women's perspectives

Key Messages

Principles

The principle of quality care for all needs to be embedded in SRMNH care provision at every level.

Policy

In order to ensure quality care, national, local and institutional policies should uphold the principles contained in the AAAQ Framework.

Practice

Midwifery practice should be evidence based, skilled and respectful so that women, their families and their communities find it acceptable.

Questions for Reflection or Review

1. Consider the Midwifery Services Framework (see Fig. 2 in Nove et al. 2018) cited below. Compare this with the AAAQ Framework (Fig. 8.1 and reflect on whether these may both contribute to universal coverage and quality care.

2. Examine the recommendations for improving quality from women's perspectives summarised in Fig. 8.2. Consider how these may be included in an audit tool to monitor acceptability and quality of care.

Additional Resources for Reflection and Further Study

Consider the AAAQ Framework detailed at: https://www.who.int/gender-equity-rights/knowledge/AAAQ.pdf?ua=1. How does this reflect the situation in a country/institution/area with which you are familiar?

Nove A, ten Hoope-Bender P, Moyo NT et al (2018) The Midwifery services framework: what is it, and why is it needed? Midwifery 57:54–58. https://doi.org/10.1016/j.midw.2017.11.003. Accessed 03 March 2020

United Nations Population Fund (2014) State of the world's midwifery: a universal pathway to women's health. A United Nations publication. Keep alert for any updated versions

World Health Organisation (2017) Optimizing the contributions of the nursing and midwifery workforce to achieve universal health coverage and the sustainable development goals through education, research and practice. Human Resources for Health Observer Series 22. World Health Organization, Geneva

References

Allen D, Gillen E, Rixson L (2009) Systematic review of the effectiveness of integrated care pathways: what works, for whom, in which circumstances? Int J Evid Based Healthcare 7:61–74

Attanasio L, Kozhimannil KB (2015) Patient-reported communication quality and perceived discrimination in maternity care. Med Care 53(10):863–871. https://doi.org/10.1097/MLR.0000000000000411

Blum LS, Sharmin T, Ronsmans C (2006) Attending home vs. clinic-based deliveries: perspectives of skilled birth attendants in Matlab, Bangladesh. Reprod Health Matters 14(27):51–60. PMID: 16713879

Bogren M, Erlandsson K (2018) What prevents midwifery quality care in Bangladesh? A focus group enquiry with midwifery students. BMC Health Serv Res 18(1):639. https://doi.org/10.1186/s12913-018-3447-5

Bream KD, Gennaro S, Mbweza E et al (2005) Barriers to and facilitators for newborn resuscitation in Malawi, Africa. J Midwifery Womens Health 50(4):329–334. PMID: 15973271

Butler M, Collins R, Drennan J et al (2011) Hospital nurse staffing models and patient and staff-related outcomes. Cochrane Database Syst Rev 7:CD007019

CARMMA/African Union (2013) The Mama Afrika Award. Advocay International. https://www.advocacyinternational.co.uk/featured-project/carmma. Accessed 28 Feb 2020

Cohen E, Jovcevska V, Kuo DZ et al (2011) Hospital-based comprehensive care programs for children with special health care needs: a systematic review. Arch Pediatr Adolesc Med 165:554–561

Currie S, Azfar P, Fowler RC (2007) A bold new beginning for midwifery in Afghanistan. Midwifery 23:226–234. PMID: 17707765

D'Ambruoso L, AAchadi E, Adisasmita A et al (2009) Assessing quality of care provided by Indonesian village midwives with a confidential enquiry. Midwifery 25(5):528–539

Fauveau V, Sherratt D, de Bernis L (2008) Human resources for maternal health: multi-purpose or specialists? Hum Resour Health 6:21. https://doi.org/10.1186/1478-4491-6-21. PMID: 18826600

Filby A, McConville F, Portela A (2016) What prevents quality Midwifery care? A systematic mapping of barriers in low and middle income countries from the provider perspective. PLoS One 11(5):e0153391. https://doi.org/10.1371/journal.pone.0153391. Published online 2016 May 2. https://www.ncbi.nlm.nih.gov/pmc/articles/PMC4852911/. Accessed 19 Feb 2020

Floyd L (2013) Helping midwives in Ghana to reduce maternal mortality. Afr J Midwifery Womens Health 7(1):34–38

Gamedze-Mshayisa DI et al (2018) Factors associated with women's perception of and satisfaction with quality of intrapartum care practices in Swaziland. Midwifery 57:32–38. https://doi.org/10.1016/j.midw.2017.10.016

de la Gente A (2008) Midwifery in the Philippines: 'a laudable service' but there are issues and challenges. Int Midwifery 4:21–23

Gibson H (2000) Training midwives in inner-city Karachi, Pakistan. Br J Midwifery 8(6):374–378

Graham WJ, Varghese B (2012) Quality, quality, quality: gaps in the continuum of care. Lancet 379(9811):PE5–PE6

Homer CSE, Castro-Lopes S, Nove A et al (2018) Barriers to and strategies for addressing the availability, accessibility, acceptability and quality of the sexual, reproductive, maternal, newborn and adolescent health workforce: addressing the post-2015 agenda. BMC Pregnancy Childbirth 18:55. https://doi.org/10.1186/s12884-018-1686-4. Accessed 26 March 2020

Jha P (2017) Two sides of a coin: quality of childbirth services provided in Indian public health facilities from the perspectives of women and their care providers. PhD thesis. Digital comprehensive summaries of Uppsala dissertations from the Faculty of Medicine 1384

Karkee R, Lee AH, Pokharel PK (2014) Women's perception of quality of maternity services: a longitudinal survey in Nepal. BMC Pregnancy Childbirth 14:45. https://doi.org/10.1186/1471-2393-14-45. https://bmcpregnancychildbirth.biomedcentral.com/articles/10.1186/1471-2393-14-45. Accessed 24 Feb 2020

Kaye D (2000) Quality of midwifery care in Soroti district, Uganda. East Afr Med J 77(10):558–561. PMID: 12862125

Kc A, Bajracharya K (2013) State of midwives in Nepal: HRH to improve maternal and neonatal health and survival. J Nepal Health Res Counc 11(23):98–101. PMID: 23787538

Ki-moon B (2013) A life of dignity for all: accelerating progress towards the MDGs and advancing the UN development agenda beyond 2015. Report of the Secretary-General. (A/68/202). United Nations, New York

Machira K, Palamuleni M (2018) Women's perspectives on quality of maternal health care services in Malawi. Int J Womens Health 10:25–34. https://doi.org/10.2147/IJWH.S144426

Maclean GD (1998) An examination of the characteristics of short-term international midwifery consultants. PhD Thesis, University of Surrey, Guildford

Maclean GD (2013) Electives and international midwifery consultancy: a resource for students, midwives and other health professionals, Tiger Stripes and Tears. Quay Books, London

Moyer C, Aborigo RA, Logonia G et al (2012) Clean delivery practices in rural northern Ghana: a qualitative study of community and provider knowledge, attitudes, and beliefs. BMC Pregnancy Childbirth 12:50. https://doi.org/10.1186/1471-2393-12-50.   PMID: 22703032

Nair M, Yoshida S, Lambrechts T et al (2014) Facilitators and barriers to quality of care in maternal, newborn and child health: a global situational analysis through metareview. BMJ Open 4:e004749. https://doi.org/10.1136/bmjopen-2013-004749

National Health Service (2018) 2017 survey of women's experiences of maternity care. Statistical release. NHS Care Quality Commission. https://www.cqc.org.uk/sites/default/files/20180130_mat17_statisticalrelease.pdf. Accessed 24 Feb 2020

Pettersson KO (2007) Major challenges of midwifery in Africa. Br J Midwifery 15(8):470–474

Pettersson KO, Johnson E, Pelembe Mde F et al (2006) Mozambican midwives' views on barriers to quality perinatal care. Health Care Women Int 27(2):145–168

Thaddeus S, Maine D (1994) Too far to walk: maternal mortality in context. Soc Sci Med 38:1091–1110. PMID: 8042057

The National Maternity Review (2016) Better births - improving outcomes of maternity services in England: a five year forward view for maternity care. https://www.england.nhs.uk/mat-transformation/mat-review/. Accessed 24 Feb 2020

Thorsen VC, Teten Tharp AL, Meguid T (2011) High rates of burnout among maternal health staff at a referral hospital in Malawi. BMC Nurs 23:9. https://doi.org/10.1186/1472-6955-10-9

Tinker A, Quinney D (1998) Team midwifery: the influence of the midwife-woman relationship on women's experiences and perceptions of maternity care. J Adv Nurs 28(1):30–35

United Nations (2015) Every woman every child: global strategy for women's, children's and adolescent's health. survive, thrive, transform (2016-2030). https://www.who.int/life-course/partners/global-strategy/ewec-globalstrategyreport-200915.pdf?ua=1. Accessed 02 March 2020

United Nations Population Fund (2014) State of the world's midwifery: a universal pathway to women's health. A United Nations publication

United Nations Population Fund (2017) In Pakistan, empowering midwives to empower women. News. https://www.unfpa.org/news/pakistan-empowering-midwives-empower-women. Accessed 14 March 2020

White Ribbon Alliance (2018a) The White Ribbon Alliance News 11 March: Swansea midwives help Zimbabwian   mums-to-be.   https://www.whiteribbonalliance.org/2018/03/11/swansea-midwives-help-zimbabwean-mums-to-be/. Accessed 02 March 2019

White Ribbon Alliance (2018b) White Ribbon Alliance year in review 2018. https://www.whiteribbonalliance.org/2019/01/17/white-ribbon-alliances-2018-year-in-review/. Accessed 02 March 2020

Windau-Melmer T (2010) Advocacy approaches to promote midwives and the profession of midwifery: brief. Health Policy Project, Washington, DC

World Health Organization (2010) Global recommendations for the retention of health workers. World Health Organization, Geneva

World Health Organization (2011) Resolution WHA64.9. Sustainable health financing structures and universal coverage. In: Sixty-fourth World Health Assembly, Geneva, 24 May 2011. World Health Organization, Geneva

World Health Organization (2014) Targets and strategies for ending preventable maternal mortality. Consensus statement of the Bangkok Consultation on Targets and Strategies for Ending Preventable Maternal Mortality (EPMM) WHO, UNFPA, USAID, MHTF, MCHIP, EPMM Working Group

World Health Organization (2016a) Availability, accessibility, acceptability, quality infographic. https://www.who.int/gender-equity-rights/knowledge/aaaq-infographic/en/. Accessed 03 March 2020

World Health Organization (2016b) Standards for improving quality of maternal and newborn care in health facilities. World Health Organization, Geneva

World Health Organization (2017) Optimizing the contributions of the nursing and midwifery workforce to achieve universal health coverage and the sustainable development goals through education, research and practice. Human Resources for Health Observer series 22. World Health Organization, Geneva

Innovations for Strengthening Global Midwifery

9

Expected Learning Outcomes

By the end of the chapter, the reader should be able to:

1. Describe some key concepts in the field of global health innovation.
2. Cite some examples of innovations in midwifery education and midwifery practice and interprofessional working.
3. Outline the process of developing, implementing and evaluating a midwifery innovation.
4. Discuss the enablers and barriers for innovations in midwifery.
5. Suggest some strategies to develop future innovations in midwifery.

9.1   What Is Health Innovation?

The Cambridge Dictionary (2020) defines innovation as 'the use of a new idea or method', whereas health innovation is 'the development or delivery of new or improved health policies, systems, products and technologies, services and delivery methods that improve people's health' (WHO 2020a). Defining features of health innovations are that they respond to unmet needs by employing new ways of thinking and working, and they add value in the form of improved efficiency, effectiveness, quality, safety and/or affordability.

Health innovation falls under the broader umbrella of social innovation which encourages new approaches to tackle issues surrounding poverty, education, health, and other human development problems by making system-level changes (Kimble and Massoud 2016). Innovations to strengthen global midwifery are, of course, health innovations. However, they are broader than this as midwifery follows a holistic model (Yanti et al. 2015; ICM 2014) drawing on social science, psychology and other disciplines. Krubiner et al. (2016) suggest that health innovations can promote women's empowerment for those working as midwives.

9.2   Policy Drivers for Innovation

In 2018, global policymakers and donors joined together in a global action plan (WHO 2018) to accelerate progress towards the health-related Sustainable Development Goals (SDGs). This action plan calls for innovative ways of working together at policy level, especially to address SDG targets where the pace of progress has not been sufficient; it also advocates for innovative approaches to programme design in fragile and vulnerable states and in disease outbreaks, such as Ebola and COVID-19. The global action plan also supports social innovation for the empowerment of people and communities as co-producers of health and suggests that innovations from the

© Springer Nature Switzerland AG 2021
J. Kemp et al., *Global Midwifery: Principles, Policy and Practice*,
https://doi.org/10.1007/978-3-030-46765-4_9

private sector and academia can be harnessed for health and health-financing. The plan acknowledges that investment is needed for sustainable scale-up of innovations, to ensure that they reach the people who need them. WHO (2020a) places special emphasis on innovations that focus on the needs of vulnerable populations; however, many health innovations are not targeted at the poorest people in the world and are unaffordable and/or unsustainable for their health systems (Barlow 2017).

Achieving the sustainable development goal (SDG) of healthy lives and well-being for all can be accelerated through innovation (WHO 2018). However, the global goal of universal health coverage (UHC) by 2030 will not be realised unless many different stakeholders work together with communities to find innovative solutions to global health challenges (Acharya et al. 2018). These health challenges are often complex; therefore, health innovation cannot be limited just to the scientific development of products and technologies. Different kinds of innovation such as business and social innovations are also required in order to reach health goals. This enables effective solutions to problems where there are systemic social and environmental issues and ensures financial sustainability to scale up new ideas (WHO 2020b; Stanford Business 2020).

UNFPA's (2019) global midwifery strategy 2018–2030 prioritises the development of innovations to improve midwifery capacity and quality of care. It promotes partnerships with the private sector on product and process innovations in midwifery, such as introducing and disseminating low-resource setting appropriate technologies, training models, products and solutions and encourages country-specific innovations in midwifery. WHO (2013a) promotes innovation to improve health professional regulation, citing the ICM's (2018) midwifery regulation toolkit an example of such an innovation. Additionally, the role of innovation is threaded through WHO's (2019) framework for strengthening midwifery education. This calls for innovative approaches and radical thinking to re-shape midwifery education for the future. WHO's seven-step plan for strengthening midwifery education mandates innovative learning techniques for student midwives, use of innovative technology such as e-learning, film, mobile phone apps and simulation, innovative financing mechanisms for strengthening midwifery education and advocacy for dedicated budgets for research and innovation. The framework also champions the role of private sector partnerships, with companies such as Laerdal Global Health (LGH), Merck for Mothers and Johnson and Johnson.

9.3 Responsible Innovation in Health

Health innovations have a poor track-record for sustainability. This may be because they are unaffordable, inaccessible or inappropriate, especially in low-resource settings (Barlow 2017). Technological innovations can contribute to spiralling healthcare costs (Kumar 2011), being quickly adopted whilst having unproven value or indeed posing a risk to health (Dixon-Woods et al. 2011). An example of this is routine continuous foetal monitoring in labour which has been shown to make no difference to infant mortality but is associated with higher rates of caesarean and instrumental births (Alfirevic et al. 2017). In the past, innovations in health care have often been driven by the producers or the financers of a particular innovation, not by the people who are going to use it (usually the healthcare professionals) or those who would benefit from it (patients or clients). This can mean the innovation is not adopted widely and is not sustainable (Ahluwalia et al. 2018). Therefore, a new approach is needed to innovations, one that is based on a real need, is affordable, fits the context, is scalable and does no harm (Bessant 2019).

Responsible Innovation in Health (RIH) is a relatively new way to frame innovation and advocates for the involvement of all stakeholders at every stage of the process for the democratisation of health technology (Silva et al. 2018; Lehoux et al. 2019; Bessant 2019; Ahluwalia et al. 2018; Westerink 2019). In RIH all stakeholders agree

…to meet a set of ethical, economic, social and environmental principles, values and requirements when they design, finance, produce, distribute, use and discard sociotechnical solutions to address the needs and challenges of health systems in a sustainable way (Lehoux et al. 2018).

RIH is essential to achieve Universal Health Coverage by 2030, for example through the development of new collaborative strategies to deal with complex issues such as the fight against HIV/AIDS, malaria and tuberculosis or antimicrobial resistance to stop the advance of drug-resistant microbes (Unitaid 2020). Silva et al. (2018) suggest five value domains for responsible innovation in health, and these are summarised in Table 9.1.

RIH embraces the additional concepts of disruptive innovation, frugal innovation and reverse (or bi-direction) innovation. 'Disruptive innovations' are ones which make products or services more accessible; they are often cheaper, simpler, smaller and more convenient to use than previous technologies. Romanzi (2015) argues that maternal and newborn health needs disruptive innovation to ensure every woman and her baby has access to high-quality maternity care to meet the sustainable development goals. Another related concept is 'frugal innovation' which offers simple and cost-effective solutions to healthcare challenges to more people with minimal use of resources (Arshad et al. 2018). 'Reverse innovation' is described as the flow of ideas from lower to higher income settings (DePasse and Lee 2013) and is discussed in Chapter 15 in relation to global midwifery partnerships. Some authors exercise caution over use of the term reverse innovation, suggesting it perpetuates a colonial world view in which the flow of information is expected to go from high-income to low-income countries (Harris et al. 2016; DePasse and Lee 2013; Kulasabanthan et al. 2017).

9.4 Innovations for Midwives and Midwifery

Midwifery innovations can be described in two ways: innovations developed by midwives or innovations developed by others for use within midwifery. Both can strengthen midwifery globally and will be featured in this section. These are summarised in Table 9.2.

Table 9.1 Value domains for responsible innovation in health (adapted from Silva et al. 2018)

Value domain	Dimension
1. Population health	• Does the innovation address a relevant health issue? • Is it ethical? • Does it promote equity?
2. Health system	• Has the process been inclusive? • Is the solution dynamic and responsive? • Can the health service provide the level of care required by the innovation?
3. Economic	• Does the innovation deliver greater value with fewer resources?
4. Organisational	• Does the business model balance value for money with a high-quality innovation?
5. Environmental	• Is the innovation and the business model eco-responsible?

Table 9.2 Summary of innovations explored in this section

Innovations in midwifery practice	1. Group antenatal care 2. Midwifery Units 3. We Care Solar Suitcase® 4. The Cradle Vital Sign Alert (VSA) device 5. Case study: The KangaWrap
Innovations in midwifery education	6. E-learning and mobile apps 7. Low-fidelity simulators for low-dose high-frequency training 8. Educational games 9. Films 10. Interprofessional education for interprofessional working for interprofessional working 11. Case study: MCAT meetings in Cambodia
Midwives' associations as innovators	12. Case study: Online voting in Bangladesh

9.4.1   Innovations in Midwifery Practice

9.4.1.1 Group Antenatal Care

Women are recommended to have a minimum of eight antenatal care (ANC) contacts during their pregnancy (WHO 2016a). This traditionally involves a schedule of one-to-one visits with a care provider (Catling et al. 2017); however, as described in Chapter 7 of this book, a new model of group antenatal care (G-ANC) known as 'CenteringPregnancy' was piloted in the United States of America (USA) in the 1990s. G-ANC puts pregnant women at the centre of service provision and fosters self-efficacy and social support, enabling women to benefit from the expertise and support of both healthcare providers and peers (Sharma et al. 2018). This is an example of disruptive innovation, which aims to provide more effective ANC by disrupting the societal and other systems and structures that drive poor health and to co-create equitable communities, building collective power (Centering Healthcare Institute 2009–2020). WHO (2016a) recognises G-ANC as having the potential to improve utilisation and quality of care for pregnant women.

9.4.1.2 Midwifery Units

A Midwifery Unit (MU) (sometimes called a birth centre) is:

> a location offering maternity care to healthy women with straightforward pregnancies in which midwives take primary professional responsibility for care. Midwifery units may be located away from (Freestanding) or adjacent to (Alongside) an obstetric service (Rocca-Ihenacho et al. 2018:7).

MUs have already been described in Chapter 7 as a model of care; however, they warrant specific exploration in this chapter as an example of an accessible and affordable midwifery innovation (Ernst and Stone 2012). WHO (2018) advocates for more holistic maternity care that promotes a positive birthing experience for women. MUs achieve this by providing a social model of care. This is described as 'bio-psycho-social model of care that addresses physical, psychological and social needs' (Rocca-Ihenacho et al. 2018:7). A

systematic review of maternal and foetal outcomes by planned place of birth (Scarf et al. 2018) concluded that outcomes in MUs, compared to obstetric units in hospitals, were improved for women, and there was no difference in neonatal outcomes; the review recommended that MUs should be scaled up. In addition to outcomes relating to safety, birth centres provide more positive experiences of maternity care for women/birthing people and cost less than traditional hospital care (Overgaard et al. 2012a, b; Macfarlane et al. 2014a, b; Rocca-Ihenacho et al. 2018). MUs can also encourage innovative ways of providing care and foster fulfilment and empowerment for midwives (Walsh 2007, 2009). However, Walsh et al. (2020) found significant obstacles to MUs reaching their full potential. These included a lack of commitment from healthcare providers to establish MUs as part of essential maternity service provision, an absence of leadership to drive change and lack of capacity and willingness to address women's information needs.

9.4.1.3 The We Care Solar Suitcase[®]

Reliable electricity and lighting in health facilities are essential for delivering high quality health care (Ouedraogo and Schimanski 2018; Rokicki et al. 2019). However, in many parts of the world midwives lack, or have intermittent supply of, electric power in their workplaces and must manage in the dark or use non-electrified light sources such as candles, torches, paraffin lamps or the light from their mobile phone (if they are able to charge it). Sometimes midwives working alone need to hold mobile phones in their mouths to keep their hands free (Fig. 9.1); this raises the risk of personal infection and inhibits verbal communication. Non-electrified light sources provide low-quality light and may emit toxic fumes or present a fire hazard. Where generators are available, they may break down, there may be no fuel to power them or facilities may have insufficient funds and/or knowledge for repair and maintenance. Lack of continuous electricity makes it impossible for midwives to provide safe, round-the-clock care or to call for help when necessary. Consequently, many health facilities are

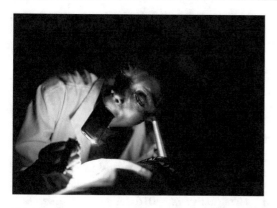

Fig. 9.1 A midwife holds a mobile phone in her mouth to provide light (used with permission)

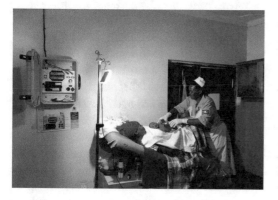

Fig. 9.2 Midwife Ariet providing care with light from a Solar Suitcase in Uganda (used with permission)

closed at night, leaving women with no access to midwifery care.

'We Care Solar Suitcase®' (Fig. 9.2) is a technological innovation that enables health facilities to provide 24-h services where there is little or no reliable source of electricity. It comprises a complete solar electric system powering customised medical lights, a foetal Doppler, mobile phones and headlamps (We Care Solar 2020; Rokicki et al. 2019). It can be equipped with additional devices such as a laptop computer programmed with educational materials and an electronic medical record information system, enabling midwives to improve the quality care they provide for women and their newborns (Kagurusi and Foulds 2020). The kit consists of a water- and-dust-tight yellow suitcase, two 100- to 250- Watt solar panels and a rechargeable battery. The suitcase becomes a cabinet that mounts to the

wall and the solar panels are secured to the health centre roof (We Care Solar 2020). The kit is low maintenance, only requiring a replacement battery every 5 years. Research from Gambia found that light from Solar Suitcases gave health workers increased confidence to manage complications, more autonomy over the quality of care and greater self-efficacy. It also enabled health workers to use both hands when providing emergency care and improved sanitation and infection control measures in health facilities (Eanelli 2019). Further research studies are ongoing to evaluate the impact of Solar Suitcases (Cohen 2018; Rokicki et al. 2019; We Care Solar 2020).

This innovation shows how the sustainable development goals are linked: goal 3 (good health and well-being for all) cannot be achieved without goal 7 (affordable and clean energy). Energy poverty and energy vulnerability have left almost one billion people without access to adequate health care in low-resource countries (Ouedraogo and Schimanski 2018). The device also shows how holistic approach can lead to synergistic effects, such as increased access and improved quality of care. We Care Solar (2015) estimated the cost of deploying a complete Solar Suitcase system at about $2500.

9.4.1.4 The Cradle Vital Sign Alert (VSA) Device

The Microlife Cradle VSA Device (Fig. 9.3), a low-cost blood pressure machine, is accurate in pregnancy and specifically designed for low-resource settings. Its traffic-light early warning system alerts midwives and other health workers to the

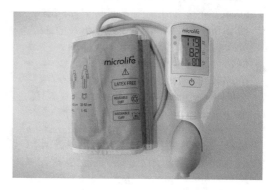

Fig. 9.3 The Cradle VSA Device

need for escalation of care for women with hyper- or hypo-tension (Cradle Trial 2020; Vousden et al. 2018). Evaluation of the Cradle VSA Device (Nathan et al. 2018) showed that it was easy to use, accurate and perceived positively by health workers. Women and their families reported that the traffic lights enabled a better understanding of their health. It encouraged them to attend their appointments and accept treatment. The Cradle VSA Device is an example of a frugal innovation that has potential to aid midwives in detecting problems, make appropriate decisions and improve outcomes for women and their newborns.

Case Study in Innovation for Midwifery Practice: The KangaWrap Project

Mothers have carried their babies in cloth wraps for centuries. Kangaroo mother care (KMC) is one of a suite of innovations in maternal and newborn care that could save millions of lives by 2030 (Batson 2016). KMC for premature babies in hospitals started in Colombia in the 1970s (Simkiss 1999) and is now recommended by the World Health Organization (WHO 2015) as a key intervention to improve pre-term birth outcomes.

In 2011 research by midwives in England demonstrated that KMC using a cloth wrap for pre-term or low-birth-weight babies in the postnatal ward setting was highly valued by parents, reduced the length of stay in hospital and improved exclusive breastfeeding rates (Gregson and Blacker 2011). However, parents found the wrap, which had been designed for baby-carrying rather than facilitating KMC, heavy and hot. Therefore, the team set out to develop the 'KangaWrap' (Fig. 9.4), a lighter, cooler option. Made from FairTrade cotton, the wrap not only promotes KMC but provides an income for women producers who might otherwise be exploited or unemployed. The wrap is now widely sold to hospitals, service users, retailers and baby-sling libraries, and the profits are used to fund maternal and child health care in developing communities through charities such as Christian Aid and Asha India (Kangawrap 2020; Christian Aid 2020).

Following the success of the Kangawrap, the same team of midwives developed the 'KangaWrap Kardi', a simple garment to help facilitate KMC in the operating theatre after caesarean section and when women are confined to bed in the postnatal ward (Gregson et al. 2016). A further research study found a trend towards increased breastfeeding rates at 48 h and 6 weeks when using the KangaWrap Kardi. The team has also developed a popular video on 'Baby friendly caesarean section birth' (Maidstone and Tunbridge Wells NHS Trust 2016), available on YouTube, demonstrating how to achieve KMC in the operating theatre. The team has been invited to share their knowledge and skills across Europe, Africa, Asia and the Middle East.

This example of reverse innovation (an approach developed in a low-resource setting and subsequently adopted in a high-resource setting) by midwives not only improves outcomes for newborns but benefits three groups of women; those giving birth, those making the wraps and recipients of maternal and child health in low-resource settings, thus contributing to gender empowerment. The project also had a positive impact on the satisfaction of the midwives and other staff involved and KMC reduced costs for the health service with shorter stays in hospital (RCM Midwives 2012).

9.4.2 Innovations in Midwifery Education

Creative and innovative teaching methods are an essential part of student-centred learning; they accommodate students' different learning styles and foster creativity in future practitioners (McCormack et al. 2014). Chapter 4 of this book, dedicated to midwifery education, contains a

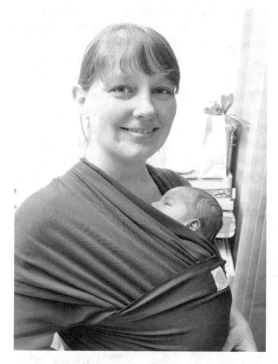

Fig. 9.4 Annie providing KMC to her pre-term son with a KangaWrap (used with permission)

comprehensive table of education models, technological advances, innovations and instructional technologies in midwifery education. Complementing that, a few educational innovations will be explored here in greater detail.

9.4.2.1 E-Learning and Mobile Apps

E-learning is cited by WHO (2018) and UNFPA (2019) as an example of innovation in midwifery education. E-learning can enable health workers to stay in their workplaces whilst learning, thus avoiding the service-gaps of traditional classroom-based teaching. It is a flexible and low-cost method of education that is user-centred and easily updated; however, it requires motivation and digital literacy from the learner and can be demanding for those providing the education (Rugeri et al. 2013). Also, in reality not every midwife has access to a smartphone, tablet or computer; therefore, over-reliance on digital learning can increase inequalities and contribute to 'digital exclusion' and 'digital poverty' (PSE 2020). Even those with access to the requisite

technology may not know how to use it. Gudgeon (2018) suggests that midwives may become disempowered and disillusioned when their working environment does not support and enable them to embrace the digital help available. Although the UK's standards of proficiency for midwives (NMC 2019) include digital skills and technological literacy as essential, these are not part of international midwifery competencies (ICM 2019a).

Arbour (2018) provides a comprehensive pocket guide to mobile applications for maternity care and midwives, mainly developed in the USA; however, she cautions that midwives can become overwhelmed with so many applications available. She suggests ensuring that apps are peer-reviewed or developed by professional sources, to practice using an app and learn its functionality, to verify the accuracy of any tools on the app (e.g. a pregnancy dating calculator), and to ensure that reliance on apps does not replace interprofessional collaboration. A description of e-learning and links to innovative mobile apps for midwives and service users can be found in Chapter 4 of this book.

9.4.2.2 Low-Fidelity Simulators for Low-Dose High-Frequency Training

Simulation is most effective within low dose, high frequency (LDHF) training, an innovative approach that employs short, targeted learning by simulation 'on the job' at repeated intervals, reinforced by structured practice settings in the workplace (Jhpiego 2013). This promotes maximum retention of clinical knowledge, skills, and attitudes (LGH 2020). A randomised controlled trial in Nigeria found that, when compared to traditional off-site lecture-style training, simulation-based LDHF training and mentoring in basic emergency obstetric and newborn care was more effective at improving health workers' skills acquisition and retention (Ugwa et al. 2020). However, the cost of simulators can be prohibitive for midwifery education institutions.

Laerdal Global Health (LGH) has developed a range of low-fidelity simulators and other products to help train and equip birth attendants and to save lives (LGH 2020). 'MamaNatalie' is used in 'Helping Mothers Survive' training programmes across 65 countries, a partnership between Jhpiego and LGH that aims to build capacity of all health workers who care for women and newborns on the day of birth and beyond. 'NeoNatalie' is used for 'Helping Babies Breathe', a newborn resuscitation training programme by the American Academy of Pediatrics, based on WHO guidelines. More than 4000 of these simulators have been donated to LGH's partners in low-resource settings through the 'buy one, gift one' scheme. When one birthing simulator is purchased for use in a high-income setting, one is donated to support the 'Helping Mothers Survive' initiative (LGH 2020). These low-fidelity simulators are supported with a range of training and therapy tools to help health workers detect and/or treat birth asphyxia (LGH 2019).

9.4.2.3 Educational Games

The use of creative teaching methods, such as games, in professional education can be motivational and enhance learning of the multiple skills and concepts needed for real-world situations; they can also encourage deeper learning by engaging the right side of students' brains (Starbuck 2006; Paz 2017). Bartels (2017) suggests that games are serious teaching tools that represent an innovative approach to teaching; they are most effective when thoughtfully designed and carefully analysed after playing and can be used for four basic purposes: discovery of new knowledge, analysis, training and education. Bartels recommends being clear about the game's objectives, choosing carefully the environment in which the game will be played, considering the players and their roles, and having a clear set of rules that mimics the processes and constraints of the system under study.

Games have their place as an innovative teaching method for midwifery. Maclean and Laisser (2020) advocate that games are cost-effective, suitable for a number of different settings, promote critical thinking and behavioural change and allow midwifery students to learn from their mistakes without endangering lives.

The Charity 'Hands on for mothers and babies' has produced the board game 'Walking with Mrs X' based on the film 'Why Did Mrs X Die, retold?' (see Chapter 2 of this book). 'Walking with Mrs. X' provides a stimulating, highly interactive and exciting approach to learning about, and promoting, safer childbirth in many different countries and contexts. An earlier version of the Mrs. X game is still available as part of WHO's Foundation Module for Safe Motherhood. WHO's (2008) midwifery education modules also include games to assist learners in managing post-partum haemorrhage, eclampsia and infection. Most recently, a series of games have been developed by the Lugina Africa Midwives Research Network (LAMRN) including a game to improve midwives' use of the partograph for charting progress in labour, a game called 'Crisis' to enhance knowledge about obstetric and neonatal emergencies and another to promote respectful care (Maclean and Laisser 2020; Lavender et al. 2019).

Games add fun to learning and enable student-led discovery (Marshall 2017; Baid and Lambert 2010). However, they must be properly evaluated and any potential actions implemented if their effectiveness is to be fully realised (Bartels 2017; Maclean and Laisser 2020).

9.4.2.4 Films

Films are not new; however, they can offer an innovative solution to the delivery of midwifery education and health worker training where there are barriers to learning such as low levels of literacy, language barriers and lack of transport (McCarthy 2017). Hall (2016) describes how films from the White Ribbon Alliance were used in the UK to teach student midwives about dignity and respectful maternity care. Teaching resources, such as films, that use real-life scenarios can help students tap into tacit knowledge and develop a deeper understanding of their own behaviours and the impact of these in practice (Dewar 2012).

Medical Aid Films (MAF) is a charity that uses film to empower health workers and communities about maternal and child health. They have produced a large number of films useful for midwifery education in many different countries, contexts and languages. Global Health Media also has an extensive collection of videos of real-life action to meet the learning needs of midwives and other health workers. The White Ribbon Alliance, a movement for reproductive, maternal and newborn health rights, also has some excellent films useful to midwifery educators.

9.4.2.5 Interprofessional Education for Interprofessional Working

Working collaboratively as part of the interprofessional healthcare team is an essential competency for midwives (ICM 2019a). However, such collaboration may be hindered by different professional cultures and stereotypes, physical distance, poor communication, gender inequity, different uses and understanding of language and poor knowledge of each other's roles and scope of practice (Romijn et al. 2017; Aquino et al. 2016; WHO 2013b). Innovative approaches are therefore essential to address these barriers and to prepare midwives for interprofessional working. WHO (2010) cite interprofessional education (IPE) as an innovative strategy to bolster the global health workforce and to prepare health workers for interprofessional working. The Centre for the Advancement of Interprofessional Education (CAIPE) defines interprofessional education as 'occasions when two or more professions learn with, from and about each other to improve collaboration and the quality of care' (CAIPE 2002).

PROMPT (PRactical Obstetric Multi-Professional Training) is an example of an innovation in interprofessional learning for midwives, obstetricians and others in the maternity care team. It started in the UK in 2006 when training for obstetric emergencies as a team was noted to significantly reduce hypoxic brain injuries and injuries after shoulder dystocia and to improve the management of emergency caesarean sections (PROMPT 2020). PROMPT has now developed a range of training packages, and the innovation has been scaled up across the UK and in many other countries and contexts, including Sierra Leone and Zimbabwe. It is cited as an example of best practice in multiprofessional obstetric training (NHSE 2016) and has been shown to improve maternal and foetal outcomes as well as saving money for health systems through reductions in litigation (PROMPT 2020).

Case Study in Innovation for Midwifery Education: Midwifery Coordination Alliance Team (MCAT) Meetings in Cambodia

In Cambodia, giving birth is traditionally known as 'chlong tonle' or 'crossing the river', a dangerous activity that can go badly wrong. In recent years, Cambodia has made impressive improvements in maternal and neonatal mortality (MOHC 2015) and has strengthened its midwives through a number of initiatives including an international midwifery association twinning partnership (RCM 2015). Recent changes in legislation mean that continuing professional development is now a mandatory requirement for midwives to renew their professional licence (Law et al. 2019) but, in the past, there was little in-service training available for midwives (URC 2019). With support from development partners, innovative multidisciplinary MCAT meetings have been taking place every quarter across all areas of Cambodia where every midwife meets with others to learn practical skills, share their experiences and receive supportive supervision (CARE Cambodia 2016). The MCAT meetings, which aim to improve teamwork, relationships and communication and to clarify roles and responsibilities, have changed midwives' and other health workers' ingrained and widely accepted practices and built their capacity to solve their own challenges. MCAT meetings have subsequently been scaled up nationally and adopted by the Cambodian Ministry of Health (URC 2019).

9.4.3 Midwives' Associations as Innovators

Professional associations have a role in promoting and diffusing innovations (Swan and Newell 1995; NAS 2005). Through bringing members together in meetings, conferences and other forums, professional associations can nourish new ideas and innovations and foster interprofessional collaboration (NAS 2005). Umbrella organisations of professional associations also have a role in promoting innovation; for example, the International Confederation of Midwives' Young Midwife Leader programme challenges young midwives to create innovative projects to address global health challenges (ICM 2019b). More information about midwifery associations can be found in Chapter 6 of this book.

Midwife twinning projects are an innovative method of empowering midwives and strengthening midwives' associations; in particular, the reciprocal aspect of twinning is considered to be innovative (Cadée et al. 2013; Ireland et al. 2015). 'twintowin' is an innovative social enterprise created by midwives that provides made-to-measure support to organisations and individuals that want to start a Twinning project (twintowin 2020). The project has developed a mobile app for twinning with support from the WeObservatory for eHealth (WeObservatory 2015). Midwives' association twinning is described in detail in Chapter 15 of this book.

Case Study of a Midwives' Association as an Innovator: Online Voting in Bangladesh

Midwifery is a new profession in Bangladesh. In 2017 the Bangladesh Midwifery Society (BMS) entered into an international twinning partnership with the Royal College of Midwives (RCM) in the UK. The partnership plan included development of a new membership data management system for BMS, and delivery of a democratic election for new executive committee members, the first since the organisation was founded. Working with a local digital technology consultant in Bangladesh, and with the RCM's data analyst in the UK, BMS developed a new online membership database which allows members to join and pay their membership fees using a mobile phone. The database, using a member's phone number as their unique identifier, was designed to include a voting function so that members could vote on any society matter remotely from a mobile phone or other device. The first remote election of officers was held in September 2018 and was hugely successful, enabling midwives from all over the country to vote democratically for their chosen leaders. It saved significant costs as every member was able to vote and did not have to travel to the capital city to do so. It was the first known example of online voting for any purpose in Bangladesh, catching the interest of news media and government. Thus, midwives led the way in a technological innovation.

9.5 Lessons in Midwifery Innovation from the COVID-19 Pandemic

At the time of writing, the world is in the midst of the COVID-19 pandemic. This has certainly posed many challenges for midwives and for the wider health sector but has also provided opportunities for innovation. Digital communication can overcome physical distancing restrictions (Farao 2020) and provide opportunity for sharing information with large numbers of people en masse. However, an 'infodemic' can also occur during a pandemic, where health professionals become saturated with large amounts of data (Zaracostas 2020). Midwives need accurate information to reduce the confusion caused by fear-based rhetoric broadcast on social media (O'Connell et al. 2020).

Midwives are at the core of the response to the pandemic (Bick 2020) and, around the world, have responded in innovative ways to challenges posed by COVID-19, offering video consultations and online clinics for women, hosting antenatal clinics in football stadiums, developing antenatal education videos accessible on popular social media sites and facilitating antenatal care groups via Zoom (Stephenson 2020; Furuta 2020). In addition to the many challenges, COVID-19 has also provided opportunities for innovation in midwifery education. In at least one setting, COVID-19 caused rapid digitalisation of curriculum and teaching, achieving more progress in the digitalisation of midwifery education in a few months than in the last decades (Luyben et al. 2020). In some places, COVID-19 has given student midwives additional clinical learning opportunities in interprofessional teams, thus enhancing their education (Luyben et al. 2020).

Professional Midwives' Associations have also demonstrated innovative responses to the pandemic. For example, in the UK the Royal College of Midwives formed an immediate collaborative partnership with the Royal College of Obstetricians and Gynaecologists. Working with an expert clinical advisory group and several midwifery professors, they provided rapid evidence reviews and clinical guidance to inform the required swift reconfiguration of maternity services to ensure that women and their families continued to receive high-quality care. In Bangladesh, where the supply of personal protective equipment for midwives was problematic, the Bangladesh Midwifery Society (BMS) joined forces with a woman's organisation to sew washable masks for midwives. The masks, displaying the BMS logo, were distributed to midwives across Bangladesh and came with instructions for use, plus information about joining the association and accessing online education resources. This initiative had the additional benefits of providing an income for the women manufacturing the masks and building stronger relationships between BMS and the women's development sector.

9.6 Challenges in Innovation for Midwives

McKellar et al. (2009) highlight that a negative culture in midwifery practice can make change and innovation difficult. They suggest that midwives may experience grief when not able to practice according to the ideals of their profession. This grief feeds negative workplace cultures and may be fuelled by the frustration, exhaustion and stress resulting from changes and innovations that have been introduced without proper evaluation of their impact on midwives' workload and experiences. This resonates with the WHO's (2016b) 'Midwives Voices, Midwives Realities' report which showed that midwives from across the world were frustrated by the realities they experience. Additionally, midwives knew what changes and innovations were required to improve the quality of care for women, but their voices were not being heard. This was attributed to gender discrimination, disrespect and lack of status. Where midwives do develop good innovations, these may not be scaled up because of midwives' lack of influence at policy level and their lack of power to influence widespread diffusion and adoption of innovations.

Identifying existing innovations can prove difficult for midwives as, if they have been published, this may be in sources from many different disciplines, making the literature searches complicated (Leyersdorff et al. 2013). Technological innovation has the potential to improve global health; however, it also brings new challenges, such as criminal activities linked to cyber and biological weapons, piracy of medical devices, fraud and theft of personal data (Ahluwalia et al. 2018). Poor regulation, in health and other sectors, also hampers innovation. It may be outdated or irrelevant, thus becoming an unnecessary burden, or may be too rigid, excessive or unresponsive (WHO 2013a; Gutiérrez-Ibarluzea et al. 2017; EC 2017).

9.7   Turning Ideas into Innovations

Health innovation is often described as linear, or as a cycle with different phases such as identifying needs and challenges, developing ideas for solutions, testing ideas, analysing solutions and supporting implementation (CHI 2016). Such linear approaches may be unhelpful and inefficient. In reality, health innovation is almost never straightforward, and the different steps overlap each other in complex ways (Gutiérrez-Ibarluzea et al. 2017; Nolte 2018). However, use of the innovation cycle may be helpful to consider how midwives might turn their own ideas into innovations.

When identifying needs and challenges, a stakeholder analysis is a good starting point as collaboration with all stakeholders is important at every stage of the innovation process (Ahluwalia et al. 2018). An example of a stakeholder analysis tool is given in the additional resources for reflection and study. Remember that collaboration may be required with stakeholders outside of health care (Leyersdorff et al. 2013) and ensure that service users participate at every stage of the project. Collaborators on the production of an innovative toolkit to reduce caesarean section rates highlighted the importance of co-production in innovation and of finding in-house solutions when change is needed (Brodick et al. 2011). Action research can provide a helpful framework for ensuring collaboration for innovations and change (McKellar et al. 2009; Kemp et al. 2018).

It is important to undertake a literature search to identify whether a similar idea or innovation already exists; this may be in a different field. Hospital, university and professional association libraries can help with literature searching. Next is the development of ideas for solutions; again, there may be a need to look outside of midwifery and health care for the solutions needed. Lateral thinking tools such as Edward de Bono's (2016) 'Six Hat Thinking' can help with finding creative approaches. When testing ideas, the people using the innovation must be the ones to test it out, and such testing must be done in real-life situations. All stakeholders should be consulted when analysing solutions; often the people most crucial to the success of an innovation are not the midwives themselves. For example, Chamberlain (2008) describes the importance of involving security guards in a maternity quality improvement project in Uganda. The last stage, supporting innovation, relies on the success of every other stage in the process. Attention to detail, getting the governance right, having the right people on board and communicating clearly will make all the difference.

Unfortunately, few healthcare innovations are successfully implemented, scaled up or sustained, and therefore, few produce real change (Zietmann et al. 2019; Geerligs et al. 2018). Côté-Boileau et al. (2019) argue that an additional 3Ss (spread, sustainability and scale-up) must be considered alongside the stages already described. The 'Diffusion of Innovation Theory' (Rogers 2003) describes how some people are more ready to adopt innovations than others. Understanding this theory and developing strategies to get the least-willing adopters on board may be important in sustaining and scaling-up midwifery innovations.

9.8   Monitoring and Evaluation of Innovations

Monitoring and evaluation are vital to the success of innovation. Regular monitoring of implementation activities gives assurance as to how the innovation is being delivered. For example, does the innovation function consistently as it should? Do the realities of practice lessen the functionality of the innovation? Is the content and the delivery of the innovation pitched correctly to get the intended result? How well are the users of the innovation delivering it? Conversely, evaluation is a periodic, in-depth analysis that attributes some output, outcome or economic value to the innovation; for example, is the intervention being used and by whom? Has it led to behaviour change? Is it cost-effective compared to existing services?

What impact is the innovation having (WHO 2016c)? Allocating sufficient budget and expertise for monitoring and evaluation is essential during the planning phase (MAMA 2018; Nolte 2018). However, it is rare to have sufficient emphasis on monitoring and evaluation (Cadée et al. 2013). In the UK, consultant midwives have a specific remit for research, evaluation and planning new services (Cooke 2018); this role could support midwife innovations in the future.

9.9   The Future of Innovation by and with Midwives

As midwives already know the solutions to providing high-quality maternity care (WHO 2016b), they must be at the table with health innovators and entrepreneurs as they design new approaches to health care (Langway 2017). High-quality midwifery leadership is essential in supporting innovation (NHS England 2016). Byrom et al. (2011) describe transformational leadership in which, through trusting her colleagues, a midwife leader can build a virtuous circle of organisational trust. This creates a spirit of positivity which allows creativity and innovation to flourish. Social franchising, where midwives can own and operate their own practices supported by a clinical franchise (e.g. promoting reproductive health and family planning services), may provide a way forward for midwifery innovation and empowerment (Krubiner et al. 2016).

Collaboration is essential, especially with maternity service users and beneficiaries. This will enable the contextual suitability of innovations and allow for the democratisation of health technology which is a key for achieving universal equitable health care (Ahluwalia et al. 2018; Mutsvangwa 2018). Guy's and St. Thomas's Charity (2020) set out five principles for involving people in health innovation, listed in Table 9.3.

Finally, supporting innovation to strengthen global midwifery and contribute to the achievement of global health goals can only happen with sufficient funding for innovations and where global markets support innovation by competitive pricing and sustained production (WHO 2018).

Table 9.3 Five principles for involving people in health innovation (Guys and St. Thomas' Charity 2016)

1. Experts are everywhere. Listen intently
2. Balance leadership with sharing power
3. Go to where people are and use a shared language
4. Involve at all stages: think 'who', 'how' and 'when'?
5. Build in appropriate time and resources on all sides

Key Messages

Principles

Innovation by midwives and for midwifery services has the potential to improve efficiency, effectiveness, quality, safety and/or affordability of maternity care. However, many innovations are not sustained in the long term. There is a supportive policy environment for innovation, and there are interesting examples from practice, education and midwifery associations across the world. Collaboration with all stakeholders, especially midwifery service users, at every stage of the process is a key to success along with robust monitoring and evaluation.

Policy

Innovation is needed to reach the health-related SDGs and to strengthen midwifery for the future. Global health policy supports innovative approaches to developing midwifery education, regulation and practice, especially for fragile and vulnerable populations. Social innovation and new forms of partnership across different sectors are encouraged and will require sufficient funding and support from global markets. Future innovations must be responsible. Midwives must have a seat at the table when new approaches are designed.

Practice

Innovation has the potential to transform midwifery practice and benefit midwives, those who work with midwives and others from different disciplines. Responsible innovation in health demands that those who will use and benefit from the innovation must be involved at every stage of the design and implementation. Innovations should be targeted at the populations who need it most. Digital innovations can make high-quality midwifery care more accessible for those with digital access. Midwives who want to turn their ideas into innovations may find the five value domains of responsible innovation to be a helpful framework.

Additional Resources for Reflection and Further Study

Read 'The art of involving people in health innovation: lessons from the frontline' by Guy's and St. Thomas' Charity https://www.gsttcharity.org.uk/what-we-do/our-strategy/convene/art-involving-people-health-innovation. Reflect on a health innovation that has been introduced in your workplace. To what extent were the 'five principles for involving people' followed in the introduction of that innovation? How could you use these five principles if you were involved in developing a midwifery innovation in the future?

Download a free paper copy (or buy a boxed set) of the board game 'Walking with Mrs. X' from Hands on for Mothers and Babies http://www.hofmab.com/board-game. Consider how you could use this with your colleagues or students to consider the barriers that women in your community or country face in accessing high-quality maternity care and how these might be overcome.

Reflect on your own digital competence. If you feel comfortable with technology and have access to it, explore some of the applications and resources mentioned in this chapter and in Chap. 4. How can you help your colleagues to improve their digital competence? If you feel digitally excluded, consider how you can address this to improve your confidence in using learning and practice technologies and innovations.

Consider whether high-frequency low-dose training could improve professional education in your workplace and familiarise yourself with some of the low-fidelity simulators developed for this purpose.

This chapter has identified that collaboration with all stakeholders is essential for successful innovation. Download a free resource on stakeholder analysis here https://improvement.nhs.uk/documents/2169/stakeholder-analysis.pdf and use it to identify the stakeholders for any idea that you might wish to develop into an innovation.

Look at MAF films at https://www.medicalaidfilms.org/watch-2/—there is an MAF film about the Cradle VSA device and many other topics of interest to midwives.

Consider how you might use these resources in your practice or teaching.

References

Acharya S, Lin V, Dhingra N (2018) The role of health in achieving the sustainable development goals. Bull World Health Organ 96:591–591A. https://doi.org/10.2471/BLT.18.221432

Ahluwalia A, De Maria C, Díaz Lantadab A (2018) The Kahawa declaration: a manifesto for the democratization of medical technology. Glob Health Innov 1(1). https://doi.org/10.15641/ghi.v1i1.507

Alfirevic Z, Gyte G, Cuthbert A et al (2017) Continuous cardiotocography as a form of electronic fetal monitoring for fetal assessment in labour. Cochrane Syst Rev. Accessed 12 Jul 2020. https://doi.org/10.1002/14651858.CD006066.pub3/full

Aquino M, Olander E, Needle J (2016) Midwives' and health visitors' collaborative relationships: a systematic review of qualitative and quantitative studies. Int J Nurs Stud 62:193–206. https://doi.org/10.1016/j.ijnurstu.2016.08.002

Arbour M (2018) Mobile applications for women's health and midwifery care: a pocket reference for the 21st century. J Midwifery Womens Health 63:330–334

Arshad H, Radic M, Radic D (2018) Patterns of frugal innovation in healthcare. Technol Innov Manag Rev 8(4):28–37

Baid H, Lambert N (2010) Enjoyable learning: the role of humour, games, and fun activities in nursing and midwifery education. Nurse Educ Today 30(6):548–552

Barlow J (2017) Managing innovation in healthcare. World Scientific, London

Bartels E (2017) Innovative education: gaming—learning at play. INFORMS 41(4) https://www.informs.org/ORMS-Today/Public-Articles/August-Volume-41-Number-4/INNOVATIVE-EDUCATION-Gaming-Learning-at-play. Accessed 11 Jul 2020

Batson A (2016) 11 health innovations to drastically cut maternal and child mortality rates. The Guardian: development 2030. https://www.theguardian.com/global-development-professionals-network/2016/oct/27/11-health-innovations-to-drastically-cut-maternal-and-child-mortality-rates. Accessed 7 Jun 2020

Bessant J (2019) Responsible innovation in healthcare: unlocking the power of users. https://disruptorleague.com/2019/10/11/responsible-innovation-in-healthcare-unlocking-the-power-of-users/. Accessed 8 Jun 2020

Bick D (2020) COVID-19: 2020 is international year of the midwife. Midwifery 85:102719

Brodick A, Mason N, Baldwin J et al (2011) Using collaborative theories to reduce caesarean section rates and improve maternal and infant Well-being. In: Byrom S, Downe S, Simpson L (eds) Essential midwifery practice: leadership, expertise and collaborative working. Wiley Blackwell, Oxford, pp 195–220

Byrom S, Byrom A, Downe S (2011) Transformational leadership and midwifery. In: Byrom S, Downe S, Simpson L (eds) Essential midwifery practice: leadership, expertise and collaborative working. Wiley Blackwell, Oxford, pp 23–43

Cadée F, Perdok H, Sam B et al (2013) 'Twin2Twin' an innovative method of empowering midwives to strengthen their professional midwifery organisations. Midwifery 29:1145–1150

CAIPE (2002) Defining inter professional education. https://www.caipe.org/about-us. Accessed 12 Jul 2020

Cambridge Dictionary (2020) Meaning of innovation in English. https://dictionary.cambridge.org/dictionary/english/innovation. Accessed 7 Jun 2020

Care Cambodia (2016) MCAT meetings giving women confidence. https://www.care-cambodia.org/singlepost/2016/02/16/The-success-of-MCAT-meeting. Accessed 12 Jul 2020

Catling C, Medley N, Foureur M et al (2017) Group versus conventional antenatal care for women. Cochrane Database Syst Rev (2). https://doi.org/10.1002/14651858.CD007622.pub3

Centering Healthcare Institute (2009–2020) About us. https://www.centeringhealthcare.org/about. Accessed 1 Jul 2020

Chamberlain J (2008) Where have all the mothers gone? Essence Publishing, Hamilton, ON

Christian Aid (2020) Trade4Life: what is a KangaWrap? https://www.christianaid.org.uk/resources/trade4life. Accessed 28 Jun 2020

Cohen J (2018) Evaluation of the impact of the 'Solar Suitcase' installation in healthcare facilities in Uganda on quality of care during labor and delivery and reliability of electricity: AEA RCT registry. https://www.socialscienceregistry.org/trials/3078. Accessed 02.07.2020

Cooke P (2018) The role of the consultant midwife in the UK. In: Rocca-Ihenacho L, Batinelli L, Thaels E et al (eds) Midwifery unit standards. City University, London

Copenhagen Health Innovation (CHI) (2016) Health innovation in CHI. https://copenhagenhealthinnovation.dk/en/health-innovation-in-chi/. Accessed 12 Jul 2020

Côté-Boileau E, Denis JL, Callery B et al (2019) The unpredictable journeys of spreading, sustaining and scaling healthcare innovations: a scoping review. Health Policy Res Syst 17:84. https://doi.org/10.1186/s12961-019-0482-6

Cradle Trial (2020) The device: the Microlife Cradle VSA. http://cradletrial.com/the-device/. Accessed 8 Jul 2020

De Bono E (2016) Six thinking hats. Penguin, London

DePasse J, Lee P (2013) A model for 'reverse innovation' in health care. Glob Health 9(1):40

Dewar B (2012) Using creative methods in practice development to understand and develop compassionate care. Int Pract Dev J 2(1):2

Dixon-Woods M, Amalberti R, Goodman S et al (2011) Problems and promises of innovations: why health-

care needs to rethink its love/hate relationship with the new. BMJ Qual Saf 20(Suppl 1):i47ei51

Eanelli BA (2019) The perceived impact of the we care solar suitcase on the quality of care health workers deliver in the Gambia. Master of Science thesis, Duke Global Health Institute. https://dukespace.lib.duke.edu/dspace/bitstream/handle/10161/18876/Eanelli_duke_0066N_15082.pdf?sequence=1&isAllowed=y. Accessed 2 Jul 2020

Ernst E, Stone S (2012) The birth centre: innovation in evidence-based midwifery care. In: Anderson B, Stone S (eds) Best practices in midwifery: using the evidence to implement change. Springer, New York

European Commission (EC) (2017) Assessing the impacts of EU regulatory barriers on innovation. Publications Office of the European Union, Luxembourg

Farao J (2020) Digital health communication in South Africa during COVID-19. Glob Health Innov 3:1. https://doi.org/10.15641/ghi.v3i1.891

Furuta M (2020) 2020 international year of midwifery—in the midst of a pandemic. Midwifery 87:102739

Geerligs L, Rankin N, Shepherd H et al (2018) Hospital-based interventions: a systematic review of staff-reported barriers and facilitators to implementation processes. Implement Sci 13:36. https://doi.org/10.1186/s13012-018-0726-9

Gregson S, Blacker J (2011) Kangaroo care in pre-term or low birth weight babies in a postnatal ward. Br J Midwifery 19(9):566–575

Gregson S, Meadows J, Teakle P et al (2016) Skin-to-skin contact after elective caesarean section: investigating the effect on breastfeeding rates. Br J Midwifery 24(1):18–25

Gudgeon J (2018) How to reach digital maturity. RCM Midwives magazine. https://www.rcm.org.uk/news-views/rcm-opinion/how-to-reach-digital-maturity/. Accessed 11 Jul 2020

Gutiérrez-Ibarluzea I, Chiumente M, Dauben HP (2017) The life cycle of health technologies: challenges and ways forward. Front Pharmacol 8:14. https://doi.org/10.3389/fphar.2017.00014

Guys and St. Thomas' Charity (2016) The art of involving people in health innovation: lessons and tips from the frontline. https://www.gsttcharity.org.uk/what-we-do/our-strategy/convene/art-involving-people-health-innovation#standard-panel-2. Accessed 10 Jul 2020

Hall J (2016) Dignity and respect in midwifery education in the UK: a survey of Lead Midwives for Education. Available at http://eprints.bournemouth.ac.uk/24740/3/Dignity%20and%20Respect%20in%20Midwifery%20Education.pdf. Accessed 08.11.2020

Harris M, Weisberger E, Silver D et al (2016) That's not how learning works—the paradox of reverse innovation: a qualitative study. Glob Health 12:36

ICM (2014) Core document: philosophy and model of midwifery care. https://www.internationalmidwives.org/assets/files/definitions-files/2018/06/eng-philosophy-and-model-of-midwifery-care.pdf. Accessed 9 Jul 2020

ICM (2018) Midwifery regulation toolkit. https://www. internationalmidwives.org/assets/files/regulation-files/2018/04/icm_toolkit_eng.pdf. Accessed 9 Jul 2020

ICM (2019a) Essential competencies for midwifery practice.   https://www.internationalmidwives. org/assets/files/general-files/2018/10/icm-competencies%2D%2D-english-document_final_oct-2018.pdf. Accessed 3 Jul 2020

ICM (2019b) 2019 Young Midwifery Leaders Programme. https://www.internationalmidwives.org/assets/files/ project-files/2019/02/final-yml-advert%2D%2D-selection-c-and-process-document.pdf. Accessed 13 Jul 2020

Ireland J, van Teijlingen E, Kemp J (2015) Twinning in Nepal: the Royal College of Midwives UK and the midwifery Society of Nepal working in partnership. J Asian Midwives 2(1):26–33

Jhpiego (2013) Low dose, high frequency: a learning approach to improve health workforce competence, confidence, and performance. https://hms.jhpiego. org/wp-content/uploads/2016/08/LDHF_briefer.pdf. Accessed 11 Jul 2020

Kagurusi P, Foulds J (2020) How solar power and advocacy brightens maternal and newborn health care in Uganda. https://www.grandchallenges.ca/2016/solar-power-advocacy-brightens-maternal-newborn-health-care-uganda/. Accessed 2 Jul 2020

KangaWrap (2020) Our story. https://kangawrap.co.uk/ our-story/. Accessed 28 Jun 2020

Kemp J, Shaw E, Nanjego S et al (2018) Improving student midwives' practice learning in Uganda through action research: the MOMENTUM project. Int Pract Dev J 8(1):7

Kimble L, Massoud MR (2016) What do we mean by innovation in healthcare? Eur Med J Innov 1(1):89–91

Krubiner C, Salmon M, Synowiec C et al (2016) Investing in nursing and midwifery enterprise: empowering women and strengthening health systems: apro landscaping study of innovations in low and middle-income countries. Nurs Outlook 64:17–23

Kulasabanthan K, Issa H, Bhatti Y et al (2017) Do international health partnerships contribute to reverse innovation? A mixed methods study of THET-supported partnerships in the UK. Glob Health 13:25

Kumar R (2011) Technology and healthcare costs. Ann Pediatr Cardiol 4(1):84–86

Laerdal Global Health (2019) Safer births: a research and development project to save lives at birth. 2019 update. https://cdn0.laerdal.com/cdn-4a257a/globalassets/lgh/ partnerships%2D%2Dprograms/safer-births/safer-births-report-screens-07.08.29.pdf. Accessed 10 Jul 2020

Laerdal Global Health (2020) Our products. https:// laerdalglobalhealth.com/products. Accessed 11 Jul 2020

Langway Z (2017) Midwives: innovators on the front lines of care. Healthy newborn network blog. https:// www.healthynewbornnetwork.org/blog/midwives-innovators-front-lines-care/.   Accessed   12   Jul 2020

Lavender T, Omoni G, Laisser R et al (2019) Evaluation of an educational board game to improve use of the partograph in sub-Saharan Africa: a quasi-experimental study. Sex Reprod Health 20:54–59. https://doi. org/10.1016/j.srhc.2019.03.001

Law K, Te V, Hill P (2019) Cambodia's health professionals and the ASEAN mutual recognition arrangements: registration, education and mobility. Hum Resour Health 17:14

Lehoux P, Silva H, Sabio R et al (2018) The unexplored contribution of responsible innovation in health to sustainable development goals. Sustainability 10(11):4015

Lehoux P, Roncarolo F, Pacifico Silva H et al (2019) What health system challenges should responsible innovations in health address? Insights from an international scoping review. Int J Health Policy Manag 8(2): 63–75

Leyersdorff L, Rotolo D, de Nooy W (2013) Innovation as a non-linear process: the scientometric perspective, and the specification of an 'innovation opportunities explorer'. Technol Anal Strat Manag 25(6):641. https://doi.org/10.1080/09537325.2013.801948

Luyben A, Fleming V, Vermeulen J (2020) Midwifery education in COVID-19- time: challenges and opportunities. Midwifery 89:102776

Macfarlane AJ, Rocca-Ihenacho L, Turner LR, Roth C (2014a) Survey of women's experiences of care in a new freestanding midwifery unit in an inner city area of London, England – 1: Methods and women's overall ratings of care. Midwifery 30(9):998–1008

Macfarlane AJ, Rocca-Ihenacho L, Turner LR, Roth C (2014b) Survey of women's experiences of care in a new freestanding midwifery unit in an inner city area of London, England: 2. Specific aspects of care. Midwifery 30(9):1009–1020

Maclean G, Laisser R (2020) The use of educational games in midwifery: an overview. Afr J Midwifery Women Health 14(1):1–10. https://doi.org/10.12968/ ajmw.2019.0003

Maidstone and Tunbridge Wells NHS Trust (2016) Baby   friendly   caesarean   birth.   https://www. youtube.com/watch?time_continue=5&v=fR-39ITbJOQ&feature=emb_logo. Accessed 29 Jun 2020

Marshall J (2017) Approaches to midwifery education. In: Hutton E, Murray-Davis B, Laufman K et al (eds) Comprehensive midwifery: the role of the midwife in health care practice, education and research. https:// ecampusontario.pressbooks.pub/cmroleofmidwifery/. Accessed 11 Jun 2020

McCarthy C (2017) Transforming midwifery education in Somaliland through film. J Womens Health 6(6):69

McCormack B, McGowan B, McGonigle M, Goode D, Black P, Sinclair M (2014) Exploring 'self' as a person-centred academic through critical creativity: a case study of educators in a school of nursing. International Practice Development Journal 4(2):1–18

McKellar L, Pincombe J, Henderson A (2009) Encountering the culture of midwifery practice on the postnatal ward during action research: an impediment to change. Women Birth 22(4):12–118

Ministry of Health Cambodia (MOHC) (2015) Success factors for women's and children's health. https://www.who.int/pmnch/knowledge/publications/cambodia_country_report.pdf. Accessed 12 Jul 2020

Mobile Alliance for Maternal Action Approach (MAMA) (2018) Lessons from country programs implementing the mobile alliance for maternal action programs in Bangladesh, South Africa, India and Nigeria, 2010–2016. https://www.mcsprogram.org/resource/mama-lessons-learned-report/. Accessed 14 Jul 2020

Mutsvangwa T (2018) Engaged scholarship for health innovation. Glob Health Innov 1(2). https://doi.org/10.15641/ghi.v1i2.686

Nathan H, Boene H, Munguambe K et al (2018) The CRADLE vital signs alert: qualitative evaluation of a novel device designed for use in pregnancy by healthcare workers in low-resource settings. Reprod Health 15:5. https://doi.org/10.1186/s12978-017-0450-y

National Academy of Sciences (NAS) (2005) The role of professional societies. Facilitating interdisciplinary research. National Academies Press, Washington, DC, pp 137–136

NHS England (2016) Better births: the national maternity review. https://www.england.nhs.uk/wp-content/uploads/2016/02/national-maternity-review-report.pdf. Accessed 13 Jul 2020

Nolte E (2018) Policy brief: how do we ensure that innovation in health service delivery and organisation and implemented, sustained and spread? WHO regional Office for Europe. https://www.euro.who.int/__data/assets/pdf_file/0004/380731/pb-tallinn-03-eng.pdf. Accessed 13 Jul 2020

Nursing and Midwifery Council (2019) Standards of proficiency for midwives. Available at https://www.nmc.org.uk/globalassets/sitedocuments/standards/standards-of-proficiency-formidwives.pdf. Accessed 08.11.2020

O'Connell M, Crowther S, Ravaldi C et al (2020) Midwives in a pandemic: a call for solidarity and compassion. Women Birth 33(3):205–206

Ouedraogo C, Schimanski N (2018) Energy poverty in healthcare facilities: a 'silent barrier' to improved healthcare in sub-Saharan Africa. J Public Health Policy 39:358–371. https://doi.org/10.1057/s41271-018-0136-x

Overgaard C, Fenger-Grøn M, Sandall J (2012a) Freestanding midwifery units versus obstetric units: does the effect of place of birth differ with level of social disadvantage? BMC Public Health 12(1):478

Overgaard C, Fenger-Grøn M, Sandall J (2012b) The impact of birthplace on women's birth experiences and perceptions of care. Soc Sci Med 74(7):973–981

Paz O (2017) What motivates adults to learn? In: Wlodkowski R, Ginsbery M (eds) Enhancing adult motivation to learn, 4th edn. Wiley, San Francisco

Poverty and Social Exclusion (PSE) (2020) Growing problem of digital exclusion. https://www.poverty.ac.uk/report-social-exclusion-disability-older-people/growing-problem-%E2%80%98digital-exclusion%E2%80%99. Accessed 11 Jul 2020

PROMPT (2020) PROMPT PRactical obstetric multi-professional training. https://www.promptmaternity.org/Default.aspx. Accessed 13 Jul 2020

RCM Midwives (2012) RCM awards: kangaroo care on the postnatal ward. RCM Midwives Mag 2:46

Rocca-Ihenacho L, Batinelli L, Thaels E et al (2018) Midwifery unit standards. https://www.midwiferyunitnetwork.org/mu-standards/. Accessed 8 Jul 2020

Rogers E (2003) Diffusion of innovation, 5th edn. Free Press, New York

Rokicki S, Mwesigwa B, Schmucker L et al (2019) Shedding light on quality of care: a study protocol for a randomized trial evaluating the impact of the solar suitcase in rural health facilities on maternal and newborn care quality in Uganda. BMC Pregnancy Childbirth 19:306. https://doi.org/10.1186/s12884-019-2453-x

Romanzi L (2015) Let's create disruptive innovation for maternal newborn health. https://www.mhtf.org/2015/10/16/lets-create-disruptive-innovation-for-maternal-newborn-health-at-gmnhc2015/. Accessed 7 Jun 2020

Romijn A, Teunissen P, de Bruijne M et al (2017) Interprofessional collaboration among care professionals in obstetrical care: are perceptions aligned? BMJ Qual Saf. https://doi.org/10.1136/bmjqs-2016-006401

Royal College of Midwives (RCM) (2015) Supporting midwifery beyond our borders: the global midwifery twinning project. https://www.rcm.org.uk/media/2389/supporting-midwifery-beyond-our-borders.pdf. Accessed 12 Jul 2020

Rugeri K, Farrington C, Brayne C (2013) A global model for effective use and evaluation of e-learning in health. Telemed J E Health 19(4):312–321

Scarf V, Rossiter C, Vedam S et al. (2018) Maternal and perinatal outcomes by planned place of birth among women with low-risk pregnancies in high-income countries: a systematic review and meta-analysis. Midwifery, 62:240–255

Sharma J, O'Connor M, Jolivet R (2018) Group antenatal care models in low- and middle-income countries: a systematic evidence synthesis. Reprod Health 15:38. https://doi.org/10.1186/s12978-018-0476-9

Silva H, Lehoux P, Miller F et al (2018) Introducing responsible innovation in health: a policy-oriented framework. Health Res Policy Syst 16:90

Simkiss D (1999) Kangaroo mother care. J Trop Paediatr 45:192–193

Stanford Business (2020) Defining social innovation. https://www.gsb.stanford.edu/faculty-research/centers-initiatives/csi/defining-social-innovation. Accessed 7 Jun 2020

Starbuck D (2006) Creative teaching: getting it right. Continuum, London

Stephenson J (2020) Midwives praised on international midwife day for 'rising to Covid-19 challenge. Nursing Times. https://www.nursingtimes.net/news/leadership-news/midwives-praised-on-international-midwife-day-for-rising-to-covid-19-challenge-05-05-2020/. Accessed 28 Jun 2020

Swan J, Newell S (1995) The role of professional associations in technology diffusion. Organ Stud 16(5):847–874

Ugwa E, Kabue M, Otolorin E et al (2020) A mixed-methods evaluation of a cluster randomized controlled trial on simulation-based low-dose, high-frequency plus mobile mentoring training versus traditional group-based training of health workers in Ebonyi and Kogi states. Nigeria BMS Health Serv Res 20:586

UNFPA (2019) Global midwifery strategy 2018–2030. UNFPA, Geneva

Unitaid (2020) Special report: innovating for universal health coverage. https://unitaid.org/innovating-for-universal-health-coverage/#en. Accessed 18 Jul 2020

URC (2019) Transforming the health workforce: developing a culture of team work and continuous quality improvement. https://www.urc-chs.com/sites/default/files/URC%20Cambodia%20HSS%20legacy%20Capacity%20v7-USAID.pdf. Accessed 12 Jul 2020

Vousden N, Lawley E, Nathan H et al (2018) Evaluation of a novel vital sign device to reduce maternal mortality and morbidity in low-resource settings: a mixed method feasibility study for the CRADLE-3 trial. BMC Pregnancy Childbirth 18:115

Walsh D (2007) A birth centre's encounters with discourses of childbirth: how resistance led to innovation. Sociol Health Illn 29(2):216–232

Walsh D (2009) Small really is beautiful: tales from a free-standing birth Centre in England. In: Floyd D et al (eds) Birth models that work. University of California Press, Berkeley, pp 159–186

Walsh D, Spiby H, McCourt C et al (2020) Factors influencing the utilisation of free-standing and alongside midwifery units in England: a qualitative research study. BMJ Open 10:e033895. https://doi.org/10.1136/bmjopen-2019-033895

We Care Solar (2015) We Care Solar Fact Sheet. http://wecaresolar.org/wp-content/uploads/2015/05/We_Care_Solar_FAQ-2015.pdf. Accessed 15 Jul 2020

We Care Solar (2020) The solar suitcase. https://wecaresolar.org/solar-suitcase/product-information/. Accessed 2 Jul 2020

WeObservatory (2015) twintowin: reciprocal development. http://www.m2025-weobservatory.org/twin-2twin.html. Accessed 14 Jul 2020

Westerink J (2019) Technology and the democratisation of healthcare. https://www.philips.com/a-w/about/news/archive/blogs/innovation-matters/20190925-technology-and-the-democratization-of-healthcare.html. Accessed 12 Jul 2020

WHO (2008) Midwifery education modules: education materials for teachers of midwifery. https://www.who.int/maternal_child_adolescent/documents/9241546662/en/. Accessed 11 Jul 2020

WHO (2010) Framework for action on interprofessional education and collaborative practice. WHO, Geneva

WHO (2013a) Transforming and scaling up health professional education and training: policy brief on regulation of health professions education. https://www.who.int/hrh/resources/transf_scaling_hpet/en/. Accessed 9 Jul 2020

WHO (2013b) Interprofessional collaborative practice in primary health care: nursing and midwifery perspectives. https://www.who.int/hrh/resources/IPE_SixCaseStudies.pdf?ua=1. Accessed 11 Jul 2020

WHO (2015) Recommendations on interventions to improve pre-term birth outcomes. https://www.who.int/reproductivehealth/publications/maternal_perinatal_health/preterm-birth-guideline/en/. Accessed 28 Jun 2020

WHO (2016a) WHO recommendations on antenatal care for a positive pregnancy experience. https://www.who.int/reproductivehealth/publications/maternal_perinatal_health/anc-positive-pregnancy-experience/en/. Accessed 1 Jul 2020

WHO (2016b) Midwives' voices, midwives' realities. Findings from a global consultation on providing quality midwifery care. https://www.who.int/maternal_child_adolescent/documents/midwives-voices-realities/en/. Accessed 5 Jul 2020

WHO (2016c) Monitoring and evaluating digital health interventions: a practical guide to conducting research and assessment. WHO, Geneva

WHO (2018) Towards a global action plan for healthy lives and wellbeing for all: uniting to accelerate progress towards the health-related SDGs. https://apps.who.int/iris/handle/10665/311667. Accessed 9 Jul 2020

WHO (2019) Strengthening quality midwifery education for universal health coverage 2030: framework for action. https://apps.who.int/iris/bitstream/handle/10665/324738/9789241515849-eng.pdf?ua=1. Accessed 9 Jul 2020

WHO (2020a) WHO Health innovation group. https://www.who.int/life-course/about/who-health-innovation-group/en/. Accessed 7 Jun 2020

WHO (2020b) Nursing and midwifery: key facts. https://www.who.int/news-room/fact-sheets/detail/nursing-and-midwifery. Accessed 12 Jul 2020

Yanti Y, Claramita M, Emilia O et al (2015) Students' understanding of 'women-Centred care philosophy' in midwifery care through continuity of care (CoC) learning model: a quasi-experimental study. BMC Nurs 14:22

Zaracostas J (2020) How to fight an infodemic. Lancet 395(10225):676. https://doi.org/10.1016/S0140-6736(20)30461-X

Zietmann A, Chen Y, Kyratsis Y et al (2019) What makes innovations both 'stick' and 'spread'? A multidisciplinary systematic review to understand implementation depth and scale-up of innovations in healthcare. Implement Sci 14:69

Part IV

The Profession of Midwifery

Professionalising Midwifery

10

Expected Learning Outcomes
By the end of the chapter, the reader should be able to:

1. Define professionalisation and consider the attributes of a profession.
2. Reflect on the global history of the development of midwifery towards professionalism.
3. Consider the influence of gender and masculinisation on the profession.
4. Discuss the influence of medicalisation of childbirth on the development of midwifery.
5. Describe the role of midwifery education in professionalising midwifery taking into consideration the perceptions of various countries and regions.
6. Consider the influence of higher education and its impact on professionalising midwifery and enhancing career progression.
7. Discuss the concept of professional identity amongst midwives.

theories form a broad framework for practice and are most likely expressing the goals and core values of the profession. In addition the researchers specify that theories and models regarding professionalism in midwifery should always include professional caring and wisdom, interpersonal competence and personal and professional development (Halldorsdottir and Karlsdottir 2011:10–11).

The Nursing and Midwifery Council in the United Kingdom (UK) has stated that 'Professionalism means something to everyone who works as a nurse or midwife. Being an inspiring role model working in the best interests of people in your care, regardless of what position you hold and where you deliver care, is what really brings practice and behaviour together in harmony' (NMC 2018:i). Furthermore, it is stated that 'Good health and care outcomes are highly dependent on the professional practice and behaviours of nurses and midwives' (NMC 2018:1). Globally, midwifery has been on a long journey of professionalisation, and there have been many obstacles in its path. Today, midwives are increasingly being recognised as expert professionals; however, there is still a way to go in many countries, and numerous examples have been provided in Chapter 8 in the context of providing quality care.

10.1 Introduction

Midwifery has been described as both a scholarly and a practice discipline which is in constant evolution (Halldorsdottir and Karlsdottir 2011). Midwifery must essentially be theory based as the

10.2 Establishing a Definition

In seeking clarity, it is prudent initially to consider the definition of what constitutes a profession. Many meanings are offered, but the one most appli-

© Springer Nature Switzerland AG 2021
J. Kemp et al., *Global Midwifery: Principles, Policy and Practice*,
https://doi.org/10.1007/978-3-030-46765-4_10

cable in this context states that a profession is 'a vocation requiring knowledge of some department of learning or science' (Dictionary.com 2020) https://www.dictionary.com/browse/profession#:~:text=noun,science%3A%20the%20profession%20of%20teaching.&text=the%20body%20of%20persons%20engaged,respected%20by%20the%20medical%20profession. Whilst professionalism has been defined as 'the standards, practice or methods of a professional as opposed to an amateur', 'to professionalise' describes the activity of 'giving a professional character or status to; or to make into or establish as a profession' (Dictionary.com 2020). The difference between an occupation and a profession has been widely debated for decades (Abbott 1988; Freidson 2001; Evetts 2003; Surbhi 2018). Lester (2014) highlights the Latin root of the word profession, namely *'profiteri'*. He emphasises that this describes the act of making a public declaration or vow and indicates that a member of a profession demonstrates a recognised commitment to acquire relevant knowledge and skills and accepts the philosophy and approach of the identified profession. Skilled midwifery falls into the category of a profession, but in doing so, there is a presupposition that certain prerequisites exist. These are summarised in Box 10.1.

Box 10.1. Characteristics of a Profession

A profession

- Requires a high degree of knowledge and expertise in a specific field.
- Requires higher education and training.
- Possesses a unique body of knowledge that is constantly updated, evidence-based and new practices can therefore evolve.
- Undertakes continuing professional development.
- Is controlled by statute.
- Has a distinct scope of practice.
- Establishes clear standards of practice that are essential and durable and can be interpreted in different situations.
- Is completely independent, autonomous.
- Is guided by ethical codes specified in a code of conduct.
- Its members demonstrate accountability.
- Has a protected title.
- Its members are respected and valued.

Derived from:
Evetts 2003; Freidson 2001; ICM 2017; Lester 2014; NMC 2018; Surbhi 2018.

In considering the professionalisation of midwifery, this can indeed be considered something of an evolutionary process gradually moving towards a highly educated, scientific and skilled profession. A professional midwife describes a practitioner appropriately qualified in the science and art of midwifery and possessing recognised competencies. In the simplest of terms, this is the contrast between the traditional birth attendant (TBA) and the internationally recognised professional midwife. In a concept analysis examining 1983 papers on the topic, Khakbazan and Ebadi (2019) concluded that the concept of professionalism in midwifery had not clearly been explained. However, it is essential in this context to explore what is known and attempt to construct a picture of the process of midwifery professionalisation in the global context.

The international Confederation of Midwives (ICM) in seeking definition has specified that midwifery is a profession and that '…only midwives practise midwifery. It has a unique body of knowledge, skills and professional attitudes drawn from disciplines shared by other health professions such as science and sociology, but practised by midwives within a professional framework of autonomy, partnership, ethics and accountability' (ICM 2017).

From amongst 13 Arab nations, 11 were found to have at least one association that included 'midwife' in its name. This is reckoned to be important for the recognition of midwifery as an independent profession (UNFPA 2015). Others may provide maternity care, and these have been discussed in Chapter 2 and the various cadres listed in Box 2.4. However, it is important to reiterate that midwifery is a unique profession.

The NMC has specified that 'Professionalism is characterised by the autonomous evidence-

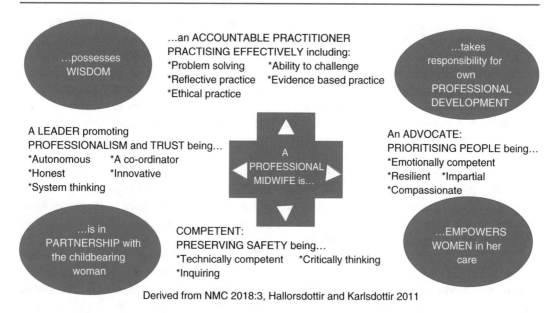

...possesses WISDOM

...an ACCOUNTABLE PRACTITIONER PRACTISING EFFECTIVELY including:
*Problem solving   *Ability to challenge
*Reflective practice   *Evidence based practice
*Ethical practice

...takes responsibility for own PROFESSIONAL DEVELOPMENT

A LEADER promoting
PROFESSIONALISM and TRUST being...
*Autonomous   *A co-ordinator
*Honest   *Innovative
*System thinking

A PROFESSIONAL MIDWIFE is...

An ADVOCATE:
PRIORITISING PEOPLE being...
*Emotionally competent
*Resilient   *Impartial
*Compassionate

...is in PARTNERSHIP with the childbearing woman

COMPETENT:
PRESERVING SAFETY being...
*Technically competent   *Critically thinking
*Inquiring

...EMPOWERS WOMEN in her care

Derived from NMC 2018:3, Hallorsdottir and Karlsdottir 2011

Fig. 10.1 The attributes of the professional midwife. (Derived from Nursing and Midwifery Council 2018:3; Halldorsdottir and Karlsdottir 2011)

based decision making by members of an occupation who share the same values and education' and that 'Professionalism in nursing and midwifery is realised through purposeful relationships and is underpinned by environments that facilitate professional practice'. Furthermore 'Professional nurses and midwives demonstrate and embrace accountability for their actions' (NMC 2018:3). A profession requires its members to practise effectively, promote professionalism and trust, prioritise people and preserve safety (NMC 2018). In the Scandinavian context, Halldorsdottir and Karlsdottir (2011) identify some key characteristics of what they regard as 'the good midwife', some of these synchronising with those later specified by the NMC. A composite picture of professionalism in midwifery is presented in Fig. 10.1 which graphically illustrates what is believed to constitute a professional midwife.

A survey amongst 1067 Turkish midwives concluded that although international professional values and codes of ethics contribute significantly to the professionalisation of midwifery, the respondents selected several preferred professional codes. These included respect for privacy, avoidance of deception, absence of conflicts of interest, reporting of faulty practices, consideration of mothers and newborns as separate beings and prevention of harm (Ergin et al. 2013). As Halldorsdottir and Karlsdottir (2011) have indicated, the professionalisation of midwifery is in a constant state of evolution and as yet what characterises the profession in one part of the globe may not necessarily do so in another; neither can it be assumed that some descriptions or definitions will remain valid over time. It is necessarily a dynamic concept.

10.3   The Development of Midwifery Professionalism Across the Globe

Midwives have served communities from the earliest times, though the process of professionalisation has emerged somewhat more slowly. Interventions from the seventeenth century onwards followed by early twentieth-century initiatives contributed to Sweden becoming a global frontrunner in establishing a skilled midwifery profession. This resulted in reducing maternal mortality. Norway and the Netherlands introduced trained midwives soon after Sweden. Early achievements in reducing the maternal death toll in Sweden were largely credited to an extensive collaboration between skilled physicians and very competent midwives who were available in the local communities. Swedish midwives were well trained in aseptic technique and taught to carry out operative procedures in the absence of physicians (Högberg 2004; De Brouwere 2007; Maclean 2017). Loudon (1992) attributes the historic decline in maternal mortality in England and Wales to an increasing number of births being undertaken by midwives and an improved standard of midwifery.

In 1925, the United States adopted a model of midwifery from Britain, which required training in both nursing and midwifery. However, primary care for childbearing women continued to be provided by some nurse-midwives but also by family nurse practitioners and physicians. Midwifery in Canada was introduced at a much later date. During the 1990s, midwifery began to be legally recognised as a profession in some Canadian provinces, and provincial or territorial legislation was introduced to regulate midwifery. Ontario and Alberta were the first provinces to implement legislation to regulate Canadian midwifery in 1994. The Canadian midwifery model aims to promote normal birth, making women the primary decision-makers and providing continuity of care from pregnancy through to the postnatal period (Mah 2013).

The professionalisation of midwifery is undoubtedly influenced by legislation which regulates practice, and this has been discussed in some detail in Chapter 5. In Japan, the greatly revered 'granny midwife' was eventually replaced by a 'medical midwife'. The Midwives' Ordinance of 1899 included a reduction in age for acceptance into midwifery training, it marked the beginning of professionalisation of midwifery in Japan but also its intermingling with nursing (Limura 2015). More recently, an 'advanced midwife' has evolved in Japan. This midwife works independent of but in harmony with physicians (Koshiyama et al. 2016). At the beginning of the twenty-first century, Australian midwives were still campaigning for a Midwives' Act. They advocated a national approach to coordinate the education of student midwives including the need to introduce competency-based practice. There was also emphasis on introducing various models of practice as well as a 3-year Bachelor of Midwifery degree (James and Willis 2001). By 2010, the Australian Health Practitioner Agency had amalgamated the national registration of health professionals across the country and introduced a separate register for midwives. However, 6 years later, it was noted that the simultaneous introduction of regulatory and legislative changes had resulted in the construction of categories within contemporary midwifery practice. These did not inevitably align with the Nursing and Midwifery Board of Australia (NMBA) requirements for re-registration (Gray et al. 2015). By 2018, the NMBA had established clear standards of practice to identify a framework for midwifery in all contexts with an emphasis placed on woman-centred care (NMBA 2018).

Although it has been recognised that progress has been made, in a study exploring the professionalisation of midwifery in Europe, Vermeulen et al. (2019) state that there remain some current areas of concern. The study involved delegates of the European Midwives' Association from 29 countries who participated in an online inquiry. It was concluded that future attempts to advance professionalisation in Europe should focus on the challenges apparent in current practice, leadership, healthcare culture and politics.

A study amongst Slovenian midwives concluded that midwifery in their country could not yet be considered a profession. Some respondents considered obstetrics to be a threat, and others perceived nursing as a challenge (Mivšek et al. 2015). The situation in Slovenia could perhaps be perceived as an example of an earlier stage of the evolutionary process of professionalisation. Midwifery in Bangladesh is another example of professionalisation in process. The establishment of a midwives' association in 2010 has helped development, and this has been assisted through a partnership with the Royal College of Midwives (RCM) in the UK since 2017. The relevance of midwifery associations is discussed in Chapter 6 and the value of partnerships in Chapter 15. Prior to 2010, midwifery was not recognised as a separate profession in Bangladesh, until the Prime Minister promoted the deployment of 3000 midwives in order to address the situation relating to poor outcomes in maternal and newborn health (MIDIRS 2017). Likewise, the Afghan Midwives' Association has played an important part in promoting the development of midwifery as a distinct profession. The emphasis is on education, registration, accreditation and career development, and there is a wide recognition both nationally and internationally of this professional association which is making a significant contribution to developing midwifery as well as promoting maternal and newborn health (AMA 2020). The Palestinian Ministry of Health has promoted the status and autonomy of women who work as professional midwives. Through a system of continuity of care in rural areas, Palestinian midwives working in urban hospitals were also given responsibility for SRMNH care in one village, providing them with a car in order to access the area. This system is reported to have enhanced the professionalisation of midwifery in the country (UNFPA 2015).

10.4   The Influence of Medicalisation and Male Gender Superiority

In the United States of America (USA), there has been a long tradition of midwives being marginalised by obstetricians. Previously most of the midwives were untrained and unsupervised and medical men viewed them as 'barbaric'. Historically, American obstetricians criticised the European practice of employing midwives and considered this reflected the backward state of those nations. However, where midwives were trained and supervised in the USA, maternal death rates were markedly reduced by comparison with those supervised by doctors. For example, in one area, the Maternal Mortality Ratio (MMR) was reduced to 150 amongst midwives' cases whilst it stood at 690 for physicians' cases (Porges 1985; Loudon 1997). In reviewing the history of midwifery in the USA, Brack (1975)

considered that childbirth was redefined as a medical rather than a social event. As a result, it is purported that the professional roles and care surrounding birth were altered and rationalised to suit medical needs. The cultural issues thought to contribute to these fundamental changes include the processes of industrialisation and urbanisation. Also 'the building of hospitals, the development of scientific knowledge and medical technology, ratios of physicians to population, and the political power of medical associations' were believed to be influential (Brack 1975:18).

In England and Wales, midwives were not regulated by law until the Midwives Act of 1902. However, interpretation and implementation of the Act were sporadic. Rivalry between general practitioners and midwives was widespread, and it was reported that the Midwives Act was used in order to harass midwives instead of inspiring improvement amongst them (Donnison 1988). At the turn of the century, Cahill (2001) reflecting on the historic male dominance and medicalisation of childbirth from the UK perspective concludes that the custom of justifying female inferiority was developed and encouraged not only through professional socialisation but also through approaches in medical education and practice. This resulted in the concept that the female body was inherently defective, and this was evident in the gender discrimination influencing a woman's place in society. The possibility of women being able to make informed choices therefore became very restricted, perpetuating the prevailing gender order. Cahill's conclusions find some resonance with those expressed by Brack (1975) concerning the American situation and cited above.

During the sixteenth century, midwifery in France was officially regarded as an occupation. The earliest formal recognition of midwifery there was as a profession supervised by the church. Midwives were expected to uphold the teachings of the church and were used as expert witnesses in cases of contested virginity, abortion, infanticide and sterility (Jones 2018). This reflects the situation of the early Swedish midwives who were licensed by the church (Högberg 2004). Sheridan (1999) concludes that in the seventeenth century the role of the French mid-wife in the medical hierarchy was bound up in state formation and consolidation. This resulted in the fact that midwives could still practise but, in the end, they were viewed as marginal to the medical community. However, French midwifery gradually transitioned into a profession, surviving the emergence of the male medical profession and eventually developing into a modern profession involved in the majority of births and supervising contemporary childbirth practices. Nevertheless, there was a history of conflict as gynaecology and obstetrics became a male-dominated profession, and in the twentieth century, along with much of Western Europe, childbirth became medicalised in hospital settings. As birth has been increasingly influenced by technology in more recent decades, it is usual for women in France to be cared for by an interdisciplinary team. French midwives complete a 4-year professional education programme and play an important part in antenatal and postnatal care too (Jones 2018).

It has been noted that between the late eighteenth and early twentieth century, there was a transition in childbirth practices from the 'wise woman' midwife to the male medical specialist across the industrialised world. In several countries, the gender-focused struggle led to a process of separation between midwifery and other branches of modern medicine. However, in Germany, midwives were actively involved in the shift away from traditional practice moving towards modern evidence-based healthcare provision. German midwives helped to protect their essential part in providing assistance to women during childbirth, and they achieved this by presenting a well-ordered voice and working together towards professionalisation (Fallwell 2013).

It has been acknowledged worldwide that around 15% of women will need obstetric interventions due to complications of pregnancy and birth, and so obstetricians have an important role to play (WHO 2017). However, at the beginning of the twenty-first century, it was asserted that in high-income countries, obstetric interventions in normal childbirth had become routine in the absence of any reliable evidence. Influencing factors in this issue have been related to medico-legal issues, private practice and omitting to wholly involve women in the decision-making process (Johanson et al. 2002). The opinion of a male midwife in the UK echoes the sentiment of Johanson et al. in stating that the male medical positivist approach concentrated on the mechanics of childbirth. This created an opportunity not only for intervening in a normal process but also to receive payment for doing so (Pendleton 2019).

The advent of male midwives in the UK was subsequent to the Sex Discrimination Act in 1976 which allowed men to be educated in the profession. Although men were limited initially in where they could practice, prejudice was gradually overcome, nonetheless male midwives still constitute a small minority of the profession (NMC 2019). In other parts of the world, male midwives have experienced a variable degree of acceptance. For example, reports from Cameroon indicate that there is a preference for a male midwife amongst Christian women who find them more attentive than their female counterparts, but Muslim women find this culturally unacceptable. However, the government was reported to be striving to educate more male midwives in order to address the acute shortage of professional midwives (Nofuru 2012). By contrast, the Ghanaian government abolished a pilot programme to train male midwives due to objection expressed by women (Suuk 2017). Undoubtedly, gender issues will to some extent continue to influence maternity care in many parts of the world.

It can be observed that obstetrics in many parts of the world is now female-dominated, but these professionals may still operate within a medical model. In this case, it needs to be asked whether it is the gender of the professional that is important or the paradigm of the profession to which they belong. It has been argued that when midwives are professionalised, they move further away from women, though this has been an area

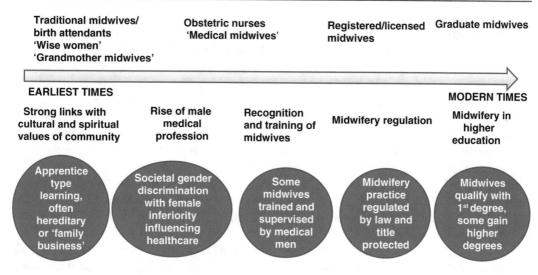

Fig. 10.2 The evolving process of midwifery professionalisation

of debate. Cronk (2010) identifying a midwife as a 'professional servant' suggests that the process of professionalisation has caused the 'servant' part of this description to be largely overlooked. The closeness and distance between mothers and midwives in this professional friendship offer variable degrees of confidence. According to Anderson (2010), the former enabling the woman to feel comfortable and the latter preventing the midwife's issues from encroaching on the woman's concerns. Nevertheless, Pairman (2010) reports that a new alliance between mothers and midwives brought about legislative changes in New Zealand and forged a 'new professionalism' which demonstrated an equitable and reciprocal relationship between mothers and midwives.

Undoubtedly, gender issues will to some extent continue to influence maternity care in many parts of the world. However, as midwifery evolves into a strong, compassionate, well-educated profession and women demonstrate preference for non-interventionist approaches, there is hope that the principles and practice associated with medicalisation of normal childbirth, and male dominance will be relegated to the history books. The concept of the dynamic and evolutionary process of professionalising midwifery discussed above is summarised in Fig. 10.2.

10.5   Educational Perspectives

It became evident during the 1980s and 1990s that across Europe, there was an increased demand by midwives for greater professionalisation of midwifery. It is considered that the 1999 Bologna Declaration reinforced professional development in midwifery education and research; however, whether this had influenced the situation in respect of practice has remained unclear (Vermeulen et al. 2019). In a study of 13 Arab countries, it was established that only two required continual professional development as a prerequisite to re-licensing. However, the midwives' associations of most countries in the region play a part in promoting professional development. In Somalia, several new midwifery schools have been opened since 2012, so that during the ensuing 3 years, it was estimated that there were to be at least 15 functioning and accredited schools in the country (UNFPA 2015). By the end of 2016, a new midwifery curriculum in Somalia was officially recognised by the International Confederation of Midwives (ICM) as meeting international standards (UNFPA 2016).

The study in Slovenia cited earlier concerning the concept of professionalisation also considered educational issues. The authors recommend that the content and structure of midwifery education should be analysed and changed. This is considered essential if a specific professional identity for midwives is to be developed. It is further considered that changes in education would result in improved socialisation and professionalism. Furthermore, it is recommended that it should be agreed between all professional groups that the scope of midwifery practice and midwife responsibilities should follow those defined in the European Union (EU) directives (Mivšek et al. 2015). The necessity of analysing and adapting midwifery education is reflected in the Icelandic context in the work of Halldorsdottir and Karlsdottir (2011:11) who maintain that in curriculum planning 'emphasis should be placed on evaluating the attitudes, interpersonal competence and self-care of student midwives and not only their cognitive and practical competencies'. Such an action is perceived as essential in preparing students for a modern midwifery profession.

The history and detail of midwifery education and higher education are discussed in some depth in Chapter 4.

10.5.1 Into Higher Education

In the study cited earlier (Vermeulen et al. 2019), most of the European countries responding reported that progress towards professionalisation of midwifery had been made as a result of moving midwifery education into higher education. The opportunities offered for postgraduate education and research had also had a positive effect in this situation. However, the loss of clinical experience and consequent expertise as midwives move into higher education presents a real threat, and this needs to be carefully managed. Efforts in the Arab region have also been enhancing the preparation of professional midwives, for example, in Lebanon the midwifery curriculum has been adapted at one university to establish a competency-based programme. In Morocco, midwives are licensed and can also qualify at a masters or doctoral level (UNFPA 2015). In parts of Africa, the opportunities offered through the

Africa Midwives Research Network (AMRN) and later the Lugina Africa Midwives Research Network (LAMRN) have made breakthroughs into higher education and the professionalisation of midwifery. The activities of these networks are discussed in Chapter 12. An evaluation of AMRN demonstrated that the emphasis placed on midwifery research and evidence-based midwifery practice had begun to transform the approach of midwives who benefited from the higher education, experience and vision displayed by the Network (Forss and Maclean 2007). The advanced international training programmes offered through AMRN had formed part of the Swedish government's commitment to an agenda providing education on gender, sexual and reproductive health and rights, professionalisation, management and evidence-based midwifery care (Sida 2009). LAMRN has continued to conduct research and improve quality in midwifery education and practice in six sub-Saharan countries. This is a partnership between Manchester University (UK) and universities with midwifery higher educational institutions in those countries, namely Kenya, Malawi, Tanzania, Uganda, Zambia and Zimbabwe. The stated goal of this multi-country partnership is 'to develop a thriving, collaborative and sustainable research network with the capacity and skills to strengthen evidence-based practice, thus improving care for women and babies' (LAMRN 2017). Undoubtedly, higher education and research go hand in hand with the professionalisation of midwifery and may be considered as catalysts in this ever-evolving process.

10.5.2 Professional Identity Amongst Midwives

In Guatemala, midwives perceive themselves as especially chosen to follow their vocation in the tradition of their predecessors. It is said of the midwife: 'She walks on foot. She crosses mountains and lakes. She carries tradition on her back and healing in her hands. She was chosen for this' (Zeltzer 2018). It may be argued that this more likely describes the TBA, but Hunter and

Warren (2013) purport that 'midwifery (is) commonly described as something someone is rather than what they do'. This combines with a sense of public service and the aspiration to contribute to the 'greater good'. They maintain that there is emphasis here on the deeply integrated professional and personal identities observed in the roles of some healthcare workers (Hunter and Warren 2013:32). This concept surely resonates with the Guatemalan philosophy of the midwife cited above. It may be asked, does vocation inevitably conflict with professionalism or is it an essential hybrid in the modern professional identity of the midwife?

Khakbazan and Ebadi (2019:LE08) in undertaking an extensive integrative literature review on the topic conclude that professionalism in midwifery comprises 'a set of personal requirements, professional requirements and intraprofessional morality'. They consider that for a midwife to maintain professionalism, she should use her personality traits, self-leadership and also 'adhere to ethical codes in direction of professional scientism, professional communication, sympathetic and trust-based interactions, patient-centered care, team-focused care, professional responsibility and commitment to the profession'. In the UK, the NMC also acknowledges that the concept of professionalism may vary amongst individuals and is influenced by their personal value system. Nevertheless, a framework has been developed which aims to strengthen and support nurses and midwives in their leadership roles, assist them in articulating their effectiveness, demonstrating accountability and meeting revalidation requirements. Also, it provides practical examples of what can be expected of these practitioners by the public (NMC 2018).

In China, the concept of hybridism has emerged where midwives have found themselves caught between two definitions. Namely 'the obstetric nurse' whose role was associated with the medical management of childbirth including risk management and 'the professional midwife' advocating natural birth. As a result of the conflicting concepts, a 'hybrid identity' was constructed. This emerged from what was described

as 'the dynamic nature of midwifery professional identity' (Zhang 2015:388).

In considering the effect of interprofessional education (IPE) on 1254 health and social care students including a small sample of midwifery candidates, Adams et al. (2006:55) consider that there were considerable differences in the perception of professional identity across the different disciplines. They identify certain variables as significant predictors of baseline professional identity. As well as the variations between the professions these included gender, previous work experience in health and social care, understanding of team working, knowledge of their profession and cognitive flexibility. Experienced midwives in Sweden reported that their professional identity had been challenged as a result of the increasing technology used in childbirth as well as the roles of other professionals involved and the demands of contemporary parents (Larsson and Aldegarmann 2009). The twenty-first century Swedish midwife undoubtedly has a differing perception of professional identity by comparison with her counterparts in the early centuries in that country, and these attributes were discussed above (Högberg 2004).

In a review of professional identities and regulation, a UK regulatory body asserts that identity matters can be complicated by factors including technology. It is maintained that 'caring values arguably have greater prominence for nursing and midwifery identity than for pharmacists, who might place greater emphasis on the "scientist" portion'. Nevertheless, it is argued that technology can enhance identity, as 'nurses take on the role of data custodians or change the nature of patient encounters or the environment in which professionals operate' (Professional Standards Authority 2016:20). Midwives in various countries have expanded their roles in response to the evolving professional situation and the changing world which surrounds them. This can be illustrated in those who train as surgical assistants and are trained to carry out caesarean sections in countries including Ghana, Ethiopia, Malawi, Mozambique and Tanzania (Pereira et al. 1996; Vaz et al. 1999; Dovlo 2004; Kruk et al. 2007). Those skilled in ultrasound

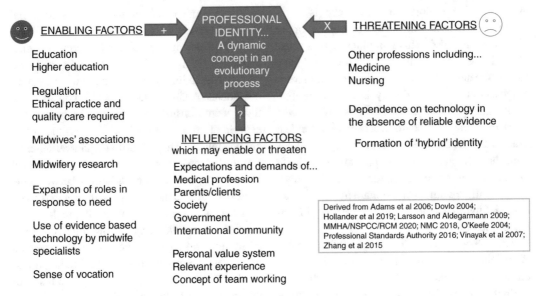

Fig. 10.3 Concepts of professional identity in midwifery. (Derived from Adams et al. 2006; Dovlo 2004; Hollander et al. 2019; Larsson and Aldegarmann 2009; MMHA/ NSPCC/RCM 2020; NMC 2018; O'Keefe 2004; Professional Standards Authority 2016; Vinayak et al. 2017; Zhang 2015)

technology (O'Keefe 2004) and others use mobile phones and tablets to transmit ultrasound readings from remote rural areas (Vinayak et al. 2017). Some midwives have become experts in counselling, psychology and mental health (MMHA/NSPCC/RCM 2020) whilst others may focus on research, epidemiology or other specialisms. A small proportion of midwives in the Netherlands, a country with a longstanding record of safe birthing and minimal intervention, identify themselves as 'holistic midwives'. These practitioners place emphasis on 'addressing a need' which they consider is not met within the organised healthcare system. They provide their clients with various options including homeopathy, herbal remedies and massage techniques (Hollander et al. 2019). Indeed, the professional identity of midwives could well be perceived to be moving with the times in this scientific and technological age whilst striving to meet varying societal needs and demands. The latter may also encompass requests for reflexology and acupuncture and some other holistic approaches cited above. Innovations in practice and how midwives are responding and using these are discussed in Chapter 9.

Figure 10.3 summarises the concepts of professional identity as identified in the literature. It needs to be appreciated that this phenomenon is dynamic and subject to change in an ever-changing world. Therefore, factors that enable may, in time and in variable situations, become threatening factors and vice versa. For example, the concept of Artificial Intelligence (AI), although offering some benefits, may place people at risk if they rely on technology for diagnosis and management of problems without consulting a medical or health professional. Every woman has the right to access the care of a professional midwife who cannot be replaced by any technological app or gadget. The concept is indeed dynamic in the evolutionary process of professionalisation.

10.6 Conclusion

Midwifery professionalisation has been perceived as an evolutionary process. The profession has transitioned from a traditional occupation to one that is highly skilled and internationally recognised. The progression has been influenced by education, higher education and research as well as the changes and demands of society and the international community. However, the professionalisation of midwifery proceeds at different rates and often in different directions in different countries. For the ultimate benefit of women and their families, the professionalisation of midwifery needs to proceed scientifically, using evidence-based skills but also clothed with compassion and respect wherever this profession is practised.

Key Messages

Principles

- The principle of professionalisation needs to be perceived as a process which is constantly evolving. Midwifery presents a dynamic situation which constantly changes at variable rates across the globe.

Policy

- As the midwifery profession constantly develops and diversifies, midwives need to be engaged at various levels of policymaking and implementation on all issues that affect childbearing women, newborns, sexual and reproductive healthcare and midwifery education and practice.

Practice

- Wherever midwives have become highly skilled professionals, they should be enabled to practice to their full capacity in political and practice environments which are enabling rather than disabling or limiting. Every woman should have access to a professional midwife who can provide skilled and respectful care.

Questions for Reflection or Review

1. Vermeulen et al. (2019) state that future attempts to advance professionalisation in Europe should focus on the challenges apparent in current practice, leadership, healthcare culture and

politics. How true do you think this could be when applied to other regions of the world? Building on these concepts can you identify approaches which could be used to accelerate progress towards professionalisation of midwifery in an area with which you are familiar?

2. The question was mooted above as to whether vocation inevitably conflicts with professionalism or whether these qualities essentially contribute to a hybrid in the modern professional identity of the midwife. How do you perceive these concepts?

3. It has been suggested that moving midwifery into higher education has enhanced the process of professionalisation in many countries. In your experience how has this move affected clinical expertise? Considering advances in this context in Lebanon cited above (UNFPA 2015), can you find other examples of ensuring that competency-based education for practice proceeds in tandem with higher education?

Additional Resources for Reflection and Further Study

Explore the Midwifery Leaders Showcase on the ICM website and consider the dynamic and diverse roles that midwives all around the world fulfil and how they make a difference. https://www.internationalmidwives.org/icm-projects/midwifery-leaders-showcase/. Accessed 2 Apr 2020

Nursing and Midwifery Council (2018) Enabling professionalism. Nursing and Midwifery Council, London https://www.nmc.org.uk/standards/guidance/professionalism/read-report/. Accessed 4 Mar 2020

References

Abbott A (1988) The system of professions. University of Chicago Press, Chicago

Adams K, Hean S, Sturgis P et al (2006) Investigating the factors influencing professional identity amongst first year health and social care students. Learn Health Soc Care 5(2):55–68

Afghan Midwives Association (2020) Strengthening Midwifery in Afghanistan: History. Afghan Midwives Association http://afghanmidwives.org/history/. Accessed 6 Mar 2020

Anderson T (2010) Feeling safe enough to let go: the relationship between a woman and her midwife during the second stage of labour. Chapter 7. In: Kirkham M (ed) The midwife-mother relationship. Red Globe Press, Macmillan International, London

Brack DC (1975) Displaced—the midwife by the male physician. Women Health 1(6):18–24. Published online 26 Oct 2008. https://www.tandfonline.com/doi/abs/10.1300/J013v01n06_04. Accessed 21 Mar 2020

Cahill HA (2001) Male Appropriation and medicalization of childbirth: an historical analysis. J Adv Nurs 33(3):334–342. https://pdfs.semanticscholar.org/e591/8d6d0b1538266ab4c351e7e7bf99613ec9b9.pdf. Accessed 21 Mar 2020

Cronk M (2010) The midwife: a professional servant? Chapter 4. In: Kirkham M (ed) The midwife-mother relationship. Red Globe Press, Macmillan International, London

De Brouwere V (2007) The comparative study of maternal mortality over time: the role of the professionalisation of childbirth. Soc Hist Med 20(3):541–562. Accessed 7 Mar 2020. https://doi.org/10.1093/shm/hkm070

Dictionary.com (2020) Professionalism; professionalise. https://www.dictionary.com/browse/professionalism?s=t. Accessed 5 Mar 2020

Donnison J (1988) Midwives and medical men: a history of the struggle for the control of childbirth. Hienemann, London

Dovlo D (2004) Using mid-level cadres as substitutes for internationally mobile health professionals in Africa. A desk review. Hum Resour Health 2:7. Accessed 24 Mar 2020. https://doi.org/10.1186/1478-4491-2-7

Ergin A, Ozcan M, Acar Z et al (2013) Determination of national midwifery ethical values and ethical codes: in Turkey. Nurs Ethics 20(7):808–818

Evetts J (2003) The sociological analysis of professionalism: occupational change in the modern world. Int Sociol 18(2):395–415

Fallwell LA (2013) Modern German midwifery, 1885–1960. (studies for the Society for the Social History of medicine, 13.) xiii + 263 pp., bibl., index. Pickering & Chatto, London. ISBN 1848934289, 9781848934283

Forss K, Maclean GD (2007) The Africa Midwives Research Network. Sida evaluation 07/16. Department for Democracy & Social Development, Stockholm

Freidson E (2001) Professionalism: the third logic. Polity, Cambridge

Gray M, Rowe J, Barnes M (2015) Midwifery professionalisation and practice: Influences of the changed registration standards in Australia. Women Birth 1:54–61. Accessed 4 Mar 2020. https://doi.org/10.1016/j.wombi.2015.08.005

Halldorsdottir S, Karlsdottir SI (2011) The primacy of the good midwife in midwifery services: an evolving theory of professionalism in midwifery. Scand J Caring Sci 25(4):806–817. https://doi.org/10.1111/j.1471-6712.2011.00886.x

Högberg U (2004) The decline in maternal mortality in Sweden. Am J Publ Health 94(8):1312–1320. https://doi.org/10.2105/AJPH.94.8.1312

Hollander M, de Miranda E, Vandenbussche F et al (2019) Addressing a need: Holistic midwifery in the Netherlands' a qualitative analysis. PLoS One. https://journals.plos.org/plosone/article?id=10.1371/journal.pone.0220489. Accessed 25 Mar 2020

Hunter B, Warren L (2013) Investigating resilience in midwifery. Final report. Cardiff University, Cardiff. http://orca.cf.ac.uk/61594/1/Investigating%20resilience%20Final%20report%20oct%202013.pdf. Accessed 23 Mar 2020

International Confederation of Midwives (2017) Definition of Midwifery. Core Document. CD2017_001 ENG. International Confederation of Midwives, The Hague, Netherlands. https://www.internationalmidwives.org/assets/files/definitions-files/2018/06/eng-definition_midwifery.pdf. Accessed 5 Mar 2020

James HL, Willis I (2001) The professionalisation of midwifery through education or politics? Aust J Midwifery 14(4):27–30. Accessed 4 Mar 2020. https://doi.org/10.1016/S1445-4386(01)80010-0

Johanson R, Newburn M, Macfarlane A (2002) Has the medicalisation of childbirth gone too far? BMJ 324(7342):892–895. https://www.ncbi.nlm.nih.gov/pmc/articles/PMC1122835/. Accessed 20 Mar 2020

Jones E (2018) Midwifery in France https://medium.com/midwifery-around-the-world/midwifery-in-france-450b3b5821e2. Accessed 11 Mar 2020

Khakbazan Z, Ebadi A (2019) Midwifery professionalism: an integrated review. J Clin Diagn Res 13(3):LE01–LE08. https://doi.org/10.7860/JCDR/2019/38209.12654

Koshiyama M, Watanabe Y, Moto-oka N et al (2016) The current state of professional midwives in Japan and their traditional virtues. Womens Health 2(1):8–10. https://openventio.org/wp-content/uploads/2017/10/The-Current-State-of-Professional-Midwives-in-Japan-and-their-Traditional-Virtues-WHOJ-2-114.pdf. Accessed 7 Mar 2020

Kruk ME, Pereira C, Vaz F et al (2007) Economic evaluation of surgically trained assistant medical officers in performing major obstetric surgery in Mozambique. BJOG 114(10):1253–1260. https://doi.org/10.1111/j.1471-0528.2007.01443.x

Larsson M, Aldegarmann U (2009) Professional role and identity in a changing society: three paradoxes in Swedish midwives' experiences. Midwifery 25(4):373–381. https://doi.org/10.1016/j.midw.2014.11.013

Lester S (2014) Professional versus occupational models of work competence. Res Post Compuls Educ 19(3):276–286. https://doi.org/10.1080/13596748.2014.920569

Limura B (2015) History of midwifery in Japan. Midwifery Today 114. https://midwiferytoday.com/

mt-articles/history-of-midwifery-in-japan/. Accessed 7 Mar 2020

Loudon I (1992) Death in childbirth. Clarendon Press, Oxford

Loudon I (1997) Midwives and the quality of maternal care. In: Marland H, Rafferty AM (eds) Midwives, society and childbirth. Debates and controversies in the modern period. Routledge, London and New York, pp 180–200

Lugina African Midwives Research Network (2017) The Lugina Africa Midwives Research Network. http://lamrn.org/aboutus/our-story/. Accessed 12 Mar 2020

Maclean GD (2017) Achieving safe motherhood globally—an historical overview. Lambert Academic Publishing, Saarbrücken

Mah L (2013) Midwifery in Canada. Birth and the Law 38–2: LawNow. https://www.lawnow.org/midwifery-canada/. Accessed 5 Mar 2020

Maternal Mental Health Alliance/National Society for Prevention of Cruelty to Children/Royal College of Midwives (2020) Specialist mental Health Midwives: What they do and why they matter. Maternal Mental Health Alliance. https://www.rcm.org.uk/media/2370/specialist-mental-health-midwives-what-they-do-and-why-they-matter.pdf. Accessed 25 Mar 2020

Midwives Information and Resource Services (2017) Partnership to strengthen midwifery in Bangladesh launched. Midirs 7 July. https://www.midirs.org/partnership-strengthen-midwifery-bangladesh-launched/. Accessed 6 Mar 2020

Mivšek P, Pahor M, Hlebec V, Hundley V (2015) How do midwives in Slovenia view their professional status? Midwifery (early online) http://www.sciencedirect.com/science/article/pii/S0266613815002260. Accessed 4 Mar 2020

Nofuru N (2012) Rise in male midwives divides clientele along religious lines in Camaroon. Global Press J. https://globalpressjournal.com/africa/cameroon/rise-in-male-midwives-divides-clientele-along-religious-lines-in-cameroon/. Accessed 21 Mar 2020

Nursing and Midwifery Board of Australia (2018) Midwife Standards for Practice. Nursing and Midwifery Board of Australia. https://www.nursingmidwiferyboard.gov.au/Codes-Guidelines-Statements/Professional-standards/Midwife-standards-for-practice.aspx. Accessed 5 Mar 2020

Nursing and Midwifery Council (2018) Enabling professionalism. Nursing and Midwifery Council. London. https://www.nmc.org.uk/standards/guidance/professionalism/read-report/. Accessed 4 Mar 2020

Nursing and Midwifery Council (2019) The NMC Register. Nursing and Midwifery Council, London. https://www.nmc.org.uk/globalassets/sitedocuments/other-publications/nmc-register-data-march-19.pdf?. Accessed 21.03.2020

O'Keefe H (2004) Specialist sonographer. The World of Irish Nursing. https://www.inmo.ie/tempDocs/Midwifery.pdf. Accessed 24 Mar 2020

Pairman S (2010) Midwifery partnership: A professionalizing strategy for midwives. Chapter 12. In: Kirkham M (ed) The midwife-mother relationship. Red Globe Press, Macmillan International, London

Pendleton J (2019) What role does gender have in shaping knowledge that underpins the practice of midwifery? J Gender Stud 28(6):629–634. Accessed 21 Mar 2020. https://doi.org/10.1080/09589236.2019.1590185

Pereira C, Bugalho A, Bergstrom S et al (1996) A comparative study of caesarean deliveries by assistant medical officers in Mozambique. BJOG 103(6):508–512. https://doi.org/10.1111/j.1471-0528.1996.tb09797.x

Porges RF (1985) The response of the New-York obstetrical society to the report by the New York Academy of Medicine on maternal mortality, 1933–34. Am J Obstetr Gynecol 152:642–649

Professional Standards Authority (2016) Professional identities and regulation: a literature review. Professional Standards Authority for Health and Social Care, London. https://www.professional-standards.org.uk/docs/default-source/publications/professional-identities-and-regulation%2D%2D-a-literature-review.pdf?sfvrsn=a7e7120_0. Accessed 23 Mar 2020

Sheridan B (1999) At birth: the modern state, modern medicine, and the royal midwife Louise Bourgeois in seventeenth-century France. Dynamis: acta hispanica ad medicinae scientiarumque historiam illustrandam 19:145–166. https://core.ac.uk/download/pdf/39076992.pdf. Accessed 11 Mar 2020

Surbhi S (2018) Difference between occupation and profession. Key differences: https://keydifferences.com/difference-between-occupation-and-profession.html. Accessed 3 Apr 2020

Suuk M (2017) Ghanaian women reject male midwives. DW made for minds: Africa: 28.02.17. https://www.dw.com/en/ghanaian-women-reject-male-midwives/a-37733547. Accessed 21 Mar 2020

Swedish International Development Agency (2009) Strengthening midwifery competence in sexual and reproductive health and services. Advanced International Training Programme, Stockholm

United Nations Population Fund (2015) Analysis of the midwifery workforce in selected Arab countries. United Nations Population Fund Arab States Regional Office. https://arabstates.unfpa.org/sites/default/files/pub-pdf/SOWMY%20ASRO%20final%20-%20English.pdf. Accessed 7 Mar 2020

United Nations Population Fund (2016) New Somali midwifery curriculum gets international recognition. News. https://somalia.unfpa.org/en/news/new-somali-midwifery-curriculum-gets-international-recognition. Accessed 23 Mar 2020

Vaz F, Bergstrom S, Vaz M et al (1999) Training medical assistants for surgery. Bull World Health Organ 77(8):688–691

Vermeulen J, Luyben A, OÇonnell R et al (2019) Failure or progress? The current state of the professionalisation of midwifery in Europe. Eur J Midwifery

3(December):22. Accessed 4 Mar 2020. https://doi.org/10.18332/ejm/115038

Vinayak S, Sande J, Nisenbaum H et al (2017) Training midwives to perform basic obstetric point-of-care ultrasound in rural areas using a tablet platform and mobile phone transmission technology—AWFUMB Coe project. Ultrasound Med Biol 43(10):2125–2132. https://doi.org/10.1016/j.ultrasmedbio.2017.05.024

World Health Organization (2017) Managing complications in pregnancy and childbirth. A guide for midwives and doctors, 2nd edn. WHO/UNFPA/UNICEF. https://apps.who.int/iris/bitstream/handle/10665/255760/9789241565493-eng.pdf?sequence=1. Accessed 20 Mar 2020

Zeltzer N (2018) A sacred calling: Midwifery in Guatemala. https://medium.com/midwifery-around-the-world/a-sacred-calling-midwifery-in-guatemala-539768907dc7. Accessed 11 Mar 2020

Zhang J (2015) Navigating the self in maternity care: how Chinese midwives work on their professional identity in hospital setting. Midwifery 31(3):388–394. https://doi.org/10.1016/j.midw.2014.11.013

Midwifery Leadership

11

Expected Learning Outcomes

By the end of the chapter, the reader should be able to:

- Define the nature of leadership.
- Distinguish leadership, management and administration.
- Outline factors impacting on leadership.
- Discuss the evolution of leadership styles.
- Elucidate emerging leadership traits and competencies relevant for the twenty-first century.
- Establish what midwifery leaders can learn from other organisations and settings, competencies that strengthen their own leadership capacity.
- Build a case for midwifery leadership and strengthening of midwifery.

11.1 The Concept of Leadership

Leadership is a concept easily used in everyday conversation but understood by a few (Bojadjiev et al. 2019). The world is rapidly changing, and it is important to determine what is required to lead in a volatile, uncertain, complex and ambiguous environment.

11.2 Leadership Management and Administration

Leadership is about providing vision, purpose and direction. It is about aligning thoughts and ideas towards the achievement of a common goal. It involves communicating and motivating others to act, and includes priority setting, analysis of situations and innovations. Leadership is about people (Rathore et al. 2017).

Management involves making decisions to achieve predetermined goals. It focuses on systems, processes, structure and goals. Management exists for operational control, monitoring performance, planning, organising, allocating resources and evaluating processes. Managers ensure that things are done right. Some authors say management is about things (USAID 2015; Management Science for Health 2015).

Administration involves operationalising organisational plans, maintaining bureaucratic policies, implementing and maintaining established rules of procedure in the best way possible, at the most appropriate time for the achievement of objectives, utilising the systems and processes mandated by management. The focus of administration is on efficiency of processes for achievement of results (Yourdictionary 2018).

Effective leaders need to develop capacities from all three areas. They must be good managers able to guide administrative processes in the

© Springer Nature Switzerland AG 2021
J. Kemp et al., *Global Midwifery: Principles, Policy and Practice*,
https://doi.org/10.1007/978-3-030-46765-4_11

ward, in the institution and nationally depending on where they work (USAID 2015; Divall 2015; Mianda and Voce 2018).

11.3 Definition and the Nature of Leadership

Hollander and Julian (1969) defined leadership as a social interpersonal influence relationship between two or more persons who depend on each other to attain certain mutual goals. So did Kanter (1982), Reid (2016) and Rathore et al. (2017). Parris and Hart (2013) and Adeyemi and Bolarinwa (2013) added the words 'to work *devotedly*' and 'to strive *willingly*' towards the achievement of objectives. Putting all these definitions together, the 'influence' is about providing vision, purpose and direction; aligning thoughts and ideas and steering people towards the achievement of a common goal. In situations of rapid change, intense competition, an explosion of new technologies, chaos, turbulence and high levels of uncertainty, leadership is critical to offer a pathway of confidence and direction, creativity and effective management of change (Bennis and Thomas 2002). In some cases, leadership involves changing people's thinking, perceptions, character and behaviour, so that they exert themselves 'willingly' in doing something(s) which they would otherwise have not done (Conger 2012). The twenty-first century turbulence and chaos has led to a rapid change in the composition of the midwifery workforce and the recipients of midwifery care. Hence, midwifery leadership needs special capabilities to respond to these changes (Bennis and Thomas 2007; Conger 2012; Lee Iacocca in Bojadjiev et al. 2017).

11.3.1 The Leadership Process

Organisations have moved away from the traditional, hierarchical structures to expanding roles of members in decision-making (Elangovan and Xie 2000; Byrom and Doiwne 2010; Carlton and Perloff 2015). Leaders more readily delegate power to different levels of the organisation (Choy et al. 2016). Midwifery leaders can learn from this trend especially in professional associations where contributing to the decision-making processes motivates and gives members a sense of belonging.

In maternal and child health (MCH) services, midwifery leaders need collaborative leadership practices to navigate the public health systems in which they work (De Pree 2006). Collaborative leadership practices involve power sharing and are process based (Clarke and Cilenti 2017). Collaborative leadership is vision based and makes it necessary and possible to convene and engage necessary stakeholders for a systems approach in solving MCH issues in the complex setting in which care is provided (Leadership Academy 2011).

11.3.2 Clinical Leadership

Mianda and Voce (2018), Jarvis and Reeves (2017) and Divall (2015) point out a gap that has persisted in midwifery leadership and clinical leadership. Emphasis has been placed on position leadership to the neglect of leadership on the bedside and in the maternity ward. In the United Kingdom, clinical leadership has been provided as an outreach activity by a District Clinical Specialist Team. This has gradually been supplemented by team leadership where every member develops some leadership capacity and exercises that during care provision. Power is shared among the team. Decision-making is by the clinicians. In addition, clinical leaders have been nurtured who have all the characteristics of a position leader. Their clinical expertise and their application of generic leadership skills to specific clinical settings differentiate them from the position leader. Self-directed learning and maintenance of clinical competence are essential for clinical leaders. The responsibilities of clinical leaders centre around organisation of care processes, ensuring better performance in the ward, well-being of women and newborn and staff, quality management and control as well as identifying best practices in care provision (Managament Science for Health 2015). They also serve as clinical mentors, facilitators of professional development of staff and building strong teams, conducive work environment and team building (Fizza et al. 2019).

11.4 Power and Leadership

Midwifery leaders need power to achieve objectives and to increase the credibility and visibility of the profession. A clear understanding and effective use of power enhance the leader's capacity to contribute to policy and engage intelligently in negotiations and advocacy settings.

Power is fluid, expendable and mostly remains potential. Power may be overt or covert, formal or informal and can be possessed by individuals or a group. Power is like a savings account. It has to be earned, saved and used well in order to last and is neutral until exercised (ICM 2014). Midwifery leaders need to recognise their power bases especially because in some countries, it takes a few years for a midwife to rise to a position of power.

11.4.1 Power Bases

Power bases are the sources of power. *Organizational or institutional* power comes from one's position in the organization giving rise to three power bases: position, reward and coercion power. *Personal* power emanates from the individual's inherent characteristics and personal traits, acquired or potential, giving rise to four power bases: referent (charismatic), expert, information and relationship power (Box 11.1).

11.4.2 Leveraging Power

Leveraging power is a skill (De Pree 2006) (Box 11.2). Technology has enabled the development of vast social networks making relationships and access to knowledge and information easier than ever before (Center for Creative Leadership 2013). Important and extraordinary, highly visible relationships can be forged with stakeholder groups in different parts of the world (Kanter 2002; Wright and Taylor 1994). Midwifery leaders should *invest* time and energy in existing relationships and creating new ones; *identify* persons to learn from and with whom to establish a relationship; *repair* damaged or neglected relationships, build trust, repair own image when needed, demonstrate confidence and develop their own brand of charisma.

With effective use of power, midwifery leaders ensure that priorities of midwifery care are heard at the right levels, that quality care is delivered and that outcomes are improved for women, newborns and families (Read 2019). Midwives need a means by which they can work in collaboration with nurses and not be subsumed in the nursing agenda (Read 2019). With adequate awareness of the power they possess, midwives can display significant leadership capabilities, authority and confidence to do things differently. As stated by Richard Buckminster Fuller:

> You can never change things by fighting the existing normal. To change something, build a new model that makes the existing one obsolete. (Read 2019:7)

> **Box 11.1. Power Bases: Brief summaries**
> **Organisational/Institutional Power**
> *Position power:* Legitimate power or authority is power bestowed on an individual by her/his position in the organization. Others accept this power and are ready and expected to submit to it. The higher a person is in the organization the more power the person has.
> *Reward power* relates to one's capacity to reward others because of control over reward mechanisms and resources (e.g. promotions, salary raise, positive appraisal). This is usually supported by the individual's position in the organization.
> *Coercive power* relates to one's capacity to make others do what they might not want to do. It is associated with the capacity to punish others. It is also related to position power but can belong to anyone (e.g. strikes, blackmail)! Coercive power is the least-leveraged source of power (Centre for Creative Leadership 2013).
> **Personal Power**
> *Referent power* is based on charisma (charismatic power) and good will generated by a leader's style or persona. A charismatic individual's character draws people, captivates and makes them want to

follow; is well liked, respected, perceived as a role model, and others are prone to consider her/his point of view. It takes time to develop, has to be earned and can be very effective in some situations. When strong enough, others may ignore the person's failures and seek her/his approval.

Relationship power is derived from the individual's relationships and networks that enable the leader to penetrate systems through formal and informal networks both inside and outside of the organization and even outside of the profession (they know people who know people). It is strengthened by the individual's integrity and positive interpersonal relationships.

Expert power emanates from the individual's expertise. The more crucial and unusual the expertise and knowledge, the greater the power. This power is sometimes "understood" from the individual's title (Professor, Doctor, Sir, etc.) and, in some cases, is reinforced by society. The individual is trusted and seen as credible because of the expertise.

Information power is when one has information valued by others. The greater difference the information makes, the more power one has over those who need it. Information power is common in scientific and technical fields and is available to anyone who seeks it through personal development.

NB: Not usually included among power bases

Personal attributes are not usually included as power bases. But there are situations when one's colour, gender, age and country of origin are power sources.

Sources: ICM Young Midwifery Leaders Programme (2014)

This agrees with Powell-Kennedy's statement that: '…leadership goes further than the common misconception of a leader as the lofty head of a group, institution or country. Rather, it is the everyday work that demonstrates strength, knowledge and ethical behaviour' (Powell-Kennedy 2011).

Box 11.2. Leveraging Power
How to gain and retain power

- Be the expert in midwifery.
- Leverage power from other sources by association or relationship.
- Invest time and energy to information, expertise and relationships.
- Identify specific persons to get to know to extend sphere of influence.
- Repair damaged relationships.
- Develop your professional presence.
- Be genuine, authentic, ethical and humble.
- Sharpen your emotional maturity, professional and psychological intelligence.
- Be helpful.
- Strive for the best without being arrogant.

Source: International Confederation of Midwives Young Midwifery Leaders Programme (2014).

11.5 Why Midwifery Needs Leadership

The midwifery workforce is getting more diverse in terms of race, gender and sexual orientation. So are its beneficiaries, presenting with different needs, concerns and personal ideologies. Given that the contexts in which midwifery care is provided are not static and in some cases are rapidly changing, the midwifery leader needs to be sensitive to diversity and the multicultural expectations and needs among the workforce and the care receivers. In situations of rapid change and stress, work and organisations become major sources of need fulfilment (Conger 2012). Hence, midwifery leaders must build the profession into communities which offer midwives a sense of identity, ownership and belonging.

In some countries, despite being key service providers, without leadership, midwives' contribution is not recognised, especially where there are severe staff shortages, weak midwifery education and weak midwifery competencies (Chapter 4). Without leadership, these and the conditions of service, the high workload and poor salaries will remain unchanged. Midwifery leadership is needed to spearhead the development of context-appropriate interventions and solutions (Robert et al. 2000).

Midwifery needs leadership in care provision to treat others as responsible, potential leaders, to earn respect and to learn to be reflective, consistent and self-disciplined (Northouse 2019). At policymaking level, the leader has to be versatile and resilient and to adopt different personae to meet the demands of each level. The midwifery leader needs to be a visionary in order to shape a vision for the profession; an optimizer to make the best of difficult situations; a builder, superconnecter, warrior, researcher and mentor (Annex 11.1).

11.5.1 Midwifery Leadership Across the World

Midwifery is at different levels of development globally. In some countries, midwives are organised in large professional associations with visible, strong and effective leadership. In some, the associations are small, weak, with no or ineffective leadership; in others the profession does not exist or is not recognised, or there is no association and therefore no leadership (see Chapter. 5 and 6). Yet by its very nature midwifery leadership should cross organisational boundaries because midwifery care is delivered by an interdependent network of organisations. Midwifery leadership should be broad based, i.e. the practice of leadership by clinicians and other frontline staff since, in many countries, it is these frontline staff that have to make decisions (Michael West et al. 2015).

11.6 The Global Leader of Midwifery

The International Confederation of Midwives (ICM) provides global midwifery leadership through supporting and representing midwives and works closely with other global bodies including United Nations agencies, other professional bodies and non-governmental organisations, bilateral and civil society groups (ICM 2019). ICM provides the midwifery voice and expertise and contributes to the global health agenda. For a detailed description of ICM, see Chapter 2.

11.7 Factors Impacting on Leadership

The hierarchical position, organisational and societal culture, gender and the age of the leader impact on leadership (Gîrneață and Potcovaru 2015). A midwifery leader in a position of power in the organisation faces different issues when leading the profession compared to a midwifery leader who is in the lower ranks of the organisation (Hochwarter et al. 2000).

11.7.1 Organisational Culture

Leadership is the most influential factor in shaping organisational culture. Organisational culture is a pattern of shared basic assumptions learned by a group, considered valid and therefore, the correct way to perceive, think and feel in relation to problems (Schein 2010; Watkins 2013). Because of these basic assumptions, where midwifery is not recognised, the mindsets in organisations impact on how midwifery leaders are perceived and determine their level of involvement in policy making bodies and activities.

11.7.2 Gender

Most midwives are women doing women's work for women and their families. Most work places are set up on male-based thinking and working philosophies (O'Sullivan 2019). Working women have to juggle family and work life (Jones et al. 2018). O'Sullivan (2019) and Xie and Zhu (2016) described Chinese women as 'Holding up half the sky', i.e. the 'Glass Ceiling' (an imaginary barrier). In some cultures, women in leadership positions are not viewed positively (O'Connor 2015; Huang and Aaltio 2014; Zhang 2005, 2010; Javalgi et al. 2011). In others they are expected to assume the greater share of the family and homelife responsibilities despite the demands of leadership (Yang 2011; Kong and Zhang 2011; Zhang and Foo 2012; Cho and Ryu 2016). Some authors posit that women tend to exclude themselves because of their social orientation, thus creating a 'psychological glass ceiling' against themselves (Austin 2009; Eagly 2015; Sandberg and Scovell 2013). Others believe that gender segregation gives women a professional advantage as they do not have to compete with men in women-only professions like midwifery (Yan et al. 2018; Alsubaie and Jones 2017). In colleges and universities, women are expected to navigate their own way to leadership (Helgesen and Johnson 2010; Wang and Cho 2013; Jones et al. 2018; Longman 2018). Midwifery leaders need to recognise and rise above these issues and to prevent the emergence of the queen bee syndrome.

Queen bee syndrome describes women who, having achieved success in male-dominated environments, perceive other women as threats and oppose their rise (Staines et al. 1973; Blau and DeVaro 2007). Midwifery leadership development should acknowledge these struggles.

11.7.3 Societal Culture

Hofstede and Minkov (Hofstede and Minkov 2010:6) described culture as:

> the collective programming of the mind that distinguishes the members of one group or category of people from others

Societal culture provides the basis for leadership styles and employee behaviours (Hofstede 1991; Dorfman et al. 2006).

Most well-researched leadership styles are based on the Western (Europe and United States of America) culture (Whitley 1994; Sørensen and Kuada 2001). Thinking has moved towards examining the concept in other cultures.

11.8 Concept of Leadership in Other Cultures

African culture is mainly based on collectivism, familism and advancing the common good (Gyekye 1997, 2010). The philosophy of 'ubuntu' encapsulated in the maxims 'I am because we are' and 'a person is a person through other persons' exhorts the exhibition of humanness, suggesting a life of positive integration with others, with communalism as a goal (Menkiti 2004; Tutu 1999; Shutte 2001; Masolo 2010). Sharing and treating everyone with respect are important values (Metz 2013, 2017, 2018; Ndlovu 2016; Ndlovu-Gatsheni and Ngcaweni 2017; Woermann and Engelbrecht 2017). Whereas western leadership has the end goal of achieving the company's objectives, African leadership has the company's objectives, the individual's goals and benefits as end goals (Fadare 2018; Kuada 2010). While Western approaches perceive human beings as resources (instruments), the African approach perceives human beings as having value in their own right (Kuada 2009; Metz 2015; Bolden and Kirk 2009).

In Mexico, Michaud et al. (2019) used Kouzes and Posner's (2012) leadership practices inventory and determined that Mexican leaders typically engage styles that involved both presenting a vision for the future and convincing employees to make this vision their own. Leaders would not engage in creative activities that deviated too far from the status quo.

In China, India and Pakistan, gender plays a big role with women in leadership being evaluated with closer scrutiny than men. In the Philippines, among the millennials,[1] age is important (Rathore et al. 2017). In Macedonia, the size of the company is important (Bonafe and Casimiro 2019).

---

[1] Millennials are those reaching adulthood in the early twenty-first century or those born between 1981 and 1986 (Oxford dictionary 2016).

In small and medium enterprises (SME) success depends on the clarity with which the leader shares the vision and motivates people towards achieving a common goal and provides direction (Bojadjiev et al. 2019; Durham et al. 1997; Mihai 2015). SMEs succeed under leadership which transforms knowledge into action, enhances autonomy and encourages cooperation among employees (Nanjundeswaraswamy and Swamy 2015; Rahman 2012; Kelchner 2016). This describes the type of leadership required to build a midwives' association (Haron 2015).

11.8.1 Multiculturalism and Leadership

Globalisation and population movements have created multicultural societies and a great diversity of beliefs and values among followers (Hofstede and Minkov 2010), challenging leaders to adapt (Eagly 2015; Bristol 2016). No one leadership approach fits all circumstances. Midwifery leaders need to be aware of these issues.

11.8.2 Age

According to Bojadjiev et al. (2017) older people can be better leaders than younger ones due to their ability to deal with and understand people in a more positive way. Younger ones are different. Table 11.1 captures some of the differences.

Table 11.1 The relationship between age and leadership behaviour

Younger leaders	Older leaders
More enthusiastic, take risks, although with some reservations	More likely to study the problems to ensure certainty and to reduce risks
More focused on new approaches	More conservative
More comfortable in turbulent and changing environments with minimal knowledge and skills in leadership and management	Wiser and have certain knowledge and skills in management and leadership
Have energy, intensity and emotional expression, when operating	More likely to maintain a modest interpersonal behaviour and to be less emotionally sensitive
Tend to emphasize short-term results with a production focus	Value good relationships as an important contributor to organisational success
Have little experience and observed to rely more on the autocratic style, move toward the democratic before finally employing the laissez-faire leadership trait	Have experience which led to development of certain attitudes and practise different leadership styles
Are somewhat self-focused	Know how to handle people during difficult times

Sources: Bojadjiev et al. (2016, 2017) Age Related Preferences of Leadership Style: Testing McGregor's Theory X and Y

fulfil these 'psychological contracts' through the way they lead.

11.8.3 Individual Expectations and Leadership

Individuals have personal and social identities which form the basis of their goals (Ashford and Cummings 1983; Lord et al. 1999). Leadership practices must align personal and organisational goals to stimulate commitment and motivation. Otherwise, individuals will find ways of fulfilling their own goals (Jackson 2004; Okpara and Wynn 2007). Personal and organisational goal alignment constitute a 'psychological' contract between the leaders and the followers (Rousseau 1990; Jackson 2004). Midwifery leaders should

11.9 Leadership Styles

Leadership styles describe how leaders exercise authority and the degree of autonomy they offer to followers. Some authors suggest that men and women lead differently (Patel et al. 2013 in Bojadjiev et al. 2017). Others feel that stereotypes may prejudice women in leadership (Kaiser and Wallace 2016). Blake and Mouton (1964), Fiedler (1967), House and Mitchell (1974), and Stogdill (1974) described behavioural approaches to leadership. Stogdill stated that leadership is situational. Fiedler's path-goal theory suggests that effective leadership provides a path to a valued goal. Characteristics of autocratic, democratic and laissez-faire leadership styles are presented in Annex 11.1. Other less discussed types are presented in Annex 11.2. Midwifery leaders need to understand these theories.

Transactional and transformational leaderships are presented in Annex 11.3. Transactional leadership focuses on exchanges of favours between leaders and followers and on reward or punishment for performance. Transformational leadership focuses on binding people around a common purpose through self-reinforcing behaviours.

Bass (1985) explained that successful leaders inspire employees to transcend themselves and do more through idealized influence, inspirational leadership, individualized consideration and intellectual stimulation. The four Is are illustrated in Fig. 11.1 and defined in Box 11.3. Midwifery leadership development programmes should consider including these concepts. Annex 11.4 presents some factors which might either neutralise or substitute leadership.

> **Box 11.3. Defining the Four Is of Transformational Leadership**
> **Idealised influence:** Leaders act as role models, are able to motivate people around a common purpose through self-reinforcing behaviours gained from successfully achieving a task and from a reliance on intrinsic rewards.
>
> **Inspirational leadership:** Leaders inspire followers by identifying new opportunities, providing meaning and challenge, and articulating a strong vision. They have positive expectations of and can convince members that they are talented and willing to work and can deliver up to their potentials.
>
> **Individualised consideration:** Leaders provide personalised consideration on individual needs for achievement, development, growth and support and adopt coaching and mentoring strategies in their relationships with followers.

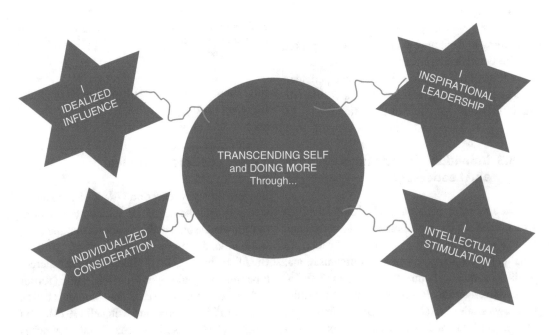

Fig. 11.1 Inspiring successful leaders "The Four 'I's". (Derived from Bass (1985))

Intellectual stimulation: Leaders are enthusiastic, optimistic, communicate clear and realistic expectations and demonstrate commitment to a shared vision. Followers are encouraged to participate in identifying required change, how to achieve it, to see deeper purpose in their work and exceed their own self-interests for the good of the organisation.

Source: Conger (2012). Leadership needs in the twenty-first century. Principles of Management.

11.10   The Leader

A leader is expected to have a certain personality, a form of persuasion and power, and the art of inducing compliance (De Pree 2006; Bass and Stogdil 1990). She/he influences diverse followers to willingly expend energy to achieve the organizational objectives (Winston and Patterson 2006); defines the vision and converts the idea into action (Bolden 2004). Midwifery leaders need capacity to do these things for them to present midwifery as one united profession. Box 11.4 presents a non-exhaustive list of selected leadership characteristics; while Box 11.5 presents what literature describes as an effective leader.

11.11   The Follower

The follower can either reject or accept a leadership activity. The follower's personality and readiness to follow determines the type of leadership style (Hollander 1964). The midwifery leader needs to be sensitive and respectful of these traits among midwives as followers.

Box 11.4. Leadership Characteristics
Leadership characteristics

- Creativity: Including generosity with ideas.
- Capacity: A jack of all trades and master in as many as possible.
- Motivation: Build on inner motivation and confidence and not be afraid of failure but confront it with gusto!
- Confidence: Willingness to take responsibility with courage, commitment.
- Ability to delegate.
- Focus on goals and keeping a clear vision.
- Ability to communicate and being a good listener, gives staff freedom of speech.
- Positive attitude, approachable and empowers others.
- Ability to inspire and nurture innovative ideas.
- Respect everyone, recognise and reward the deserving.
- Sense of humour, honesty and integrity and emotionally involved.
- Competent in own filed, knows own job and the job of those they lead.
- Gives the team members a sense that they are safe.
- Works as hard as everyone else.

Sources:
Raju and Arcand (2019). 10 ways to become a better leader at work. Work-it-Daily   https://www.workitdaily.com/10-ways-become-better-leader.   Accessed November 2019.
Deen and Keuhn (2019). 10 Characteristics of a great leader https://www.workitdaily.com/what-makes-a-good-leader. Accessed November 2019.
Byrom and Downe (2010) 'She sort of shines': midwives' accounts of 'good' midwifery and 'good' leadership. Midwifery (2010) 26, 126–137.

Box 11.5. An Effective Leader

An effective leader

- Is a difference-maker between success and failure.
- Knows the way, shows the way and goes the way.
- Has a futuristic vision and is positive.
- Knows how to turn his ideas into success stories and is oozing with confidence.
- Takes a little more than his share of blame and a little less than his share of credit (Arnold S. Glasson).
- Does not hesitate to challenge the status quo.
- Ready to ditch the traditional mind set to achieve what others have not yet achieved.
- Allows common people to achieve uncommon results (Andrew Carnegie).

Source: Mike Myatt (2019). Traits of ineffective leaders. https://www.n2growth.com/6-traits-of-ineffective-leaders/. Accessed November 2019.

11.12 Midwifery Leadership Development

The twenty-first century demanded strong, versatile, resilient leaders capable of leading in challenging circumstances (Conger 1993). Leaders needed to be:

- *Strategic opportunists*: To find strategic opportunities.
- *Globally aware*: To cope with environmental demands for flexibility and learning.
- *Sensitive to diversity:* To deal with a racially, gender, sexual orientation diverse workforce and membership.
- *Interpersonally competent*: To be aware of and sensitive to multi-cultural needs and expectations.

- *Builders of an organisational community*: Where work and organisations serve as major sources of identity and fulfilment of needs and members develop a sense of ownership and identity.

Inclusive leadership (Box 11.6), plus effective communication, credibility, being inspirational, fostering acceptance of goals, and being wise, knowledgeable and intelligent should be included in midwifery development programmes. Acts of transformational leadership are highly relevant given their effectiveness in a variety of settings and cultures (Brubaker 2013).

A midwifery leadership development programme should ensure the development of confidence and leadership skills in real-work settings and the creation of leadership teams and networks. Midwifery leadership programmes should move away from heroic leadership based on innate qualities to a set of behaviours that can be developed to produce authentic leaders (Jaye 2017).

Box 11.6. The Six Cs of Inclusive Leadership
- Commitment to people's unique contribution.
- Courage to challenge the status quo about deeply held and ingrained beliefs, attitudes and behaviours.
- Cognizance of bias: Making a deliberate effort to prevent own bias from influencing decisions.
- Curiosity: Having hunger for other perspectives to minimise own blind spots.
- Cultural intelligence: Recognise how cultural stereotypes influence one's expectations of others.
- Collaboration: Enable individuals to express their opinions without fear of judgement or retribution.
  Source: Sherwin D. (2019). Success by Design: The 6 Cs of inclusive leadership. https://www.printmag.com/imprint/the-six-cs-of-creative-leadership/. Accessed November 2019.

Authentic leadership is when the individual seeks to be reflective and develops a high level of self-knowledge to understand others with whom the individual works and to operate and engage in an honest transparent manner, providing reassurance and direction particularly in difficult situations (Ross-Davie et al. 2016). The impact of gender, age, culture, organisational politics and societal culture should be included (Eagly and Carli 2003a, b). Prospective midwifery leaders need capacity to deal with and rise above gender issues. Female midwifery leaders require effective strategies to deal with work–family conflict and to dissipate the 'glass ceiling' in many settings (Cameron and Quinn 2011; Halverson and Tirmizi 2008).

Jackson (2004), Kuada (2006) and Bolden and Kirk (2009) introduced the ideas of cross-vergence or hybridization, suggesting that leadership development must be built on ideas from many cultures and the multifaceted nature of the factors impacting on leadership practices. Midwifery leadership programme developers need evidence on these concepts including concepts on orgnasational politics (Ferris and Hochwarter 2011) for programmes to enhance the individual midwifery leader's intelligence, emotional and political quotients (Owen 2017). Additionally, for successful leadership development, the programme must include different aspects of teaching and learning including education, coaching and quality improvement to enable participants to learn and then embed whatever key leadership behaviours they will have learnt (Ross-Davie et al. 2016).

The National Health Services of the United Kingdom has developed a leadership framework made up of seven domains for leadership in clinical settings—the Clinical Leadership Framework and Medical Competency Framework (NHS Leadership Academy 2012). This is a useful tool for those developing leadership in the clinical settings. Midwifery also needs leadership at regional and global levels. The competencies for these individuals who have to lead and represent midwifery outside the midwifery settings are much broader as described above Forbes (2018).

11.13 Strengthening Midwifery and Leadership

The ICM Leadership Programme's vision is:

> …a future where women, their newborn and families are healthy and receiving optimum midwifery services because the midwifery profession is strong and well led and taking the lead in provision of services within the context of their countries. (ICM 2014)

To achieve this vision, midwifery leaders must be primary advocates for women and their families, chart the way and strengthen midwifery by contributing to global health policy. This implies having midwives holding key positions in global bodies dealing with midwifery and reproductive health; driving change in social, political and cultural arenas; promoting the profession and making midwives and midwifery visible; and acting as inspiring role models for midwives globally (ICM 2014).

Midwifery leadership is needed in research to produce evidence and new knowledge in care provision and workforce development to match the increasingly changing and expanding role of midwives and provide policymakers with a vision, a strategic path, a set of priorities and a range of suggestions and adaptable strategies for action to improve health, address health inequalities and ensure the health of future generations. WHO Regional Office for Europe (2015) in 'Health 2020' (Box 11.7) described midwives as 'a vital resource for health' and as having key and increasingly important roles to play in society's efforts to tackle the public health challenges of the twenty-first century (WHO 2015).

Box 11.7. The Aims of the European Policy Framework: Health 2020

Health 2020, the European health policy framework and strategy, aims to improve the health and well-being of populations, reduce inequalities and ensure people-centred health systems. In order to support the realization of the Health 2020 goals, the European strategic directions for strengthening nursing and midwifery towards Health 2020 was developed guiding Member States and the WHO Regional Office to mobilize the potential of the nursing and midwifery workforce. This European compendium was produced to provide operational examples of the new nursing and midwifery roles and new service delivery models currently being employed across the region. The case studies directly relate to the priority areas in Health 2020 and exemplify the types of activities needed to fully implement the objectives within the Strategic Directions framework.

Source: WHO European Region (2015) Nurses and Midwives A vital resource: European compendium of good practices in nursing and midwifery towards Health 2020 goals.

Effective leadership makes midwives associations the voice of midwifery. In midwifery education, leadership guides education institutions and programmes based on global guidelines and advocates for resources for the production of competent midwives who provide respectful midwifery care. The ICM brings together leading experts in education, regulation and research into Standing Committees which keep their fingers on the pulse of global health issues and the contribution of midwives. This global leadership needs to be owned, valued and supported by all midwives.

'In practice, effective leadership will provide oversight, advocacy for quality, respectful midwifery care provision and demonstration and promotion of examples of value-added midwifery interventions in addressing people's health needs' (WHO 2015:1). Effective midwifery leaders contribute to workforce development, evidence-based recruitment, deployment and retention of the workforce and discourage the belief that the least qualified members of the healthcare team should work closest to where women live (WHO 2008; Adhikari 2018), thus inadvertently exonerating governments from and perpetuating the lack of development of badly needed facilities and infrastructure in rural areas. Without water, electricity and other modern amenities (internet, housing, transport and communication systems), women cannot enjoy the care of professionals considered highly qualified.

11.14 Putting It All Together

No one leadership style fits all situations. Leaders need to be discerning enough to know when to change styles. Global events have challenged leadership styles. Neither the Western, the African, nor the Asian approaches to leadership fit because populations and organisations consist of neither purely African, Western (European and American) nor Asian cultures. Leaders need characteristics that enable them to function in all settings.

Midwifery leaders need to represent midwives on the decision-making table and provide a vision and a path to help individual midwives to develop an identity. Big midwives' associations can learn from the corporate world and adapt some of the approaches to midwifery leadership. The Pakistani example showed that female leaders and female followers are unique and need leaders who understand gender dynamics (Rathore et al. 2017). Smaller associations can learn from the Macedonian SME example (Bojadjiev et al. 2017) as they attempt to pull midwives together into a coherent professional group.

Existing leaders must coach, mentor, support and nurture colleagues into the profession. They must guide care processes, support colleagues to love and value the profession and the women they care for; use transactional approaches to provide order and structure to the work and be transformative enough to enable others to be creative, share ideas and continue to learn, as well as nurture and develop resilience in midwives in times of stress. They must be able to use collaborative leadership approaches to navigate the health systems in which they work and for them to manage to work with multiple stakeholders most of whom are neither midwives nor healthcare providers. Team leadership is effective in clinical settings, with clinical leaders who are experts in their field and who can get their hands dirty when needed.

Older leaders should support and guide younger leaders using their experience and analytic approach to issues. Cultural sensitivity must be one of the hallmarks of midwifery leadership in order to lead a profession that respects diversity among its members and care receivers.

11.15 Conclusion

Research on leadership and leadership styles continues. Midwifery research should contribute to these studies and guide the profession in developing its future leaders with a clear vision of what the future holds and to share that vision effectively enough for all midwives to want to follow.

Key Messages
- **Principles**
- Leadership and leadership styles should take into consideration the culture and other characteristics of the followers.
- **Policy**
- Governments and key stakeholders should support the development of midwifery leadership in order to organise and enhance the quality of midwifery services as well as contribute to the development and management of the health workforce.
- **Practice**
- Midwifery leaders should take on the responsibility of quality assurance as well as ensure the adoption and adaptation of evidence-based practice in service provision.

Questions for Reflection
1. Some text in this chapter suggests that it is easier for midwives to take on leadership because midwifery is mainly a female profession. Midwives as women do not have to compete with men. Discuss this statement giving your opinion for and against it.
2. A number of authors were quoted stating that most leadership concepts are derived from the West and attention has turned to other regions and cultures. Examine the impact of culture and context on leadership with this thought in mind. How does this impact on midwifery care provision and health services in general?
3. Rapid change and global events are stated as having posed a challenge on leadership. Identify three such events and/or changes and highlight how they have impacted on midwifery leadership and care provision (do not forget pestilences such as Ebola, COVID-19, among others).

Annex 11.1: Characteristics of Leadership Personae Required by Midwifery Leaders

Persona	Characteristics
Visionary	• Capable of shaping a vision for those who cannot see the possibilities • Thinks big and conceptualises ideas to motivate others to action • Sees the end before the beginning and able to assess from a bird's eye view • Has a long-term mindset and plots his course accordingly
Optimizer	• Assesses, analyses and maps out improvements that directly save or make money. (In health we do not make money but life and positive health outcomes) • Some people rely on to make sound decisions • Assesses a situation and immediately sees ways of improving health outcomes • Gains satisfaction from knowing her work makes a difference or makes the business more profitable

Persona	Characteristics
Builder	• Executes on a plan managing all aspects, keeping it on time under budget • Specialist in own field with a lot of hands-on experience • Executes on a plan and works through road blocks to completion • Likes to focus on ways to do things better, faster and cheaper
Educator	• Closes gaps in knowledge and ensures staff is clear of their roles and goals • Good at organising thoughts into oral or written communication to motivate and train others • Takes control of an idea and chooses the right method for communicating it • Excels at word play and uses communication skills to guide conversations
Super-connector	• Builds relationships with all types of professionals to improve business • Known for extended network of contacts and circle of influence • Identifies and outs two network connections together as a way to help them each to move towards their own goals • Actively seeks and nurtures new relationships, never worrying about whether has too many connections
Warrior	• Goes the extra mile and volunteers to do the tough work when things are challenging • Loyal and passionate about people and the ideas she believes in • Stays strong and carries on with the mission when others give up • Enjoys starting new projects and welcomes the work that goes with it
Researcher	• Gathers data and information to assist in better design and decision • Detail oriented and structured in the work efforts • Assesses and locates the right information and resources needed to complete a project • Enjoys getting things organised and building routines for consistency
Mentor	• Coaches performance and helps others develop their own skill • Seen as thought leader and highly successful in own profession • Coaches others to new levels of awareness and performance

Source: Types of leaders: Workitdaily-Leadership personae (2019)

Annex 11.2: Traditional Styles of Leadership

Autocratic Leadership Style

In the autocratic leadership style, the leader brings all the decisions and orders to the group. Group members' behaviour is controlled through punishment reward and arbitrary rules. There is no room for members' initiative and creativity. The leader, in general, is arrogant, proud and egotistical. This leadership style is useful in situations where there is little time for group decision-making or where the leader is the most knowledgeable member within the group and in times of crisis (Khan et al. 2015). The benefit of autocratic leadership is that it is incredibly efficient (Amanchukwu et al. 2015).

Democratic Leadership Style

The democratic style focuses on group relationships and the sensibility of people in the organization. Team members take responsibility for their behaviour. It encourages professional competence prompts quality assuring behaviour (Cummingham et al. 2015:34). Group members can express their feelings, ideas and give suggestions. The leader proposes ideas, is patient, confident and friendly and offers guidance to the members. The leader perceives her/himself as a member of the group and allows sharing ideas from other members of the group. Group members are involved in the decision-making process, although the leader has the last word (Khan et al. 2015). This results in increased motivation, creativity and confidence among group members. The main disadvantage is that extended time is required to move forward (Amanchukwu et al. 2015). It is most suitable for small- and medium-sized groups where the leader can focus on developing highly driven, smaller teams (Fiaz et al. 2017:147). This style is particularly recommended in cases of innovative organizations or projects which require cooperation between various units (Mohuidin 2017:26–27).

Laissez-Faire Style

The laissez-faire leadership style is characterized by a lack of real leadership, where every team member can do what he/she wants. There is a disregard of supervisory duties and lack of guidance given to subordinates, which later results in low productivity, resistance to change and low quality of work (Murnigham and Leung 1976). The team members are not only involved in the decision-making process, but they are also responsible for making the final decision, although the full responsibility goes to the leader. Suitable for situations where employees are highly educated and they are confident enough to bring the right decision. They know how to deal with a specific task and how to use the strategies in order to complete the same task (Khan et al. 2015).

Source: Conger (2012). Leadership in the twenty-first Century.

Annex 11.3: Other Less-Talked-About Leadership Styles

- *Supportive leadership*—Leadership that demonstrates concern for the well-being and personal needs of members. A supportive leader is friendly, approachable and considerate to individuals. Supportive leadership is especially effective when members are performing boring, stressful, frustrating, tedious, unpleasant or difficult tasks. Supportive leadership can reduce anxiety, increase confidence, increase satisfaction and determination to do well in individuals with low self-esteem.
- *Directive leadership*—At times, effective leaders set goals and performance expectations, let organizational members know what is expected, provide guidance, establish rules and procedures to guide and direct work, and schedule and coordinate the activities of members. Directive leadership is called for when role ambiguity is high. Removing uncertainty and providing needed guidance can increase members' effort, job satisfaction and job performance.
- *Participative leadership*—At times, effective leaders consult with group members and consider their opinions and suggestions when making decisions. Participative leadership is effective when tasks are unstructured, when leaders need help in identifying work procedures and where followers have the expertise to provide this help.
- *Achievement-oriented leadership*—At times, effective leaders set challenging goals, seek improvement in performance, emphasize excellence and demonstrate confidence in organizational members' ability to attain high standards. Achievement-oriented leaders capitalise on members' needs for achievement and use goal-setting theory to great advantage.
- *Complexity theory of leadership is based on the idea that lead*ership is part of a dynamic and evolving pattern of behaviours and complex interactions among various players, producing power structures and networks of relationships (Schneider and Somers 2006). It states that no single leader can determine the path of the organization; the capacity of each leader depends on his/her position within the complex network of relationships within the organization and her/his capability to distribute resources and emotional support (Ardichivili and Manderscheid 2008).
- *Authentic leadership theory focuses attention on leaders' self-awareness and self-regulated positive behaviours and their tendency to exhibit transparent and ethical behaviours* (Avolio et al. 2009) *which encourage openness and the desire to share informa*tion among followers and the leader.
- *Servant leadership theory*—A derivative of the authentic leadership is the servant and coach leadership theory based on the devolution of power to follower. Leaders see themselves as stewards, serving their followers and enhancing their contribution to fulfilling organizational objectives.

Source: Conger 2012: Leadership in the twenty-first Century

Annex 11.4: Transformational and Transactional Leadership Styles

Transformational Leadership

Transformational leadership involves binding people around a common purpose through self-reinforcing behaviours gained from successfully achieving a task and from a reliance on intrinsic rewards. There are six dimensions of transformational leadership. These are intellectual stimulation, articulating a vision, appropriate role model, and expectations of high performance, group goals and individualized support (Edwards et al. 2016; Speitzer et al. 2005:212).

Transformational leaders act as role models and are able to motivate and inspire their followers by identifying new opportunities, providing meaning and challenge, and articulating a strong vision for the future (Barling et al. 2000; Khaliq et al. 2017). They are enthusiastic and optimistic, communicate clear and realistic expectations and demonstrate commitment to a shared vision. The leader's responsibility is to convey and communicate a clear vision with clear explanation why and what type of change is necessary (Bass 1999). Followers are encouraged to participate in identifying required change and how to achieve it (Bass 1997), to see deeper purpose in their work and exceed their own self-interests for the good of the organisation and to consider the needs of others over their own, share risks with others and conduct themselves ethically. Transformational leaders provide personalised consideration on individual needs for achievement, development, growth and support and adopt coaching and mentoring strategies in their relationships with followers (Bass and Steidlmeier 1999; Dong et al. 2017; Brodbeck et al. 2002) and have positive expectations of the team members (Ogbonnaya and Nielsen 2016). The leader is naturally enthusiastic and capable of convincing members that they can deliver up to their potentials because she/he believes they are talented and willing to work and utilises whatever rewards are available (Ahmad et al. 2014). This highly motivates and inspires the team members.

Transactional Leadership

Transactional leaders are very consistent in accomplishing the organization goals and objectives made by either the leaders themselves or the top management. Their prime concern is the accomplishment of task by all means through reward and punishment strategy (Tremblay et al. 2013). The leader makes explicit agreements with the team members about the rewards if they adhere to the policies and the punishment if they fail to do so. The promise of reward and the fear of punishment thus drive the efforts and commitment of the employees and the leader keeps tag of each individual's performance purpose. For an organization, this style maybe useful to keep every working unit in the organization on track (Vera and Crossan 2004).

Source: Conger (2012). Leadership needs in the twenty-first century. Principles of Management.

Annex 11.5: Substitutes and Neutralisers of Leadership

There are some situations that challenge leadership however well it is exercised. Discuss substitutes for leadership and neutralisers of leadership. Substitutes for leadership are those situations where the role expectations, motivation of organisational members, and some group members characteristics render leadership irrelevant. One example given is when a highly skilled expert performs her/his work according to her/his own standards without needing any outside prompting. A leader is not needed to motivate this person. In some situations, the work itself is motivating. For example, when it involves solving of an intricate problem or when it is familiar and well structured, it is intrinsically satisfying and therefore renders the leader irrelevant. In other situations, the organisational rules are so clear and specific that workers know exactly what is expected of them and do not need help from outside. These situations substitute for leadership.

Neutralisers are situations that prevent the leaders from exercising their authority the way they would like to. Examples include computer-paced activities which prevent the leader from initiating structure or behaviour to either speed up or slow down the process. Some organisations' labour conditions and terms do not allow the leader to reward people according to performance or be creative in correcting issues. Instead rewards could be based on seniority and years of work irrespective of quality of work, and disciplinary rules are laid down and have to be followed despite the leaders' desires. This tends to be common in the civil service. So, there is not external motivation from the leader to enhance production. This brings up the issue that allowing oneself to be led is a choice. Individual can resist the efforts of leader, and it is up to the leader to identify what would be neutralising her/his leadership attempts and develop an effective way of dealing with the situation should leadership be needed.

Source: Conger (2012). Leadership needs in the twenty-first century. Principles of Management.

Additional Materials

Divall B (2015) A rock and hard place: challenges for midwifery leadership. ACM2015 Oral Presentations/Women and Birth 28S(2015):S7–S32

Edwards N, Kaseje D, Kahwa E et al (2016) The impact of leadership hubs on the uptake of evidence-informed nursing practices and workplace policies for HIV care: a quasi-experimental study in Jamaica, Kenya, Uganda and South Africa. Implementation Science (2016 11:110. https://doi.org/10.1186/s13012-016-0478-3

Jarvis D, Reeves P (2017) Enabling BME Nurse and Midwife Progression into Senior Leadership Positions. NHS England. Version 1.0. December 2017

Kouzes JM, Posner BZ (2012) The leadership challenge: how extraordinary things happen in organizations. Leadership Challenge, San Francisco, CA

Leadership Academy (2011) Leadership framework: a summary. NHS Leadership Academy, 2011

Stogdill RM (1963) Manual for the leader behavior description questionnaire. Ohio State University, Columbus, OH

References

Adeyemi TO, Bolarinwa R (2013) Principals' leadership styles and student academic performance in secondary school in Ekiti State, Nigeria. International journal of academic research in progressive education and development 2(1) ISSN: 2226-6348

Adhikari S (2018) Task shifting: what is task shifting and why is it needed? Glob Health. https://www.publichealthnotes. Accessed 12 Jan 2020

Alsubaie A, Jones K (2017) An overview of the current state of women's leadership in higher education in Saudi Arabia and a proposal for future research directions. Administrative Sciences 7(4):36. ISSN 2076-3387. https://doi.org/10.3390/admsci7040036

Amanchukwu RN, Stanley GJ, Ololude NP (2015) A review of leadership theories, principles and styles and their relevance to educational management. https://doi.org/10.5923/j.mm.20150501.02

Ardichivili A, Manderschied SV (2008) Emerging practices in leadership development:an introdcution. Advances in Developing Human Resources. SAGE Journals

Ashford SJ, Cummings LL (1983) Feedback as an individual resource: personal strategies of creating information. Organ Behav Hum Perform 32:370–398

Austin LG (2009) What's holding you back?: eight critical choices for women's success. Basic Books, New York

Avolio BJ, Walumbwa FO, Weber TJ (2009) Leadership:current theories, research and future directions. Annual Review of Psychology Vol 60:421–449

Barling J, Slater F, Kelloway K (2000) Transformational leadership and emotional intelligence: an exploratory study. Leadership and Organisational Development Journal 21(3):157–161

Bass BM (1985) Leadership and performance beyond expectations. The Free Press, New York

Bass BM, Stogdil RM (1990) Handbook of leadership, vol 11. Free Press, New York

Bass BM (1997) Does the transactional-transformational leadership paradigm transcend organisational and national boundaries? American Psychologist. 52(2):130

Bass BM (1999) Two decades of research and development in transformational leadership. European Journal of Work and Organisational Psychology. 8(1):9–32

Bass BM, Steidlmeier P (1999) Ethics, character and authentic transformational leadership behaviour. The Leadership Quarterly 10(2):181–217

Bennis WG, Thomas RJ (2002) Geeks and geezers: how era, values and defining moments shape leadership. In: Smith DN, Suby-Long S (eds) Advancing women in leadership: women leaders and narratives: the power of reflecting on purpose and career. Harvard Business School Press, Boston, MA

Bennis WG, Thomas RJ (2007) Leading for a lifetime: how defining moments shape the leaders of today and tomorrow. In Smith DN, Suby-Long S (2019) Advancing women in leadership: women leaders and narratives: the power of reflecting on purpose and career. Boston, MA: Harvard Business School Press

Blake RR, Mouton JS (1964) The Managerial Grid, Gulf, Houston, TX. Blanchard, K. (2007), Leading at a Higher Level, FT Press, Upper Saddle River, NJ

Blau FD, DeVaro J (2007) New evidence on gender differences in promotion rates: An empirical analysis of a sample of new hires. Ind Relat 46(3):511–550. https://doi.org/10.1111/j.1468-232X.2007.00479.x

Bojadjiev M, Hristova S, Mileva I (2019) Leadership styles in small and medium sized business: evidence from Macedonian Textile SMEs. https://www.researchgate.net/publication/335171216. Accessed 8 Feb 2020

Bojadjiev M, Kostovski N, Krlui-Handjiski V et al. (2017) Organisational culture and strategic alignment in fast moving consumer goods company. Annual of ISPJR, 41(1):45–56

Bojadjiev M, Stefonovska-Petkoska M, Krlui-Handjiski V et al. (2016) Age related preferences of leadership style:testing McGregor's Theory X and Y. Journal of Management Research, 8(4). https://doi.org/10.5296/jmr.v8i4.10088

Bolden R (2004) What is leadership? University of Exeter Centre of leadership studies. https://www.researchgate.net/publication/29810622. Accessed 8 Feb 2020

Bolden R and Kirk P (2009) Cultural perspectives: African leadership surfacing new understandings through leadership development. Int J Cross-cult Manag 9(1):69–86

Bonafe CA, Casimiro R (2019) The intersectionality between gender and generation: millennial women leadership. Garcia Memorial Research Medical Center, Nueva Ecija University of Science and Technology, Cabanatuan City, Philippines. Accessed 10 Mar 2020. https://doi.org/10.5296/jpag.v9i2.14610

Bristol G (2016) Why diversity in the workplace is imperative. Entrepreneur. https://www.entrepreneur.com/article/270110. Accessed 16 Nov 2019

Brodbeck FC, Frese M, Jowidan M (2002) Leadership made in Germany. Low on compassion, high on performance. The Academy of Management Executive 16(1):16–29

Brubaker TA (2013) Servant leadership, Ubuntu, and leader effectiveness in Rwanda. Emerging Leadership Journeys 6(1):114–147

Byrom S, Doiwne S (2010) 'She sort of shines': midwives' accounts of 'good' midwifery and 'good' leadership. Midwifery 26:126–137

Cameron KS, Quinn RE (2011) Diagnosing and changing organizational culture, based on the competing values framework. Jossey-Bass, San Francisco, CA

Carlton DW, Perloff JM (2015) Modern Industrial Organization, Global edition. Higher education, 4th edn. Pearson, Cham. https://www.pearson.ch/HigherEducation/Pearson/EAN/9781292087856/Modern-Industrial-Organization-Global-Edition. Accessed 12 Apr 2020

Center for Creative Leadership (2013) Leadership development: results that matter. Online leadership learning. https://www.cclorg/. Accessed 20 Mar 2020

Cho T, Ryu K (2016) The impacts of family-work conflict and social comparison standards on Chinese women faculties' career expectation and success, moderating by self-efficacy. Career Dev Int 21(3):299–316. https://doi.org/10.1108/CDI-11-2015-0146

Choy J, McCormack D, Djurkovic N (2016) Leader-member exchange and job performance: the mediating roles of delegation and participation. J Manag Dev 35(1):104–119

Clarke AN, Cilenti D (2017) Developing collaborative maternal and child health leaders: a descriptive study of the National Maternal and Child Health Workforce Development Center. Maternal Child Health Journal 22:17–23. https://doi.org/10.1007/s10995-017-2399-4

Conger JA (1993) Leadership needs in the 1st Century. In Principles of Management McGill University. https://opentextbc.ca/principlesofmanagementopenstax/chapter/leadership-needs-inthe-21st-century/#ch13rfin-109

Conger JA (2012) Leadership needs in the 21st century. Principles of Management BC Open textbooks. https://opentextbcca/principlesofmanagementopenstax/chapter/leadership-needs-in-the-21st-century/. Accessed 16 Nov 2019

Cummingham J, Salomone J, Wielgus N (2015) Project management leadership style: a team member's perspective. International Journal of Global Business. 8(2):27–54

De Pree M (2006) Leadership is an art. Kindle edition. https://www.amazon.com/Leadership-Art-Max-Depree-book/dp/B0053CT29A/ref=sr_1_1?_encoding=UTF8&qid=1578302739&refinements=p_27%3AMax+Depree&s=digital-text&sr=1-1

Divall B (2015) Negotiating competing discourses in narratives of midwifery leadership in the English NHS. Midwifery 31(2015):1060–1066

Dong Y, Bartol KM, Zhang Z-Xue, Li C (2017) Enhancing employee creativity via individual skill development and team knowledge sharing: Influences of dualfocused transformational leadership. Journal of Organizational Behavior 38 (3):439–458

Dorfman P, Howell JP, Hibino S et al (2006) Leadership in Western and Asian countries: commonalities and differences in effective leadership practices. In: Pierce J, Newstrom J (eds) Leaders and the leadership process. McGraw-Hill, New York

Durham CC, Knight D, Locke EA (1997) Effects of leader role, team-set goal difficulty, efficacy, and tactics on team effectiveness. Organ Behav Hum Decis Process 72(2):203–231

Eagly AH (2015) Foreword. In: Ngunjiri FW, Karen A, Longman KA et al (eds) Women and leadership around the world. Information Age, Charlotte, pp ix–xiii

Eagly AH, Carli LL (2003a) Finding gender advantage and disadvantage: systematic research integration is the solution. Leadersh Q 14(6):851–859. https://doi.org/10.1016/j.leaqua.2003.09.003

Eagly AH, Carli LL (2003b) The female leadership advantage: an evaluation of the evidence. Leadersh Q 14(6):807–834. https://doi.org/10.1016/j.leaqua.2003.09.004

Eagly AH, Johannesen-Schimdt MC, van Engen M (2003) Transformational, transactional, and laissez-faire leadership styles: a meta-analysis comparing women and men. Psychol Bull 129(4):569

Edwards N, Kaseje D, Kahwa E et al (2016) The impact of leadership hubs on the uptake of evidence-informed nursing practices and workplace policies for HIV care: a quasi-experimental study in Jamaica, Kenya, Uganda and South Africa. Implementation Science 11:110. https://doi.org/10.1186/s13012-016-0478-3

Elangovan AR, Xie JL (2000) Effects of perceived power of supervisor on subordinate work attitudes. Leadership & Organization Development Journal 21(6):319–328

Fadare S (2018) Leadership styles and effectiveness among Sub Saharan African employees. The Journal of Value Based Leadership. 11 2:11. https://scholar.valpo.edu/jvbl/vol11/iss2/11/. Accessed 8 Mar 2020

Ferris GR, Hochwarter WA (2011) Organisational politics. In: Ferris GR, Treadway DC (eds) Politics in organizations: theory and research considerations 2012. American Psychology Assoiation, Washington, DC, pp 3–26

Fiedler FE (1967) A theory of leadership effectiveness. McGraw-Hill, New York, NY

Fiaz M, Qin S, Ikrama A et al. (2017) Leadership styles and employees' motivation: a team meber perspective from an emerging economy. Journal of Developing Areas. 51(4). https://doi.org/10.1353/jda.2017.0093

Fizza K, Rathore K, Qaisar A (2019) Relationship of benevolent leadership and organizational citizenship behavior: Interactional effect of perceived organizational support and perceived organizational politics. Pakistan Journal of Commerce and Social Sciences (PJCSS) 13(2):283–310

Forbes (2018) Leadership: 8 essential qualities that define great leadership. https://www.forbes.com/sites/kimberlyfries/2018/02/08/8-essential-qualities-that-define-great-leadership/#2707dea73b63

Gîrneață A, Potcovaru M (2015) The influence of organisational culture in increasing the performance of textile and clothing companies. in The 4th Multidisciplinary Academic Conference in Prague, Czech Republic. Proceedings of he 4th MAC

Gyekye K (1997) Tradition and modernity: Philosophical reflections on the African experience. Oxford University Press, New York

Gyekye K (2010) African ethics. In: Zalta E (ed.). Stanford Encyclopedia of Philosophy. https://plato.stanford.edu/entries/african-ethics/. Accessed 12 Dec 2019

Halverson CB and Tirmizi SA (Eds) (2008) Effective multicultural teams:theory and practice. Springer Science and Business Media, 6 June 2008

Haron H (2015) Corporate social responsibility: a review on definitions, core characteristics and theoretical perspectives. Mediterranean Journal of Social Sciences 6(4):83–95. https://doi.org/10.5901/mjss.2015.v6n4p8

Helgesen S, Johnson J (2010) The female vision: women's real power at work. Berrett-Koehler, San Francisco

Hochwarter WA, Witt LA, Kacmar KM (2000) Perceptions of organizational politics as a moderator of the relationship between consciousness and job performance. J Appl Psychol 85(3):472–478

Hofstede G (1991) Cultures and organisations: software of the mind. McGraw-Hill Book Company, London

Hofstede GJ, Minkov M (2010) Cultures and organizations—software of the mind: intercultural cooperation and its importance for survival. McGraw-Hill, New York

Hollander EP (1964) Leaders, groups and social influence. In: Pearce CL, Conger JA (eds) Shared leadership: reframing the hows and whys of leadership 2003. Oxford University Press, New York

Hollander EP, Jullian JW (1969) Contemporary trends in analysis of leadership process. Psychological Bulletin 7(5):387–397

House RJ, Mitchell TR (1974) Path-goal theory of leadership. J Contemp Business 86

Huang J, Aaltio I (2014) Guanxi and social capital: networking among women managers in China and Finland. Int J Intercult Relat 39:22–39

International Confederation of Midwives (2014) Curriculum of the young midwifery leaders programme. https://www.internationalmidwives.org. Accessed 10 Nov 2019

International Confederation of Midwives (2019) International Confederation of Midwives website. https://www.internationalmidwives.org/Who we are

Jackson T (2004) Management and change in Africa: a cross-cultural perspective. Routledge, London

Jarvis D, Reeves P (2017) Enabling BME nurse and midwife progression into senior leadership positions. NHS England Version 10, December 2017

Javalgi RG, Scherer R, Sanchez C et al (2011) A comparative analysis of the attitudes toward women managers in China, Chile, and the USA. Int J Emerg Mark 6(3):233–253

Jaye N (2017) Authentic leadership: George B in Finding Your True North. Leadership, Management & Communication Skills CFA Institute. https://blogscfainstituteorg/investor/2017/08/15/authentic-leadership-bill-george-on-finding-your-true-north/. Accessed 11 Nov2019

Jones K, Ante A, Longman KA et al (eds) (2018) Perspectives on women's higher education leadership from around the world. Administrative Sciences. MDPI, Basel, Beijing, Barcelona, Belgrade

Kaiser RB, Wallace WT (2016) Gender bias and substantive differences in ratings of leadership behavior: toward a new narrative. Consulting Psychology

Journal: Practice and Research 68(1):72–98. https://doi.org/10.1037/cpb0000059

Kanter RM (1982) Dilemmas of managing participation. Organ Dyn 11(1):527

Kanter RM (2002) Strategy as improvisational theatre. Sloan Manag Rev 43(2):76–81

Kelchner L (2016) Multicultural instructional design: concepts, methodologies, tools and applications: top ten negotiation skills http://smallbusinesschroncom/top-ten-effective-negotiation-skills/. Accessed 10 Dec 2019

Khaliq AA, Arshad R, Syed S (2017) Relationship of charismatic leadership, leadership effectiveness and team performance in employees of a microfinance bank of Lahore. sci. Int. (Lahore), 28(5):65–72

Khan SM, Khan I, Quereshi Q et al. (2015) The styles of leadership: a critical review. Public Policy and Administration Research. 5(3)

Kong D, Zhang JJ (2011) The research on Chinese ancient management philosophies' similarities with contemporary human resources management thoughts. Chin Manag Stud 5(4):368–379

Kuada J (2006) Cross-ultural interactions and changing management practices in Africa: a hybrid management perspective. African Journal of Business and Economic Research Vol 1 No.1 96–113

Kuada J (2009) Gender, social networks and intrepreneurship in Ghana. Journal of African Business vol 10 no.1 85–103

Kuada J (2010) Culture and leadership in Africa: a conceptual model and research agenda. Research Gate https://www.researchgate.net/publication/46545466. Accessed 11 Dec 2019

Kouzes J and Posner B (2012) The leadership challange. How to make extraordinary things happen in organisations.San Francisco, CA: The leadership challange-A Willy Brand

Leadership Academy (2011) Leadership framework: a summary. NHS Leadership Academy, London

Longman K (2018) Women in leadership: the future of Christian higher education. https://www.research-gate.net/publication/334349370. Accessed 16 Dec 2019

Lord RG, Brown DJ, Frieberg SJ (1999) Understanding the dynamics of leadership: the role of follower self-concepts in the leader/follower relationship. Organ Behav Hum Decis Process 78(3):167–203

Management Science for Health (2015) Leadership. Management and governance for midwifery managers. Amref Health Africa Virtual Training School, Nairobi. Kenya

Masolo DA (2010) Self and community in a changing world. University of Indiana Press, Bloomington

Menkiti I (2004) On the normative conception of a person. In: Wiredu K (ed) A companion to African philosophy. Blackwell, Oxford, pp 324–331

Metz T (2013) The Western ethic of care or an Afro-communitarian ethic? Finding the right relational morality. Journal of Global Ethics 9:77–92

Metz T (2015) How the West was one: the Western as individualist, the African as communitarian. Educ Philos Theory 47:1175–1184

Metz T (2017) Managerialism as anti-social: Some implications of ubuntu for knowledge production. In: Cross M, Ndofirepi A (eds) Knowledge and change in African Universities, vol 2. Sense Publishers, Rotterdam, pp 139–154

Metz T (2018) An African theory of good leadership. https://www.researchgate.net/publication/328981934. Accessed 12 Dec 2019

Mianda S, Voce AS (2018) Midwife conceptualizations of clinical leadership in the labor ward of district hospitals in KwaZulu-Natal, South Africa. Journal of Healthcare Leadership 10:87–94

Michaud J, Lituchy TR, Acosta M et al (2019) Effective Leadership in Mexico: an extension of the LEAD project. Journal of African Business 20(1):72–90. https://doi.org/10.1080/15228916.2019.1583936

Mihai M (2015) Processing–formulation–performance relationships of polypropylene/short flax fibre composites. J Appl Polym Sci 132(9):3–6

Mohuidin ZA (2017) Influence of leadership styles on employees' performance: evidence from literature. Journal of Marketing Management. 8(1):18–30

Murnigham JK, Leung TK (1976) The effects of leadership involvement and the importance of the task on subordinate performance. Organisational Behaviour and Human Performance. 17:299–310

Myatt M (2019). Traits of ineffective leaders. https://www.n2growth.com/6-traits-of-ineffective-leaders/. Accessed November 2019

Nanjundeswaraswamy TS, Swamy DR (2015) Quality of work life: scale development and validation. Int J Caring Sci 8(2):281

Ndlovu PM (2016) Discovering the spirit of Ubuntu leadership. Macmillan Palgrave, London. https://doi.org/10.1057/9781137526854

Ndlovu-Gatsheni S, Ngcaweni B (eds) (2017) Nelson Rolihlahla Mandela: decolonial ethics of liberation and servant leadership. Africa World Press, Trenton, NJ

Northouse PG (2019) Introduction to leadership: concepts and practice. SAGE, PG Northouse

O'Connor P (2015) Good jobs—but places for women? Gend Educ 27(3):304–319

O'Sullivan K (2019 "Holding up Half the Sky"—Women and the Glass Ceiling at a University in China. Department of Student Recruitment, Admissions & Services, Niagara College KSA, Al Majma'ah, Kingdom of Saudi Arabia

Ogbonnaya C, Nielsen K (2016) Transformational leadership, high performance work practices, and an effective organization. Academy of Management, New York

Okpara JO, Wynn P (2007) The effect of culture on job satisfaction and organizational commitment: a study of information system managers in Nigeria.

African Journal of Business and Economic Research 2(2/3):9–36

Owen J (2017) Global teams: how the best teams achieve performance. Pearson Education, Harlow

Parris RAW, Hart P (2013) The Oxford handbook of political leadership. OUP, Oxford

Patel G (2013) Gender differences in leadership styles and the impact within the corporate boards. The Commonwealth Secretariat, Social Transformation Programmes Division, London

Powell-Kennedy H (2011) Foreword. in Essential midwifery practice: Leadership, expertise and collaborative working. by Soo Downe, Sheena Byrom and Louise Simpson. Wiley-Blackwell. Blackwell publishing ltd

Rahman MA (2012) A comprehensive model of 21st century leadership. Bangladesh Journal of MIS 2,3,4,&5(1) ISSN 2073-9737 https://www.researchgate.net/publication/257351407_A_Comprehensive_Model_of_21st_Century_Leadership

Rathore K, Chaudhry AK, Nauman A (2017) The influence of leadership styles on employees performance perceptions of organizational politics: A study of telecom sector in Pakistan. International Journal of Management Research and Emerging 7(1): 106–140

Read J (2019) The profile of professional midwifery leadership in England. British Journal of Midwifery 2019 27(2):120–128

Reid J (2016) The effects of leadership styles and budget participation on job satisfaction and job performance. Asia-Pacific Management Accounting Journal 3(1):21–46

Robert C, Probst TM, Martocchio JJ et al (2000) Empowerment and continuous improvement in the United States, Mexico, Poland, and India: predicting fit on the basis of the dimensions of power distance and individualism. J Appl Psychol 85:643–658

Ross-Davie M, Stevenson R, Maynor K (2016) The development, implementation and evaluation of a leadership programme for midwives. Evidence Based Midwifery 14(3):87–93

Rousseau DM (1990) New hire perceptions of their own and their employer's obligations: a study of psychological contracts. Journal of Organizational Behaviour 11:389–400

Sandberg S, Scovell N (2013) Lean in: women, work and the will to lead. Random House, New York

Schneider H, Somers M (2006) Organisations as complex adaptive systems: implications of complexity theory on leadership research. The Leadership Quarterly 17(4):351–65

Schein EH (2010) Organizational culture and leadership, 4th edn. Jossey-Bass, San Francisco, CA

Shutte A (2001) Ubuntu: an ethic for the new South Africa. Cluster Publications, Cape Town

Speitzer GM, Perttula KH, Xin K (2005) Traditionality matters: an examination of the effectiveness of transformational leadership in the United States and Taiwan. Journal of Organisational Behaviour 26(3): 205–227

Sørensen OJ, Kuada J (2001) Institutional context of Ghanaian firms and cross-national inter-firm relations. In: Jacobsen G, Torp JE (eds) Understanding business systems in developing countries. Sage, New Delhi, pp 163–201

Staines G et al (1973) The queen bee syndrome. In: Tavris C (ed) The female Experience. CRM Books, Del Mar, CA, pp 34–56

Stogdill RM (1974) Handbook of leadership: a survey of theory and research. The Free Press, New York, NY

Tremblay M, Vandenberghe C, Doucet O (2013) Relationship between leader- contingent and non-contingent reward and punishment behaviours and subordinates' perception of justice and satisfaction, and evaluating the moderating influence of trust propensity, pay level and role ambiguity. Journal of Business Psychology 28(2):233–249

Tutu D (1999) No future without forgiveness. Random House, New York

USAID (2015) Leadership, management and governance for midwifery managers. updated in 2015. Amref Health Africa Virtual Training School. Nairobi

Vera D, Crossan M (2004) Strategic leadership and organisational learning. Academy of Management Review. 29(2):222–240

Wang W, Cho T (2013) Work-family conflict influences on female's career development through career expectation. Journal of Human Resource and Sustainability Studies 1(3):43–50. https://doi.org/10.4236/jhrss.2013.13007

Watkins MD (2013) What is organizational culture? And why should we care? Harvard Business Rev. https://hbr.org/2013/05/what-is-organizational-culture. Accessed Nov 2019

West M, Armit K, Eckert R et al (2015) Leadership and leadership development in health care: the evidence base. Center for Creative Leadership, Kings Fund

Whitley R (ed) (1994) European business systems: firms and markets in their national contexts. Sage, London

Winston BE, Patterson K (2006) An integrative definition of leadership. Int J Entrep Business Innov 6(2): 6–66

Woermann M, Engelbrecht S (2017) The Ubuntu challenge to business: from stakeholders to relation holders. Journal of Business Ethics 1(1):1–18. https://doi.org/10.1007/s10551-017-3680-6

World Health Organization (2008) Task shifting: global recommendations and guidelines. WHO, Geneva

World Health Organization Regional Office for Europe (2015) Nurses and midwives: a vital resource for health. WHO European Region, Copenhagen

Wright PL, Taylor DS (1994) Improving leadership performance: interpersonal skills for effective leadership (2nd ed.) Prentice Hall, Hemel Hempstead, Herts

Xie Y, Zhu Y (2016) Holding up half of the sky: women managers' view on promotion opportunities at enterprise level in China. Journal of Chinese Human Resource Management 7(1):45–60. https://doi.org/10.1108/JCHRM-11-2015-0015

Yan S, Wu Y, Zhang G (2018) The gender difference in leadership effectiveness and its Sino-US comparison. Chin Manag Stud 12(1):106–124. https://doi.org/10.1108/CMS-07-2016-0148

Yang Y (2011) Gender and engineering career development of hotel's employees in China. Systems Engineering Procedia 1:365–371. https://doi.org/10.1016/j.sepro.2011.08.055

YourDictionary (2018) Definition of adminsitration

Zhang L (2005) The particular career experiences of Chinese women academics. In F Du, X Zheng, and LY Tachakkayo (Eds) Women's studies in China: mapping the social, economic and policy changes in Chineses women's lives. (p77–114) Seoul: Ewha Women's University Press

Zhang L (2010) A study on the measurement of job-related stress among women academics in research universities of China. Front Educ China 5:158–176. https://doi.org/10.1007/s11516-010-0011-4

Zhang Y, Foo SF (2012) Balanced leadership: perspectives, principles and practices. Chin Manag Stud 6(2):245–256. https://doi.org/10.1108/17506141211236686

Strengthening Midwifery Research

12

Expected Learning Outcomes

By the end of the chapter, the reader should be able to:

1. Discuss how research is a fundamental component of midwifery education and practice.
2. Consider why a gap persists between dissemination of research and implementation of the findings and how this could be addressed.
3. Describe the ways in which research evidence is obtained.
4. Outline the structures that comprise network theory.
5. Give examples of national, regional and global midwifery research networks and how they influence education and practice.
6. Identify international priority areas for the development of midwifery research and discuss how these vary across different regions.
7. Discuss the potential benefits of high-quality midwifery research and its implications in the context of improving health care for women and newborns.

12.1 Research: An Indispensable Professional Pillar

Midwifery is an age-old art deeply rooted in the traditions of many cultures, but it has evolved into a highly skilled profession as it is increasingly recognised that 'midwives save lives' (PMNCH 2011; UNFPA 2014; WHO 2018a; Barnes 2019) and of course this is crucial in the context of reducing maternal and perinatal mortality and promoting health and well-being across the world. The International Confederation of Midwives (ICM) states categorically that 'Research is the foundation of midwifery's Three Pillars and ongoing education and research are the lifeblood of any vibrant profession' (ICM 2019).

Whilst midwifery is recognised as an evidence-based profession, concern has been expressed about why research is not always embraced by midwives and applied in education and practice. This is a widespread issue affecting nurses, midwives and other healthcare professionals and extends over a considerable period of time (Glacken and Chaney 2004; Hommelstad and Ruland 2004; Kajermo et al. 2010; Khammarnia et al. 2015; Yahui and Swaminathan 2017). International and interprofessional collaboration on research and the challenges in its implementation in midwifery are clearly important, but these may vary

© Springer Nature Switzerland AG 2021
J. Kemp et al., *Global Midwifery: Principles, Policy and Practice*,
https://doi.org/10.1007/978-3-030-46765-4_12

considerably in different contexts. In a study considering the progress of midwifery research across two decades in four countries, namely Austria, Germany, The Netherlands and Switzerland, it was noted that research had developed as a context-specific phenomenon influenced by the following factors:

> … the history and character of midwifery in the country,
> … the initiatives of individual midwifery researchers,
> … alliances with other professions and
> … the transition of midwifery programmes into higher education.
> (Luyben et al. 2013:6)

The authors conclude that although there appeared to be a common vision shared amongst these countries, midwifery research was closely related to the national character of midwifery practice and education. Looking ahead, it was recommended that the further development of midwifery as an academic discipline needed to take these issues into account (Luyben et al. 2013).

These matters bear some relevance to those raised by Hunter (2013) who describes a 'Black Box' which appears to exist between dissemination of research findings and possible implementation. She identifies various issues that may influence whether evidence is put into practice, and these may act as barriers or as facilitators. These are summarised in Table 12.1. Hunter stresses that in order to optimise the introduction of evidence into practice, researchers need to pay

attention to these processes; furthermore, strategies used to disseminate findings should attempt to reduce the gap between researchers and implementers.

Attitudes affecting how evidence-based practice is perceived are obviously not confined by international borders, nor to a single profession. The question remains as to how to inspire more midwives to be research-aware and research-active. Traditional versus evidence-based practice remains a challenge in many and various parts of the world. A study in Iran reflects the situation, revealing that midwives' attitudes to evidence-based practice varied considerably, some perceiving it as useful, improving outcomes and promoting woman-centred care whilst others described it as 'a waste of time', increasing workload and preferring to stick to traditional approaches (Azmoud et al. 2018). This would appear to suggest, in harmony with Luyben et al. (2013) and Hunter (2013), that the context within which the midwife is educated and practices are crucial determinants of the outcome in this complex situation. The influence of midwifery leaders and the role of midwifery associations in championing research are surely key issues in promoting quality research and in accepting the importance of evidence-based midwifery practice and these have been explored in Chapters. 6 and 11 respectively.

12.2 Research and Midwifery Education and Practice

In the context of basic and ongoing midwifery education, ICM describes midwifery as:

> …a profession in its own right, with a unique body of knowledge, skills and behaviours… continuing…
>
> …much of the knowledge and competencies are based on evidence resulting from research by midwives and others. (ICM 2014:1)

Evidence-based practice has become the norm in contemporary professional midwifery, and so research can rightly be described as an indispensable part of midwifery education.

Table 12.1 Inside the 'Black Box': the factors that may influence implementation of evidence

Characteristics of the evidence, including: …its robustness …its accessibility	Context into which the evidence is to be introduced including: …resource implications …organisational readiness to change
The significance of the evidence to the holders of authoritative knowledge	Potential users: Who will use the evidence? How does it fit with other sources of knowledge?

Derived from Hunter (2013:80)

12.2.1 Evidence-Based Midwifery Education and Practice

Evidence-based medicine has been defined as:

> …the conscientious, explicit and judicious use of current best evidence in making decisions about the care of individual patients.
> (Sackett et al. 1996:71)

Whilst evidence-based healthcare has been perceived as:

> …a strategy and a set of tools which enable a practitioner to be aware of and locate the available evidence, judge its strength and soundness and be in a position to apply it in practice.
> (Siwha and Roth 2004:48)

Evidence-based midwifery care therefore is a crucial tool in promoting safe childbirth globally and must always rely on reliable research. Evidence needs to be robust. The research process utilises systematic strategies to investigate questions, then collect and analyse data so that findings can be validated.

12.2.2 Intuition and Research

Intuition has been acknowledged as an indispensable aid in midwifery practice (Olsson and Adolfsson 2011; Muoni 2014) and could be described as a midwife's sixth sense. It may be mooted that intuition is incompatible with scientific research, yet it was Albert Einstein who said that he believed in intuition and inspiration. Claiming that imagination is more important than knowledge, Einstein proceeds to reason that:

> …knowledge is limited, whereas imagination embraces the entire world, stimulating progress, giving birth to evolution. It is, strictly speaking, a real factor in scientific research. (Einstein and Shaw 2009:97)

Little wonder then that it has been proposed more recently that:

> …personal experience and knowledge are an additional source of evidence as these should inform practice and research at every level.
> (Siwha and Roth 2004:49)

Tradition, of which there is no shortage surrounding childbirth, can be challenged or reinforced through reliable research. Intuition can be processed likewise.

12.2.3 Research as a Basis for Determining a Model of Care

As research took a firm place in professional midwifery practice, it was considered that research evidence could be instrumental in addressing the issue of midwife-led care as opposed to obstetric-led care (Renfrew 1997; Wickham 2000; Munro and Spiby 2001, 2010; Brucker and Schwarz 2002; Bogdan-Lovis and Sousa 2006). The essential issues concerning the various models of practice are discussed in detail in Chapter 7, but evidence is still sought in order to offer women the most appropriate care during their birthing experience in the situation in which they find themselves.

12.2.4 International Research Priorities and Midwifery Research

Considering the international research priorities identified and discussed below (see Table 12.3), it would seem that across the world midwives are still struggling to promote normal birth which suggests that there remains a vacuum in usable evidence that is sufficiently convincing to change policy and practice to achieve that. Maybe this emphasises the need for evidence-based advocacy (Nanda et al. 2005), and this issue is discussed in Chapters. 1 and 2 in respect of the Millennium Development Goals (MDGs), and this approach to advocacy is highlighted again in Chapter 14 in respect of international consultancy.

However, drawing on evidence from a study undertaken by the World Health Organization (WHO) as well as the 2014 Lancet Series on Midwifery, Kennedy et al. (2018) conclude that research priorities in future concerning maternal and newborn health should focus on:

> …quality care that is tailored to individuals, weighs benefits and harms, is person-centered, works across the whole continuum of care,

advances equity, and is informed by evidence, including cost-effectiveness. (Kennedy et al. 2018:222)

The authors identify three inter-related research themes in this context, namely:

> …examination and implementation of models of care that enhance both well-being and safety;
> …investigating and optimizing physiological, psychological, and social processes in pregnancy, childbirth, and the postnatal period; and
> …development and validation of outcome measures that capture short and longer term well-being. (Kennedy et al. 2018:222)

12.2.5 Categories of Research Evidence

Research evidence has been categorised into a hierarchy (Fig. 12.1) even though systematic reviews and meta-analyses lie at the tip of the hierarchy, every piece of evidence needs to be critically examined to assess its reliability, validity and relevance to the clinical issue under review. For this reason, critical thinking and research evaluation are requisite components of a midwife's education. It has further been suggested that many midwives prefer the term 'evidence-informed' to 'evidence-based', sug-

gesting that this encompasses a woman's right to choose (van Wagner 2017).

12.3 Research Networks

Networking has become a popular activity whether on a face to face level, facilitated through conferences or workshops or the ever-expanding possibilities offered by the internet, including webinars, Skype, Zoom, WhatsApp or other emerging technologies. Research networks have become a valuable resource to enhance professional practice as well as an indispensable tool to academics.

In considering research networks, it is helpful to first explore briefly how networks are defined and how they may be constructed. In this context, a network essentially denotes an organisational structure that is not formally ordered. It generally describes a formation of people who share a profession or a common cause. However, in examining a network, it can be noted that it comprises a structure of some kind with different interconnected parts. Networks may vary in their *size* and in their other properties described as *'configuration'* and *'connectedness'* (Nohria and Eccles 1992).

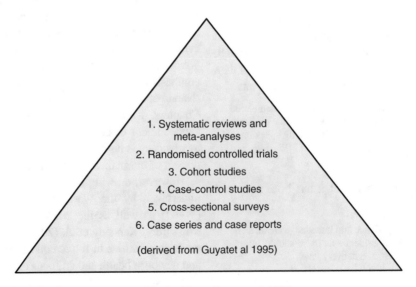

Fig. 12.1 A hierarchy of research evidence. (Derived from Guyatt et al. 1995)

Four possible network *configurations* have been described; these are hierarchical, centred, dispersed and clustered (Fig. 12.2).

Connectedness describes the number of links connecting the network units. Networks may be loosely connected or richly connected (Fig. 12.3).

12.3.1 The Importance of Networks in Research

Some researchers propose that richly coupled networks may have definite advantages in coordinating behaviour and consequently in responding to opportunities or threats (Perrow 1986; Porter 1990; Piore 1990). But in the context of sociological network theory, it has also been mooted

that weak ties provide valuable insights into the nature of co-operation occurring between a larger number of acquaintances regarded as 'weak ties'. However, it is reckoned that the former will exhibit greater collective innovativeness, cohesiveness and adaptability (Granovetter 1973). In the context of a major analysis of networks within Sector Wide Approaches (SWAp) development programmes in Africa, Forss et al. (2000:2) identify six roles that exist within networks; these they labelled 'visionary, network builder, financier, operator, controller and facilitator'. The researchers suggest that mapping out networks can help analyse whether there are too many actors in a particular role and establish if some roles are neglected. They advise that characteristically some network maps indicate that there are

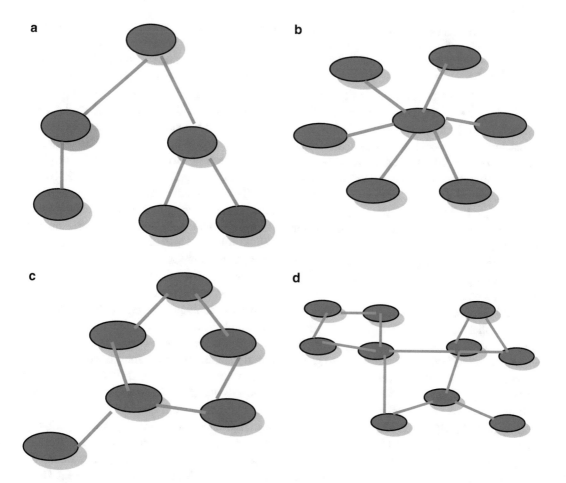

Fig. 12.2 Examples of network configurations. (**a**) Hierarchical. (**b**) Centred. (**c**) Dispersed. (**d**) Clustered. (Derived from Forss et al. (2000) and reproduced with author's permission)

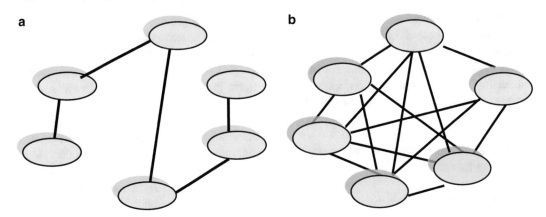

Fig. 12.3 Showing different 'connectedness' in networks. (**a**) A loosely coupled network. (**b**) A richly coupled network. (Derived from Forss et al. (2000) and reproduced with author's permission)

several actors in the visionary roles, many in controller roles, but few in the operative role, concluding that:

> …All actors concerned would benefit if less of the network roles depended on personal inclination and chance, and more on policy and planning. (Forss et al. 2000:3)

It may well be a consideration as to whether this is the case in the context of professional research networks in general and midwifery networks in particular and may reflect the issues raised by Hunter (2013) and discussed above. It could be advantageous if research networks were less hierarchical (Fig. 12.2a) and more richly coupled (Fig. 12.3b). Maybe if more midwives in clinical practice were active members of research networks, this may help to bridge the dissemination–implementation gap. Possibly the research network type plays a part here and could be added to Hunter's black box.

In this context, it is worthy of note that the WHO Collaborating Centres provide major opportunities for research networking across the world. More than 800 centres in 80 countries participate as World health Organization Collaborating Centres (WHOCCs) (WHO 2018b), 43 of these are designated as centres for Nursing and Midwifery (WHO 2020). WHOCCs may carry out research for WHO, assist with dissemination of information, offer technical advice to WHO and provide training courses (WHO 2018b).

12.3.2 Examples of Research Networks

Research networks amongst professionals have evolved across countries and across regions and continents. Perhaps one of the earlier formalised midwifery research networks was established in Africa. The Africa Midwives Research Network (AMRN) emanated from a regional workshop in 1993 with the rationale of 'enhancing the quality of midwifery care in Africa' whilst strengthening and empowering African midwives in their professional capacity (Maclean and Forss 2010:e1). AMRN was initially supported by the Swedish International Development Co-operation Agency (Sida) involving a technical collaboration with the Karolinska Institute (KI) in Stockholm. Thirty-two countries were reported as originally forming the network, though just seven were regarded as active members; these were Eritrea, Kenya, Mozambique, Tanzania, Uganda, Zambia and Zimbabwe (Maclean and Forss 2010:e3). AMRN was formally evaluated and described as a fairly small, dispersed, loosely connected network (see Figs. 12.2c and 12.3a). The major achievements of AMRN were clearly identified as creating a network that had shown a remarkable resilience and continuity over a period of 15 years at the time of evaluation. The work of AMRN was considered highly relevant in the context of the Millennium Development Goals (Forss and Maclean 2007:34).

AMRN initiated the *African Journal of Midwifery and Women's Health* which helps to disseminate research evidence across the continent and beyond and promote safe evidence-based midwifery care (AJM 2017). This network made a valuable contribution to midwifery in Africa where it was maintained for more than two decades and the lessons learned were eventually inherited by a new network, the Lugina Africa Midwives Research Network (LAMRN). LAMRN was named in honour of the late Dr. Helen Igobeko Lugina, whose dedicated service to the field of midwifery in Africa saw her make significant contributions in training, research and policy advocacy. LAMRN has been supported from the British Department for International Development (DFID) with the leadership of midwives from the University of Manchester, England. The network's activities seek to advance the original ideals of the founding champions of AMRN whilst also tackling newer challenges in six countries, namely Kenya, Malawi, Tanzania, Uganda, Zambia and Zimbabwe. LAMRN's aim is:

> …to serve as a base for sharing information, strategies and solutions based on scientific evidence for provision of quality midwifery care in the region. (LAMRN 2019)

The priority areas that have been identified for LAMRN activities are summarised in Box 12.1.

LAMRN has become involved in a major research project in collaboration with The University of Manchester and the National Institute of Health Research (NIHR), UK. The research is investigating and then seeking ways to prevent stillbirth, promote evidence-based intrapartum care and ensure humane and respectful care for bereaved parents (LAMRN 2019; NIHR 2020). LAMRN has also developed and researched the effectiveness of educational games in midwifery designed to address specific issues relating to promoting high-quality care. These include intrapartum care, emergency obstetric and neonatal care and respectful care (Lavender and Omoni 2019; Laisser et al. 2019; Maclean and Laisser 2020).

In the *United States (USA)*, the American College of Nurse-Midwives (ACNM) organises a series of research interest groups. These aim to facilitate relevant research and connect individuals with others working with similar areas of interest in midwifery. The ACNM research interest groups' objectives are summarised in Box 12.2.

Box 12.1. The Priority Areas of LAMRN

- Supporting senior midwifery partners to develop research leadership skills.
- Working with midwives in target countries to identify country-level maternal health research priorities.
- Providing training midwives for six countries to improve evidence-based practice skills.
- Developing a mentorship system for midwives to develop research projects in priority areas such as reduction of obstructed labour or postpartum haemorrhage.

LAMRN.org (2019)

Box 12.2. ACNM Research Interest Groups'
. **Objectives**

1. Foster broad-based midwifery research by supplementing the Research Advisory Networking (RAN) begun by the International Confederation of Midwives (ICM).
2. Promote opportunities for multi-site U.S.-based research.
3. Support potential mentoring relationships between new and experienced researchers by providing another mechanism for identification individuals involved in midwifery research and in specific areas of investigation.
4. Provide a service to ACNM members and other researchers that facilitates rapid identification and contact between individuals of similar researcher interests to more effectively stimulate and support coordination of midwifery-focused research.

ACNM (2019)

Spread widely across the USA with networking facilitated at least initially via the internet, this would appear to be a large clustered network (Fig. 12.2d) linking midwives with common specialised interests and expertise. The connectedness within such a network would inevitably vary with time, the extent of existing common interest and the personnel involved. Other midwifery associations around the globe provide members with resources and relevant guidance in promoting evidence-based care for women and their families.

The Doctoral Midwifery Research Society (DMRS) represents a global network offering membership to:

> ...all registered, certified or licenced midwives, nurse-midwives or obstetric nurses, doctors or allied health professionals from within higher education and practice development who hold a doctoral degree or are currently studying towards a doctoral degree from any institution worldwide.
> (Doctoral Midwifery Research Society 2020)

There are also opportunities for associate and affiliated membership. This organisation provides opportunity for all concerned with maternal and newborn health to network and to facilitate the global dissemination of relevant research.

12.4 Promoting and Facilitating Midwifery Research Around the World

In order to promote and disseminate research the International Confederation of Midwives (ICM) has established a research network facilitated by a Research Standing Committee. The role of this committee is summarised in Box 12.3.

Box 12.3. The ICM Research Standing Committee
- Identifies midwifery research in progress and takes part in the discussions to develop the ICM research strategy.
- Creates communication networks between researchers working in reproductive health and midwifery.

- Maintains a database of researchers which acts as a source of information and support.
- Recommends to the ICM Board, Executive Committee and Council, activities, priorities, strategies and practices for midwifery research throughout the world.
- Reviews abstracts submitted for peer-review.
- Plans the Committee's involvement in each ICM congress and facilitates research workshops at these.
- Provides a resource of expert midwifery research workers for access by ICM if required.
- (ICM 2018)

Various countries promote and support research through their universities and professional associations, mostly the network structures and organisation are insufficiently described to be classified here; however, a few examples are cited below. The *New Zealand* College of Midwifery aims to 'promote collaboration and facilitate liaison' between their members undertaking research both nationally and internationally and to facilitate collaborative research between multidisciplinary groups and researchers (NZCM 2019). The *Australian* College of Midwives facilitates links between members on innovation and research (ACM 2019). The Dutch midwives' professional association facilitates what is termed: 'a first line network for midwifery research'. This is shared in collaboration with several midwives' and medical groups including the Royal Dutch Organization of Obstetricians and aims 'to stimulate and where possible facilitate midwifery science in the *Netherlands*' (KNOV 2013). The European Midwives Association supports research from European Union (EU) countries and extends to addressing the global problem of maternal and infant mortality and morbidity (EMA 2019).

In addition to numerous journals publishing relevant research, the Royal College of Midwives (RCM) in the *United Kingdom* regularly publishes a research journal entitled *Evidence-Based Midwifery* (RCM 2019) working closely with midwifery academics and the RCM's appointed midwifery professors to support midwifery research studies throughout the UK and further afield.

Nursing and midwifery research activity in *Arab countries* has been perceived as an important indicator of the quality of healthcare services provided as well as the status of the respective professions. According to Sweileh et al. (2019), nursing and midwifery research had markedly increased between 1950 and 2017 and improved dramatically in the period 2012–2017. Through analysing almost 3000 documents, it was concluded that *Jordan* ranked first in research output followed by *Saudi Arabia, Egypt* and *Lebanon.*

A review of midwives' perceptions of and participation in research revealed that very few research programmes in *France* examined any aspects of midwifery. This paucity is seen as a major barrier to the involvement of midwives in research. The situation is linked to a shortage of adequate and specialised French journals publishing midwifery topics. This is a matter of concern particularly in the context of Francophone Africa where maternal mortality ratios tend to be very high (Goyet et al. 2018:109).

An increasing number of educational institutions around the world are including research skills and the opportunity to develop research projects in their undergraduate midwifery programmes, and some of these are illustrated in Table 12.2 along with other research initiatives.

Table 12.2 Global glimpses into enhancing research skills and evidence-based practice

The challenge in Chile	*Changing concepts in Australia*
In recent years, universities in Chile have included research skills development in most curricula for professional degree programmes. Therefore, a research unit was established within the Midwifery Department. Both students and their teachers rated the experience of acquiring research skills through the curriculum positively. It was concluded that this enabled them to acquire competencies and confidence in their research skills. It is also considered that midwives were well prepared to participate as active members in multidisciplinary research teams needed to successfully implement evidence-based practice change (Bonilla et al. 2018)	A university in Australia exploring the negative attitudes of postgraduate nursing and midwifery students towards research concluded that a 'Community of Inquiry' offered promising potential. The 'Community' comprised 'an online teaching, learning, thinking, and sharing space'. This was produced by combining three domains, namely teacher presence, social presence and cognitive presence comprising critical thinking. The intellectual and professional communities formed through using such a framework appeared promising in that students also showed interest in undertaking research themselves (Mills et al. 2016:39)
Incentives in Ireland	*Insights from Asia*
After a comparatively recent move of midwifery education into universities in Ireland, there were ambitious plans to develop the research ability of all academics. There were also aims to improve external research funding and to increase peer-reviewed publications and conference presentations. Provision for sabbatical leave and allowing periods of reduced teaching commitments enabled staff to pursue doctoral studies. Some incentive was offered through allowing for conference and research expenses related to the academics' research output of publications, conference presentations and external funding submissions during the preceding year. The set goals were surpassed, and it was concluded that 'strong research leadership, generous support and liberal encouragement can change a predominantly teaching-focused culture to one of academic research excellence'. It is believed that the increasing expertise in research should lead to an improved education of nursing and midwifery students and ultimately to a better provision of care (Begeley et al. 2014)	More than 1300 midwives from central Asian countries comprising Kyrgyzstan, Tajikistan and Uzbekistan have completed practical training in evidence-based approaches to preventing and treating postpartum haemorrhage, neonatal resuscitation and essential newborn care In Bangladesh, a new generation of midwifery faculty has been built up through a progressive programme of higher education. This is believed to be contributing towards bridging higher education and research (at graduate and undergraduate levels) with policy, regulation and practice. It has been credited with creating a work culture in which research findings can be seen as key for the improvement of academic and health systems Also in Bangladesh, 'standard operating procedure' now involves the provision of evidence-based respectful care by midwives as independent practitioners or as part of a multi-disciplinary team (Kolfenbach and Birdsall 2015; Bogren et al. 2017; DGNM 2017)

In **Chile** it is believed that the absence of training in research poses a serious constraint hampering scientific and technological development. This problem is stated to be a common feature shared with other Latin American countries (Bonilla et al. 2018:60). This finds congruence with a scoping review to discover nurse and midwife led published research which reported a lack of midwifery-related research in both **Latin America** and the **Caribbean** (Iribarren et al. 2018).

12.5 Priority Areas for the Development of Midwifery Research

Midwifery has evolved as a skilled and indispensable profession in the context of global health. Furthermore, it has been acknowledged that quality care is essential to facilitate a safe passage through childbirth for the woman and her baby (UNFPA 2014; WHO 2018a). It therefore stands to reason that much research needs to be undertaken in order to seek the best way forward. Priorities must always be identified. In 2014 an online survey was undertaken through first approaching the ICM Research Advisory Networking members who then disseminated a questionnaire to a wider midwifery research interest group. Respondents were asked to grade the importance of research priorities and provide further suggestions. The topics offered were gleaned from previous scoping exercises and a literature review. Originating from 37 countries, 271 respondents completed the questionnaire. These included 'midwifery practitioners, researchers, lecturers and service providers'.

The findings of the survey are summarised in Table 12.3. These are being used to establish priorities and to inform ICM of the most appropriate research strategy in the development of its research agenda (Soltani et al. 2016). Inevitably each of the priority areas cited above demand sub-dividing into numerous practice areas, each requiring investigation in countless environments and in diverse situations.

Table 12.3 Identified research priorities

Top 3 important themes globally:
1. Promotion of normal birth
2. Prevention of maternal and fetal/neonatal morbidity and mortality
3. Psychosocial aspects of maternity care

Greatest priority in *'more resourced regions'*:
…promotion of normal birth

Greatest priority in *'less resourced locations'*:
…prevention of maternal and fetal/neonatal morbidity and mortality

(Derived from Soltani et al. 2016)

Unarguably, each of these priorities falls in line with the Sustainable Development Goals (SDGs) which are discussed in Chapter 1, and more specifically, they relate to SDG 3 aiming to achieve 'good health and well-being'. In essence, research priorities would seem to enshrine values that are becoming increasingly entwined with woman-centred, holistic care which provides skilled assistance for women and their families wherever they may be. WHO (2019a, b) advocates not only physical safety but promotion of perinatal mental health since almost 20% of women suffer some kind of mental or emotional ill health in the time surrounding birth. This topic is explored in more detail in Chapter 2.

From a survey undertaken across southern and eastern African countries, midwifery topics identified as critical research priorities included HIV/AIDS, tuberculosis, maternal health and mortality, infant mortality and obstetric emergencies (Sun et al. 2015). It is proposed that the shortage of nurse and midwifery researchers in many African countries means that identification of clinical nursing and midwifery research is of the highest priority for the region in order to improve health outcomes (Sun et al 2015:466). In an extensive review of research literature, Sun and Larson (2015:116) conclude that the most published research related to that which had received greatest funding and issues surrounding the human immunodeficiency virus (HIV) had taken priority in that respect. However, the study revealed that there was a considerable gap between the needs and problems encountered in health care and the emphasis of the majority of clinical nursing research. This regional study, to a large extent, echoes the opinions expressed in the international survey cited above (Soltani et al. 2016).

12.6 The Benefits of High-Quality Midwifery Research

Without doubt, high-quality research has the potential to improve the lives and health of women, newborns and their families. According to the study undertaken to inform ICM cited above (Soltani et al. 2016), it became very clear that midwives across the world work in diverse settings. Limited resources and staff shortages are believed to have influenced the priorities they identified. Whereas in some regions, particularly in Africa, the HIV epidemic has coloured the picture, in other areas obesity has become a health challenge influencing some of the priorities for public health research and expenditure, not least that of maternity care.

In attempting to utilise evidence-based strategies that will benefit women and their families, it would seem fundamental to address those deficiencies that have already been uncovered that influence the working practice of midwives. In a combined statement issued by WHO, ICM and the White Ribbon Alliance (WRA) in the context of providing professional support, it has been stressed that:

> …To improve working conditions for midwives and quality of care for women and newborns, midwifery professionals need salaries that adequately reflect the level of their skills and responsibilities, health insurance and social security systems, professional support networks, good living environments, and counselling services. (WHO 2016a)

The largest ever global survey of 2470 midwifery personnel from 93 countries highlights critical issues in the provision of quality midwifery care. It defines the barriers as well as possible solutions to improving care for women, newborns and their families. The study concludes that:

> …The active involvement of midwifery personnel, at all levels, in the development of the research and guidance, is crucial to building long-term leadership and capacity. The research findings are further needed to develop guidance to clarify midwifery roles and responsibilities within health systems and services. (WHO 2016b:67)

At a global summit organised by 'Women Deliver', it was stressed by many midwives and global experts that an enabling environment to allow midwives to practice to their full scope of practice and a functional health infrastructure were essential in the context of providing woman centred continuity of care (Barnes 2019). The concepts of continuity of care and of respectful care are discussed in Chapter 7, and there is considerable evidence that where the latter does not exist, women will not seek skilled attendance (Bowser and Hill 2010; Abuya et al. 2015). Furthermore, disrespect and abuse has been associated with provider stress and burnout (Burrowes et al. 2017; Ndwiga et al. 2017). Women and midwives must surely form an indivisible part of the same equation in aiming to achieve a childbirth experience that is both safe and satisfying. What affects midwives, affects women. Midwives can only provide evidence-based respectful skilled care if they are equipped and enabled to do so. Nothing less should be acceptable across the world stage.

12.7 Conclusion

Research, especially high-quality research, places midwifery on a par or in equal standing with other professions. This occurs through having its own body of knowledge and evidence collected in a manner befitting midwifery practice, that is the woman as a human being rather than an entity to be studied. Hence the unique approach of midwifery researchers in asking different questions which elicit the humanness of women and their families. Other professions may call it soft evidence, but women are complex humans living in complex environments and experience more affective and psychological disruption or enhancement rather than purely physical quantitative experiences. Midwifery research acknowledges this and therefore is often qualitative though there is also obviously room for quantitative research and randomised controlled trials.

Midwifery research offers another pathway for professional development which caters for the analytically minded and academically inclined midwives as well as being critical to evidence-based practice. The former currently involves a relatively small number of the profession, but they are greatly needed and valued. However, as indicated earlier, more midwives need to become research-aware and research-active. The development of midwifery as a profession and the diversity amongst its practitioners is discussed in Chapter 10. Lastly, midwifery research has weaned midwifery education and practice away from using results from research conducted by other professional groups. Instead, midwifery can collaborate and compare findings with other professionals rather than completely depend on them.

Key Messages

Principles

The principle of reliable research must form the foundation of the modern midwifery profession across the globe providing safe, skilful, sensitive and satisfying care to women and their families everywhere.

Policy

Evidence-based practice should be enshrined in policy at local, national and global levels; it should constantly be reviewed in line with current advances in research undertaken for and by midwives.

Practice

The need for evidence-based practice is undeniable, and midwives are best placed to be the visionaries, controllers and operators within research networks and every practice domain.

Questions for Reflection or Review

1. Considering the principles of network theory explained above, examine a research or other professional network with which you are familiar and consider its size, configuration and connectedness. Describe the strengths of the network and what they offer. Are there enough persons at the operative level and does the network depend on inclination and chance rather than on policy and planning?

2. Identify some examples of improved outcomes where evidence-based maternity care is considered normal practice.

3. It has been suggested above that 'women and midwives must surely form an indivisible part of the same equation'. Think about the ideal equation which you consider balances the needs of both women and midwives to facilitate the best possible outcome.

Additional Resources for Reflection and Further Study

Visit the website of the Lugina Africa Midwives Research Network (LAMRN) at: http://lamrn.org/ Examine the ambitions and achievements of this network and consider how such a network may be replicated in other regions.

Explore the website of the Journal of Asian Midwifery (JAM) at: https://ecommons.aku.edu/jam/ Reflect on the aims and scope of the journal and consider its role in promoting midwifery research and enhancing evidence-based practice.

Readers may wish to compare and contrast the activities of the two structures described above and consider what strengths could be gleaned from both in order to establish a wider network for undertaking and disseminating midwifery research.

World Health Organization (2019) Setting the research agenda: read about the current and ongoing research priorities in maternal, newborn and adolescent health at: https://www.who.int/maternal_child_adolescent/research/en/. Recent research publications are regularly updated here too.

Soltani H, Low LK, Duxbury A et al (2016) Global midwifery research priorities: an international survey. Int J Childbirth 6(1):5–18 Consider these in the context of your own practice and experience

In the context of global research priorities, explore what the National Institute of Health Research (NIHR) Global Health Research Group are doing to address stillbirth and perinatal mortality in Sub-Saharan Africa: https://sites.manchester.ac.uk/stillbirth-prevention-africa/. Accessed 23 Oct 2019.

References

Abuya T et al (2015) Exploring the prevalence of disrespect and abuse during childbirth in Kenya. PLoS One 10(4):e0123606. Accessed 3 Oct 2019. https://doi.org/10.1371/journal.pone.0123606

African Journal of Midwifery (2017) African J Midwifery & Women's Health. MA Healthcare. http://www.magonlinelibrary.com/toc/ajmw/current. Accessed 12 Mar 2020

American College of Nurse-Midwives (2019) Midwifery Research Interest Groups. American College of Nurse Midwives. http://www.midwife.org/Midwifery-Research-Interest-Groups. Accessed 15 Oct 2019

Australian College of Midwives (2019) Research and innovation: Australian College of Midwives: https://www.midwives.org.au/interest-group/research-and-innovation. Accessed 15 Oct 2019

Azmoud E, Aradmehr M, Dehghani F (2018) Midwives' attitude and barriers of evidence based practice in maternity care. Malay J Med Sci 25(3):120–128. https://doi.org/10.21315/mjms2018.25.3.12

Barnes S (2019) Empowered midwives could save lives. New Security Beat, Wilson Center, Environmental Change and Security. https://www.newsecuritybeat.org/2019/08/empowered-midwives-save-lives/. Accessed 16 Oct 2019

Begeley C, Mccarron M, Huntley-Moore S et al (2014) Successful research capacity building in academic nursing and midwifery in Ireland: an exemplar. Nurse Educ Today 34(5):754–760

Bogdan-Lovis E, Sousa A (2006) The contextual influence of professional culture: certified nurse-midwives' knowledge of and reliance on evidence-based practice. Soc Sci Med 62(11):2681–2693

Bogren M, Doraiswamy S, Erlandsson K (2017) Building a new generation of midwifery faculty members in Bangladesh. J Asian Midwives 4(2):52–58

Bonilla H, Ortiz-Llorens BM et al (2018) Implementation of a programme to develop research projects in a school of midwifery in Santiago. Chile Midwifery 64:60–62

Bowser D, Hill K (2010) Exploring evidence for disrespect and abuse in facility-based childbirth: report of a landscape analysis. USAID-TRAction Project, University Research Corporation, LLC, and Harvard School of Public Health, Bethesda, MD. http://www.tractionproject.org/sites/default/files/Respectful_Care_at_Birth_9-20-101_Final.pdf

Brucker M, Schwarz B (2002) Fact or fiction? International Confederation of Midwives Triennial Conference Proceedings. Austria, Vienna

Burrowes S, Holcombe SJ, Jara D et al (2017) Midwives' and patients' perspectives on disrespect and abuse during labor and delivery care in Ethiopia: a qualitative study. BMC Preg Childbirth Open Access 17:263. https://bmcpregnancychildbirth.biomedcentral.com/articles/10.1186/s12884-017-1442-1. Accessed 8 Oct 2019

Directorate General of Nursing and Midwifery (2017) National Guidelines for Midwives, Directorate General of Nursing and Midwifery, Bangladesh. http://dgnm.gov.bd/cmsfiles/files/SOP%20for%20Midwives.pdf. Accessed 23 Oct 2019

Doctoral Midwifery Research Society (2020) DMRS background and membership. https://www.doctoralmidwiferysociety.org/. Accessed 3 Jun 2020

Einstein A, Shaw GB (2009) Einstein on cosmic religion: and other opinions and other aphorisms. Dover, New York

European Midwives Associations (2019) EU Research. European Midwives Association. http://www.europeanmidwives.com/eu/eu-research. Accessed 15 Oct 2019

Forss K, Maclean G (2007) Evaluation of the Africa midwives research network. A study commissioned by the Swedish International Development Cooperation Agency. Sida, Stockholm

Forss K, Birungi H, Saasa O (2000) Sector wide approaches: from principles to practice. A study commissioned by the Department of Foreign Affairs, Dublin, Ireland. Final report 13/11/2000 Andante – tools for thinking AB. https://www.researchgate.net/publication/252177958_Sector_wide_approaches_from_principles_to_practice. Accessed 26 Oct 2019

Glacken M, Chaney D (2004) Perceived barriers and facilitators to implementing research findings in the Irish practice setting. J Clin Nurs 13(6):731–740. Accessed 3 Jun 2020. https://doi.org/10.1111/j.1365-2702.2004.00941.x

Goyet S, Sauvegrain P, Schantz C et al (2018) State of midwifery research in France. Midwifery 64(101–109):2018

Granovetter M (1973) The strength of weak ties. Am J Sociol 78:1360–1380

Guyatt GH, Sackett DL, Sinclair JC et al (1995) Users' Guides to the Medical Literature: IX. A Method for Grading Health Care Recommendations. JAMA 274(22):18001804. Accessed 16 Oct 2019. https://doi.org/10.1001/jama.1995.03530220066035

Hommelstad J, Ruland CM (2004) Norwegian nurses' perceived barriers and facilitators to research use. Assoc Perioper Reg Nurs J 79(3):621–634. https://doi.org/10.1016/S0001-2092(06)60914-9

Hunter B (2013) Implementing research evidence into practice some reflections on the challenges. Evid Based Midwifery 11(3):76–80

International Confederation of Midwives (2014) Basic and ongoing education for midwives: position statement. strengthening midwifery globally: PS2008_001 V2014. International Confederation of Midwives, The Hague. https://www.internationalmidwives.org/assets/files/statement-files/2019/06/basic-and-ongoing-education-for-midwives-eng-letterhead.pdf. Accessed 15 Oct 2019

International Confederation of Midwives (2018) Research Standing Committee: https://www.internationalmidwives.org/our-work/research/research-standing-committee.html [last accessed 09.11.2020]

International Confederation of Midwives (2019) Research: Midwifery led research. International Confederation of Midwives, The Hague. https://www.internationalmidwives.org/our-work/research/. Accessed 23 Oct 2019

Iribarren S, Larsen B, Santos F et al (2018) Clinical nursing and midwifery research in Latin American and Caribbean countries: a scoping review. Int J Nurs Pract 24(2):e12623. Accessed 18 Oct 2019. https://doi.org/10.1111/ijn.12623

Kajermo KN, Boström A-M, Thompson DS et al (2010) The BARRIERS scale—the barriers to research utilization scale: a systematic review. Implement Sci 32(5):1–22. https://doi.org/10.1186/1748-5908-5-32

Kennedy HP, Cheyney M, Dahlen H et al (2018) Asking different questions: research priorities to improve the quality of care for every woman, every child. Lancet Glob Health. Revised May 2018. https://onlinelibrary.wiley.com/doi/pdf/10.1111/birt.12361. Accessed 28 May 2020

Khammarnia M, Haj Mohammadi M, Amani Z et al (2015) Barriers to implementation of evidence-based practice in Zahedan teaching hospitals, Iran, 2014. Nurs Res Pract:1–5. https://doi.org/10.1155/2015/357140

Kolfenbach M, Birdsall K (2015) (2015) international cooperation: strengthening midwifery in Central Asia. J Asian Midwives 2(2):57–61

Koninklijke Nederlandse Organisatie van Verloskundigen (KNOV) (2013) Midwifery Research Network, Dutch Midwives Association. https://www.knov.nl/vakkennis-en-wetenschap/tekstpagina/117-2/midwifery-research-network/hoofdstuk/45/midwifery-research-network/. Accessed 15 Oct 2019

Laisser R, Chimwaza A, Omoni G et al (2019) Crisis: an educational game to reduce mortality and morbidity. Afr J Midwifery Women Health 13:1–6. https://doi.org/10.12968/AJMW.2018.0025

Lavender T, Omoni G, Laisser et al (2019) Evaluation of an educational board game to improve use of the partograph in sub-Saharan Africa: a quasi-experimental study. Sex Reprod Healthc (20) 54–59

Lugina African Midwives Research Network (2019) The Lugina Africa Midwives Research Network. http://lamrn.org/. Accessed 4 Jun 2020

Luyben A, Winjen H, Oblasser C et al (2013) The current state of development of midwifery and midwifery research in four European countries. Midwifery 29(5):417–424. Accessed 1 Jun 2020. https://doi.org/10.1016/j.midw.2012.10.008

Maclean GD, Forss K (2010) An evaluation of the Africa midwives research network. Midwifery 26:e1–e8

Maclean G, Laisser R (2020) The use of educational games in midwifery. Afr J Midwifery Women Health 14(91):1–10

Mills J, Yates K, Harrison H et al (2016) Using a community of inquiry framework to teach a nursing and midwifery research subject: an evaluative study. Nurse Educ Today 43:34–39

Munro J, Spiby H (2001) Evidence into practice for midwifery-led care: part 2. Br J Midwifery 9:771–774

Munro J, Spiby H (2010) The nature and use of evidence in midwifery care: evidence-based midwifery. https://www.researchgate.net/publication/242188203_1_The_Nature_and_Use_of_Evidence_in_Midwifery_Care. Accessed 28 May 2020

Muoni T (2014) Decision-making, intuition and the midwife: understanding heuristics. BJM 20(1). Published Online: 16 Aug 2013. Accessed 26 Oct 2019. https://doi.org/10.12968/bjom.2012.20.1.52

Nanda G, Switlick K, Lule E (2005) Accelerating progress towards achieving the MDG to improve maternal health: a collection of promising approaches. Health, Nutrition & Population Discussion Paper. The International Bank for Reconstruction and Development/The World Bank, Washington, DC, p 20433

National Institute of Health Research (2020) Stillbirth prevention in sub-Saharan Africa. The National Institute of Health Research and University of Manchester. https://sites.manchester.ac.uk/stillbirth-prevention-africa/. Accessed 4 Jun 2020

Ndwiga C, Maingi G, Serwanga J et al (2017) Exploring provider perspectives on respectful maternity care in Kenya: "Work with what you have". Reprod Health 14:99. Accessed 8 Oct 2019. https://doi.org/10.1186/s12978-017-0364-8

New Zealand College of Midwives (2019) Research: New Zealand College of Midwives. https://www.midwife.org.nz/midwives/research/. Accessed 15 Oct 2019

Nohria N, Eccles RG (eds) (1992) Networks and organisations: structure, form and action. Harvard Business School Press, Boston

Olsson A, Adolfsson A (2011) Midwife's experiences of using intuition as a motivating element in conveying assurance and care. Health 3:453–461. Accessed 26 Oct 2019. https://doi.org/10.4236/health.2011.37075

Perrow C (1986) Complex organisations: a critical essay. Random House, New York

Piore MJ (1990) Fragments of a cognitive theory of technological change and organizational behaviour. In: Nohria N, Eccles RG (eds) Networks and organisations: structure, form and action. Harvard Business School Press, Boston

Porter ME (1990) The competitive advantages of nations. Free Press, New York

Renfrew MJ (1997) The development of evidence-based practice. Br J Midwifery 5(2):100–104

Royal College of Midwives (2019) Evidence-based midwifery. Royal College of Midwives publications. https://www.rcm.org.uk/publications. Accessed 26 Oct 2019

Sackett DL, Rosenberg WM, Gray JA et al (1996) Evidence-based medicine: what it is and what it isn't. Editorial: BMJ. Accessed 16 Oct 2019. https://doi.org/10.1136/bmj.312.7023.71

Siwha J, Roth C (2004) Evidence-based practice. Ch 4. In: Henderson C, Macdonald S (eds) Mayes Midwifery. Bailliére Tindall, Edinburgh

Soltani H, Low LK, Schuiling KD et al (2016) Global midwifery research priorities: an international survey. Int J Childbirth 6(1):5–1

Sun C, Larson E (2015) Clinical nursing and midwifery research in African countries: a scoping review. Int J Nurs Stud 52(5):1011–1016

Sun C, Dohrn J, Klopper H et al (2015) Clinical nursing and midwifery research priorities in eastern and southern African countries: results from a Delphi survey. Nurs Res 64(6):466–475

Sweileh WM, Al-Jabi SW, Zyoud SH et al (2019) Nursing and midwifery research activity in Arab countries from 1950 to 2017. [Review]. BMC Health Serv Res 19(1):340. Accessed 18 Oct 2019. https://doi.org/10.1186/s12913-019-4178-y

The Partnership for Maternal Newborn & Child Health (2011) A Global Review of the Key Interventions Related to Reproductive, Maternal, Newborn and Child Health (RMNCH). Geneva, Switzerland: PMNCH.

United Nations Population Fund (2014) State of the world's midwifery: a universal pathway to women's health. A United Nations publication, New York

van Wagner V (2017) Midwives using research: evidence-based practice and evidence-informed midwifery. Chapter 12. In: Comprehensive midwifery: the role of the midwife in health care practice, education and research. Press Books, Open Library. https://ecampusontario.pressbooks.pub/cmroleofmidwifery/chapter/midwives-using-research-evidence-based-practice-evidence-informed-midwifery/. Accessed 28 May 2020

Wickham S (2000) Evidence-informed midwifery 3: evaluating midwifery evidence. Midwifery Today Autumn:45–46

World Health Organization (2016a) WHO and partners call for better working conditions for midwives. World Health Organization, Geneva. https://www.who.int/news-room/detail/13-10-2016-who-and-partners-call-for-better-working-conditions-for-midwives. Accessed 16 Oct 2019

World Health Organization (2016b) Midwives' voices, midwives' realities. Findings from a global consultation on providing quality midwifery care. Originally published under ISBN 978 92 4 151054 7. World Health Organization, Geneva. https://apps.who.int/iris/bitstream/handle/10665/250376/9789241510547-eng.pdf;jsessionid=6F7EFCDDC808DE4828446A6FF8B7844B?sequence=1. Accessed 4 Jun 2020

World Health Organization (2018a) Midwives are essential to the provision of quality of care in all settings, globally. World Health Organization, Geneva. International Day of the Midwife 2018: https://www.who.int/news-room/commentaries/detail/midwives-are-essential-to-the-provision-of-quality-of-care-in-all-settings-globally. Accessed 16 Oct 2019

World Health Organization (2018b) World Health Organization Collaborating Centres: fact sheet. https://www.who.int/docs/default-source/documents/about-us/factsheetwhocc2018.pdf?sfvrsn=8c7166ee_2. Accessed 3 Jun 2020

World Health Organization (2019a) Maternal mental health. Sexual and reproductive health. World Health Organization, Geneva. https://www.who.int/mental_health/maternal-child/maternal_mental_health/en/. Accessed 12 Apr 2019

World Health Organization (2019b) Comprehensive mental health action plan 2013–2020. World Health Organization, Geneva. https://www.who.int/mental_health/action_plan_2013/en/. Accessed 12 Apr 2019

World Health Organization (2020) World Health Organization news-room fact sheet: nursing and midwifery. https://www.who.int/news-room/fact-sheets/detail/nursing-and-midwifery. Accessed 3 Jun 2020

Yahui HC, Swaminathan N (2017) Knowledge, attitudes, and barriers towards evidence-based practice among physiotherapists in Malaysia. Hong Kong Physiother J 37:10–18

Part V

Midwifery Across the Globe

Midwifery in Humanitarian and Emergency Settings

13

Expected Learning Outcomes

By the end of the chapter, the reader should be able to:

1. Describe different types and stages of humanitarian and crisis settings.
2. Articulate the specific challenges for women's and newborn's health in emergency settings.
3. Demonstrate awareness of international humanitarian standards and the Minimal Initial Service Package for sexual and reproductive health in humanitarian settings.
4. Explain the role of, and challenges for, midwives in providing high-quality maternal and newborn care in crisis situations.
5. Identify gaps in their own knowledge and skills in relation to midwifery care in humanitarian settings and develop a personal action plan to address these.

13.1 Background to Humanitarian and Emergency Settings

Despite global development and economic growth, humanitarian need is also increasing. Globally, there are 131.7 million (or 1 in 70) people affected by crisis, necessitating humanitarian assistance (UNOCHA 2018). Conflict is the biggest driver of crisis, with the latest available figures reporting 68.5 million people displaced by conflict; however, natural hazards also contribute, exacerbated by climate change and population growth (UNOCHA 2018; ISAC 2015). Most humanitarian crises are not caused by any single factor or event, but by the interaction between natural hazards, conflict and vulnerability (UNOCHA 2018). Infectious diseases with the potential to cause epidemics and pandemics, such as Ebola, SARS and COVID-19, also cause local or global crises and threaten global health security (WHO 2019a; Flahault et al. 2016). Climate change is contributing to the increasing numbers of displaced people across the world via several mechanisms. Environmental changes can create competition between humans and animals for dwindling habitat and resources; this increases the opportunity for zoological viruses to enter human populations and cause outbreaks of infectious disease (UNFPA 2-19b). At the time climate change is also increasing food insecurity as global weather patterns become more erratic. Drought, fires and flash-floods disrupt the food chain and force displacement as populations, for example in Guatemala and Venezuela, leave their homes in search of food and alternative livelihoods (Steffens 2018). In some cases, for example in the Sahel, Afghanistan and Yemen, these disruptions to climate change exacerbate political tensions and contribute to the

© Springer Nature Switzerland AG 2021
J. Kemp et al., *Global Midwifery: Principles, Policy and Practice*,
https://doi.org/10.1007/978-3-030-46765-4_13

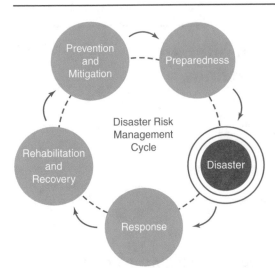

Fig. 13.1 The disaster risk management cycle (UNOOSA 2020)

escalation of armed conflicts. In a global health crisis, defenses are only as effective as the weakest link in any country's health emergency preparedness and response system (WHO 2019a).

Nothing lays bare inequality and discrimination like a disaster (Mizutori 2020). Poverty is both a driver and a consequence of disaster (Prevention Web 2015). Where natural disasters occur in countries already vulnerable through conflict, this causes additional challenges (CRED 2019). The INFORM (2020) global risk index shows how a combination of exposure to hazards, vulnerability and coping capacity results in countries becoming quickly overwhelmed by humanitarian crises and disasters (UNFPA 2019b). This clearly demonstrates that the poor are disproportionately affected by and during disasters. Women and children are especially vulnerable; UNFPA (2019a) estimates that more than half of maternal deaths occur in emergency or fragile settings. Similarly 5 out of 10 countries with the highest neonatal mortality rate are in a acute or protracted humanitarian emergency.

Crisis situations can last for long periods of time; the average humanitarian crisis lasts for more than 9 years (UNOCHA 2018). Crises are often followed by displacement and migration that threaten the health and well-being of women, children and adolescents; one billion people have been estimated to be migrating within and/or

between countries around the world (PMNCH 2019). Disasters are described in different stages: prevention, mitigation and preparedness, disaster response, and rehabilitation and recovery. This is known as the disaster risk management cycle and is illustrated in Fig. 13.1 (UNOOSA 2020). However, it is rare that crises take a straight path from emergency, through stability, recovery and onto development. They are mostly complex, with varying degrees of improvement or deterioration that can last decades (IAWG 2018a, b). Protracted crises in many countries are leading to a new urgency for collaboration and development efforts, known as the Humanitarian Development Nexus (OXFAM 2019).

13.2 Terminology Used in Humanitarian and Emergency Settings

The humanitarian workforce has become increasingly professionalised in recent years (ELRHA 2014). This is reflected in the proliferation of terminology used in humanitarian settings, requiring its own 61-page 'glossary of humanitarian terms' (Relief Web 2008). This can be bewildering for midwives and others who find themselves as first responders in crises. Table 13.1 summarises essential terminology and definitions.

13.3 Coordination of Efforts in Humanitarian Settings

Effective coordination of humanitarian relief is essential in ensuring that help quickly gets to those who need it. The Office for the Coordination of Humanitarian Affairs (OCHA) of the United Nations (UN) Secretariat is responsible for this coordination role, and works through an Inter-Agency Standing Committee with representatives from different UN agencies. Non-governmental organisations (NGOs) and the private sector also have an important role to play in the coordination of humanitarian relief (UNOCHA 2017, 2020a) along with governments, donor organisations and, sometimes, the military.

Table 13.1 Terminology used in humanitarian and emergency settings

Asylum seeker	Someone fleeing their own country and seeking sanctuary in another country, applying for asylum: the right to be recognised as a refugee and receive legal protection and material assistance
Complex emergency	Humanitarian crisis in a country, region or society where there is total or considerable breakdown of authority resulting from internal or external conflict and which requires an international response that goes beyond the mandate or capacity of any single and/or ongoing UN country programme
Crisis	A situation that is perceived as difficult. A crisis may not be evident, and it demands analysis to be recognised. Conceptually, it can cover both preparedness and response
Disaster	A situation or event, which overwhelms local capacity, necessitating a request to national or international level for external assistance
Disaster mitigation	The lessening or minimising of the adverse impacts of a hazardous event
Disaster preparedness	Pre-disaster activities, geared to helping at-risk communities safeguard their lives and assets by being alert to hazards and taking appropriate action in the face of an imminent threat or the actual onset of a disaster
Disaster response	The organisation and management of resources and responsibilities for dealing with all humanitarian aspects of emergencies
Disaster risk	The potential loss of life, injury, or destroyed or damaged assets which could occur to a system, society, or a community in a specific period of time, through the combination of hazard, exposure and capacity
Emergency	A managerial term describing a state, demanding decision and follow-up in terms of extraordinary measures
Epidemic	The occurrence in a community or region of cases of an illness, specific health-related behaviour or other health-related events clearly in excess of normal expectancy
Humanitarian	The promotion of human welfare
Humanitarian assistance	Aid to a stricken population that complies with the basic humanitarian principles of humanity, impartiality and neutrality
Humanitarian Development Nexus	The work needed to coherently address people's vulnerability before, during and after crises
Internally displaced person (IDP)	Someone forced to flee their home but who has never crossed an international border
Migrant	A person who moves away from his or her place of usual residence, whether within a country or across an international border, temporarily or permanently, and for a variety of reasons. An umbrella term, not defined under international law
Pandemic	The worldwide spread of a new disease
Recovery	Decisions and actions taken after a disaster with a view to restoring or improving the pre-disaster living conditions of the stricken community, whilst encouraging and facilitating necessary adjustments to reduce disaster risk
Refugee	Someone who has been forced to flee his or her country because of persecution, war or violence
Stateless person	Someone who is not a citizen of any country
Vulnerability	The degree to which a socio-economic system is either susceptible or resilient to the impact of natural hazards and related technological and environmental disasters

WHO 2010, 2020; IOM 2020; Relief Web 2008; UNOOSA 2020; IFRC 2018; UNHCR 2020; OXFAM 2019

Historically, humanitarian aid has often had a short-term focus and been poorly coordinated. In 2017 the UN and the World Bank set out a 'New Way of Working' (UNOCHA 2017), recognising that humanitarian and development actors, governments, NGOs and private sector actors all contribute to the 'humanitarian-development-peace nexus'. This new way of working focuses on the work needed to coherently address people's vulnerability before, during and after crises, by meeting immediate needs whilst taking steps to address systemic causes of conflict and vulnerability and supporting the peace that is essential for sustainable development (OXFAM 2019).

The COVID-19 pandemic has changed the way humanitarian action is organised, as agencies addressed the need for social distancing during relief distributions and faced challenges such as how to provide safe places for women and children in crisis using virtual technologies (UNOCHA 2020b).

13.4 Healthcare in Humanitarian Crises

The goals of the 2030 Agenda for Universal Health Coverage apply whether people are living in stability or in crisis (WHO 2019b). Humanitarian crises have immense short- and long-term health impacts (Kohrt et al. 2019). Emergencies rarely occur in settings with no pre-existing health system; where a system is weak, it may need to be strengthened or developed. However, delivery of healthcare can be very challenging in crisis settings with regular health systems frequently destroyed or disrupted; in some circumstances, health care must even be provided at sea or once individuals are brought ashore (Kohrt et al. 2019; Sphere 2018). Additionally, population data, essential for planning appropriate health care, can be difficult to gather in emergencies. Aside from initial life-saving health care following trauma, injury or infectious disease outbreaks, crisis-affected populations will have pre-existing health conditions requiring urgent and ongoing; age, gender, disability, HIV/TB status, poor mental health, linguistic or ethnic identity can further influence needs and may be significant barriers to accessing care (Kohrt et al. 2019; Sphere 2018).

The Sphere (2018) humanitarian charter states that everyone has the right to timely and appropriate health care, and a handbook sets out minimum standards for health care in humanitarian contexts. These standards identify seven areas of essential healthcare and five different health system categories. These are listed in Table 13.2.

Table 13.2 Health systems and essential health care in humanitarian settings

Health system categories	Areas of essential health care
1. Health service delivery	1. Communicable diseases
2. Health workforce	2. Child health
3. Essential medicines and medical devices	3. Sexual and reproductive health
4. Health financing	4. Injury and trauma care
5. Health information	5. Mental health
	6. Non-communicable diseases
	7. Palliative care

(Sphere 2018)

13.5 Rights in Humanitarian Settings

All people affected by disaster or conflict have a right to life with dignity, the right to receive humanitarian assistance and the right to protection and security (Sphere 2018). Sexual and reproductive health is a human right for all people, including those living in humanitarian settings; it is an essential, non-negotiable component of every humanitarian response (IAWG 2018a, b; UNFPA 2019a). The ambitious global 2030 agenda of 'leaving no one behind' will only be achieved if this includes provision of universal access to sexual and reproductive health and rights for populations in humanitarian and fragile contexts or crisis situations (UNFPA 2019a). Reproductive health, family planning services and protection from violence saves lives in emergencies; they are as essential as food and shelter (UNFPA 2019a). In addition to sexual and reproductive rights, women in crisis situations have the right to Respectful Maternity Care (White Ribbon Alliance 2019; Manning and Schaaf 2018). Health workers also have rights that should be upheld, even in crisis situations; these include the right to safe and decent working environments and freedom from discrimination, coercion and violence (WHO 2016). Violence against health care workers in conflict is increasing around the world; as health workers are predominantly female they are additionally vulnerable to violence (Safeguarding Health in Conflict Coalition 2020). Humanitarian crises often exacerbate human rights concerns, and deteriorating human rights situations can in themselves trigger crises (UNOHCHR 2019).

13.6 What Do Women and Their Newborns Need in Humanitarian Settings?

Humanitarian crises take a disproportionate toll on women and girls. However, only comparatively recently have women's needs and vulnerabilities received the same level of attention as the need for food and shelter in humanitarian emergencies (UNFPA 2019b). One in four people affected by crisis are women and girls of reproductive age (15–49 years) who require access to sexual and reproductive health services (UNFPA 2019a). However, in times of crisis, access to high-quality sexual, reproductive, maternal and newborn health services may be unavailable, increasing the risk of still births, maternal and neonatal mortality and morbidity and the prevalence of unwanted pregnancies (Sphere 2018). Despite recent investment in reproductive health in humanitarian emergencies, focus on maternal and newborn care for the mother and baby during childbirth remains inadequate with inconsistence service provision across different humanitarian contexts (IAWG 2019). In countries with ongoing emergencies, more than 500 women and girls have been reported to die every day during pregnancy and childbirth (UNFPA 2019b).

Conflicts and disasters exacerbate gender inequalities and elevate risks of sexual violence, including exploitation and abuse, due to breakdown of protection systems and an environment of impunity where perpetrators are not held accountable (Sphere 2018; UNFPA 2019a). At least one in five women refugees in complex humanitarian settings has experienced sexual violence although the real figure is likely to be much higher as many incidents go unreported and data are difficult to track (Sphere 2018; UNOCHA 2020). Displaced young people are especially vulnerable; during humanitarian cri-

ses, being young and female is one of the greatest risk factors for violence and death (UNFPA 2019a). Furthermore, women are at risk because they will often prioritise the needs of children, friends and neighbours over their own (UNFPA 2019a).

Women in all settings in all countries want respectful, kind and personalised maternal and newborn health services, delivered by knowledgeable, skilled and culturally sensitive health professionals who inspire trust (Renfrew et al. 2014). To reduce maternal and newborn mortality in humanitarian settings, women and their families must have improved access to high-quality comprehensive sexual and reproductive health services, skilled care during labour and childbirth, and access to quality emergency obstetric and newborn care (IAWG 2019). Women should have access to high quality care by a midwife regardless of their refugee status (ICM 2017).

13.7   Core Documents for Women's and Newborns' Health in Crises

Core documents and standards have been developed over the past two decades to inform the provision of care to, and with, those affected by crisis (Fig. 13.2).

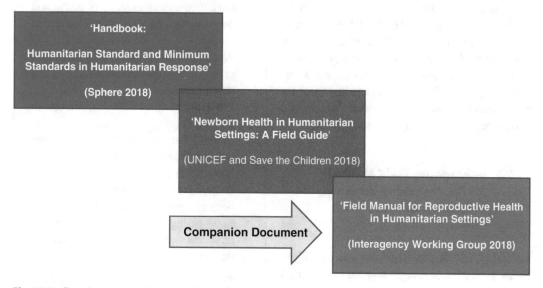

Fig. 13.2 Core documents to inform healthcare for women and newborns in crises

13.7.1 Sphere Humanitarian Standard and Minimum Standards in Humanitarian Response (Sphere 2018)

Sphere, a network of humanitarian organisations, has developed a rights-based framework, known as 'The Sphere Handbook', designed for use by practitioners involved in planning, managing or implementing a humanitarian response. The handbook can also be used for advocacy to improve the quality and accountability of humanitarian assistance and is increasingly being used by governments, donors, the military and the private sector to help them in working constructively with humanitarian organisation (Sphere 2018).

The handbook contains the humanitarian charter, protection principles to inform any humanitarian response, the core humanitarian standard comprised of nine commitments and four technical chapters, each including minimal standards for four sectors. The standards address: water supply, sanitation and hygiene (WASH), food security and nutrition, shelter and settlement, and health. Within the over-arching Sphere standard for health, there is a sexual and reproductive health standard which states that 'people have access to healthcare and family planning that prevents excessive maternal and newborn morbidity and mortality' (Sphere 2018). Of relevance to midwives, the handbook also contains standards for sexual violence and clinical management of rape, HIV and palliative care.

Since these four core standards do not cover every aspect of humanitarian assistance, in partnership with Sphere, other organisations have developed complementary standards including those for child protection, inclusion for older people and those with disabilities and economic recovery.

13.7.2 Interagency Field Manual for Reproductive Health in Humanitarian Settings (IAWG 2018a, b)

In 1991, UNHCR published the first guidelines for the protection of refugee women written from within a human rights context and taking note of women's and girl's gender-specific needs. In 1995, many different humanitarian and other organisations formed an Interagency Working Group which published the first field manual for reproductive health in emergency situations. This group has continued to grow and with a current membership of over 450 agencies and has authored the 'Interagency field manual for reproductive health in humanitarian settings', last issued in 2018. This manual acknowledges that the provision of comprehensive and high-quality Sexual and Reproductive Health (SRH) services requires a multisectoral, integrated approach and that affected communities should be involved in every phase of action from needs assessment, programme planning, programme implementation and evaluation (IAWG 2018a, b). The interagency manual sets out the Minimum Initial Service Package (MISP) for SRH in crises situations. The MISP itself is a health standard within the Sphere Minimum Standards in Humanitarian Response (Sphere 2018). Box 13.1 summarises the key actions considered relevant in crisis situations.

Box 13.1. Key actions in sexual and reproductive health in crises situations

- Clean and safe delivery, essential newborn care and emergency obstetric and newborn care services to be available at all times.
- Establish a 24/7 referral system with effective communication and transportation.
- Provision of clean delivery packages to all visibly pregnant women.
- Consult the community to understand local preferences, practices and attitudes towards contraception.
- Involve men and women, and adolescent boys and girls privately and separately.
- Long-acting reversible and short-acting contraceptive methods available on demand.

Box 13.2. Signal functions of emergency obstetric and newborn care (WHO 2009)

Basic emergency obstetric and neonatal care (minimum five facilities per 500,000 people)	Comprehensive emergency obstetric and neonatal care (minimum one facility per 500,000 people)
1. Administer parenteral antibiotics 2. Administer uterotonic drugs 3. Administer parenteral anticonvulsants for preeclampsia and eclampsia 4. Manually remove the placenta 5. Remove retained products 6. Perform assisted vaginal delivery 7. Perform basic neonatal resuscitation	Perform signal functions 1–7, plus: 8. Perform surgery (e.g. caesarean section) 9. Perform blood transfusion

A basic emergency obstetric care facility is one in which all functions 1–7 are performed. A comprehensive emergency obstetric care facility is one in which all functions 1–9 are performed

---

To prevent avoidable maternal and newborn mortality and morbidity in humanitarian settings the MISP calls for Basic Emergency Obstetric and Newborn Care (BEmONC) and Comprehensive Emergency Obstetric and Newborn Care (CEmONC) (see Box 13.2) to be available at all times in humanitarian settings. These two levels of care include seven (BEmONC) and nine (CEmONC) 'signal functions'; these are the key medical interventions that are used to manage the direct obstetric complications that cause the vast majority of maternal deaths around the globe and also include newborn resuscitation. Signal functions for inpatient care of small and sick newborns are also currently under development (Moxon et al. 2019). Globally, WHO (2009) suggests that approximately 5–15% of births will require surgical intervention such as caesarean section and 9–15% of newborns will require life-saving emergency care. Therefore, an effective referral system with functional communication and transportation between basic and comprehensive care facilities is also essential to enable access to these life-saving services (Sphere 2018). In addition to the signal functions, the MISP also includes the prevention of sexual violence and assistance to survivors, the provision of sexual and reproductive health services such as family planning and access to safe abortion and post-abortion care, and reduction in the transmission of HIV.

13.7.3 Newborn Health in Humanitarian Settings: a Field Guide (UNICEF and Save the Children 2018)

Another document, Newborn Health in Humanitarian Settings: A Field Guide (UNICEF and Save the Children 2018) is a companion to the interagency manual, providing information related specifically to newborn care during the neonatal period. This guide is supported by the multi-agency Roadmap to Accelerate Progress for Every Newborn in Humanitarian Settings 2020–2023 (Save the Children et al. 2019) and promotes the provision of skilled care at birth, preferably in a healthcare facility, for all newborns. The field guide details clinical and technical guidance for providing newborn care in humanitarian settings, centred on preventing and treating the three main causes of newborn mortality: direct preterm complications, severe infection and intrapartum-related complications. It also presents strategic considerations for broader programme development, service integration and coordination within humanitarian settings. These strategic considerations include the appointment of a lead agency for the SRH response in an emergency, the implementation of a situation analysis with use of the findings to implement the SRH response plan and the development of monitoring and evaluation plans with relevant experts and stakeholders. It is essential that programming interventions are based on keeping a mother and her baby together and that the principles of quality, equity and dignity apply to both (White Ribbon Alliance 2019).

Box 13.3. Essential Newborn Care in all Settings

- Thermal care (delay bathing, keep the baby dry and warm, skin-to-skin contact).
- Infection prevention (clean birth practices, handwashing, cord care, skin and eye care).
- Feeding support (immediate and exclusive breastfeeding).
- Monitoring (for infection or other conditions necessitating referral).
- Postnatal care (first 24 h most critical; aim for three home visits in the first week)

Derived from: Inter-agency Working Group on Reproductive Health in Crises 2018a, b; WHO 2014.

13.8 The Role of the Midwife in Disasters and Emergencies

Skilled midwives could avert a total of 83% of all maternal deaths, stillbirths and neonatal deaths (Homer et al… 2014). However, as discussed in Chapters 1–3 of this book, the unique contribution of midwives has only recently been internationally acknowledged as focus was previously on skilled birth attendants and competence in the 'signal functions'. Hobbs et al.'s (2019) scoping review of in 36 low and middle income countries found 102 unique cadre names identified for those providing 'skilled attendance' at birth with large variations in competency. In all settings, including humanitarian crises, the midwife is the most appropriate healthcare professional with defined competencies in delivering skilled care to women during pregnancy, childbirth and the postnatal period; midwives should be considered as essential health workers providing a critical service to childbearing women and their

babies (WHO 2019c; ICM 2020), not only competent in the emergency signal functions but able to provide the full range of maternal, newborn, adolescent, sexual and reproductive health services. Midwives are key to supporting the goals of Universal Health Coverage in emergencies as they often live close to affected communities and are the first point of contact, especially in remote or isolated areas (WHO 2019c). Midwifery competencies (ICM 2018) include being able to accompany women through pregnancy, childbirth and the postnatal period, no matter what the circumstances (WHO 2019c). A recent systematic review of the role and scope of midwives in humanitarian settings (Beek et al. 2019) found that midwives, as frontline health workers with geographic and social proximity to the communities they serve, are uniquely positioned during a crisis. . However, the same study reported gaps in international guidance for midwives in humanitarian settings, especially in the mitigation and preparedness, and recovery phases of a response. Miyake et al. (2017) found that community midwifery programmes in fragile and conflict-affected countries were weakened by inappropriate recruitment and training, lack of support and general insecurity. The World Health Organization (2019c) states that there is an urgent need to examine and develop the role of midwives in humanitarian settings.

13.8.1 Coordination of Midwifery in Crises

Leadership and coordination are vital in a humanitarian health response (Sphere 2018). WHO (2019c) has called for midwifery leadership to be included within the national emergency cluster and other key coordination mechanisms appropriate to the context. At the onset of a humanitarian situation, there will usually be a lead organisation for the sexual and reproductive response (UNICEF and Save the Children 2018). The number and profile of available health workers, including midwives, should match the population and service needs (Sphere 2018). Midwives should engage in partnership with communities, especially women's groups, community leaders, community health workers and young people to identify needs, barriers to care and context-specific solutions (Sphere 2018).

People should have access to free priority health care (Sphere 2018), and maternity services should be prioritised as an essential core health service (ICM 2020). However, during the 2020 COVID-19 pandemic, it was reported that restrictive practices were introduced in maternal and newborn care, limiting women's decisions and rights of women and newborn infants, including restrictions on the place of birth, continuity of care and mother–baby contact (Renfrew et al. 2020). Protocols for pregnancy and childbirth during emergencies must be evidence-based and uphold the human rights of all women and their newborns (ICM 2020). Sexual and reproductive health care such as family planning, emergency contraception and abortion services should also remain available as core health services (Sphere 2018). Abortion is needed even in settings where it is restricted (Guttermacher 2020) but safe abortion services are rarely addressed in humanitarian settings (IPPF 2015). Where possible, continuity of midwifery care should be encouraged and provided; in a pandemic, this will reduce the number of caregivers in contact with the woman and her birth partner and decrease the chances of disease spreading in hospitals (ICM 2020).

Midwives work best within an enabling environment (WHO 2019c). In settings with a functional supply chain midwives and other maternity care providers may be able to access special supplies to support their role, such as the Inter-Agency Emergency Reproductive Health kits (IARH). These kits are globally standardised, pre-packed, and available for immediate dispatch in event of an emergency. The kits, usually managed and distributed by UNFPA (2019a, b), contain all of the life-saving medicines, devices and commodities/supplies necessary to implement the MISP. Direct Relief, a non-governmental organisation, is working with the ICM to supply 'Midwife Kits' which contain the 59 essential items a midwife needs to perform 50 facility-based safe births in almost any environment (Direct Relief 2020). Newborn Supply Kits are also available to complement the reproductive health kits (IAWG 2018c).

Humanitarian settings are not immune from accountability and international standards and norms (Schaaf et al. 2020). Therefore midwives and other health workers in crisis situations must present themselves as neutral and impartial. They should support existing health systems and use national standards and protocols where possible. Midwives should contribute to health management information systems (HMIS) and other routine health surveillance systems, taking appropriate data protection measures (Sphere 2018). During disease outbreaks such as Ebola or COVID-19, midwives should follow international guidance from organisations such as WHO and engage with their own professional association and the ICM for support. International midwives who volunteer in humanitarian settings require comprehensive preparation and support, in addition to skilled translators where required (O'Mally Floyd 2013). More information on international volunteering can be found in Chapters 14 and 15 of this book.

13.8.2 The Role of Professional Midwives' Associations in Crisis Situations

Professional midwives' associations are not humanitarian organisations. However, they often have branches or networks of midwives across a country or region and are well connected with national and local health systems and communities. Moreover, they have working knowledge of local culture and language, unlike many foreign humanitarian organisations. In fragile situations, such as Afghanistan and Yemen, even nascent midwives' associations have proven to be inportant advocates and sources of information for members. Therefore, with the right support, midwifery associations can play an important role during crises situations, and they must be fully involved in disaster preparedness, harm reduction and rapid response to disasters/emergencies. However, midwives are often not included in emergency preparedness and response planning at local, national and international level (ICM 2014a). ICM (2014a) advises its member midwife associations to ensure that midwives participate and take up their role in disasters and emergencies and to systematically train midwives to be effective in crisis/emergency situations. Beek et al. (2019) call upon the international agencies to play their part in ensuring that midwives and national midwives' associations can take their place in high-level disaster preparedness, response planning and coordination activities, and to provide technical guidance.

Unfortunately crises can leave professional associations struggling to respond, especially if they have experienced damage to offices and staff or had officers made homeless, injured or sick, or have been forced to migrate (Kemp et al. 2017; Health Cluster/UNFPA 2018). During the COVID-19 pandemic, most midwives' associations, like many other organisations, had to adopt social distancing measures, becoming almost fully virtual. Communication systems can be fractured in emergencies, with disruptions to power supplies and networks. Despite these difficulties, many midwives' associations have stepped up to respond with a speed and efficiency suggestive of much larger and well-resourced organisations. Two such case studies are shared at the end of this chapter.

13.8.3 Educating and Preparing Midwives for Their Role in Emergencies

This chapter has demonstrated how midwives can provide an essential role in meeting the care needs of women, adolescents and newborns during humanitarian crises. However, despite the growth in such crises globally, midwives are neither sufficiently prepared nor educated for this role (Beek et al. 2019). WHO (2019c) has called for emergency preparedness and response to be embedded in midwifery curricula. Global competencies for midwives (ICM 2018) include all seven signal funtions of basic emergency obstetric, essential newborn care and care for small and sick newborns, underpinned by respectful maternity care. However, IAWG (2019) recommends further building the capacity of midwives through training and mentoring approaches to ensure they are equipped for their role in humanitarian emer-

gencies. In addition to competence in signal functions, midwives require resilience to work in challenging settings; however, Williams (2020) questions whether resilience can be taught in midwifery education. Fred and Kernohan (2015) found that preparedness of midwives for their role in humanitarian response depended on both intrinsic factors such as flexibility and humility, and external factors such as education, aqusition of local language skills and understanding of infrastructural challenges. These issues need to be embedded within the midwifery curriculum. Midwifery education may take place in the context of a crisis; Renfrew et al. (2020) noted that during the 2020 COVID-19 pandemic, student midwives were learning in a context of altered priorities; this could influence the care they provide for women and their families in the long-term. Therefore, it is imperative for educators and professional associations to take particular care of students who are working in frontline care, to be alert for moral distress and to support their mental health needs.

Humanitarian crises, though extremely challenging, can provide opportunity for midwifery education to flourish. Prior to the war in Syria, the Syrian health system did not support autonomous normal midwifery, and many midwives themselves were unaware of the core competencies of midwifery practice. UNFPA, galvanised by national and local level support, are working with Syrian colleagues and other strategic partners to implement a programme to build a new cadre of healthcare providers, with the aim that they will eventually become fully trained midwives as defined by the ICM standards (Health Cluster/UNFPA 2018).

13.8.4 Impact of Emergencies on Midwives

The ICM has recognised the courage of midwives who in the most difficult of circumstances continue to provide care for women and their newborn (ICM 2014a, b). However, in crises situations midwives may themselves become the victims of war, civil unrest, natural disasters or infectious diseases. They may be killed, raped, maimed and suffer the loss of family members (ICM 2014a, b); they may lose their homes or family members from storms or earthquakes (Cuesta et al. 2018; Kemp et al. 2017). Stress, burnout and post-traumatic stress disorder are commonly reported in studies of healthcare workers in pandemics and major national/global emergencies; fear, uncertainty and moral distress are common (Hunter et al. 2020). Midwives are better able to provide quality midwifery care and to have a sense of personal well-being, if they feel well supported (Hunter et al. 2020). Midwives have the right to a safe and respectful working environment, including sanitation and access to necessary personal protective equipment (International Confederation of Midwives 2020). Midwives also have the right to freedom from all kinds of discrimination, coercion and violence (WHO 2016). Renfrew et al. (2020) state that in a crisis situation there must be no trade-off between protecting the health and well-being of midwives and other health workers, and the rights of women and babies. Box 13.4 provides suggestions for supporting midwives' well-being in emergency situations.

13.9 Disaster Mitigation and Preparedness

The impact of disasters on women and newborns can be reduced by preparedness and resilience-building efforts; this includes ensuring that laws, policies, protocols, coordination mechanisms and communication channels are in place prior to a disaster, and pre-positioning live-saving to support the implementation of the MISP and priority maternal and newborn health interventions (IAWG 2019). Midwives have unique skills and knowledge and are often geographically and socially close to communities (Beek et al. 2019), so it is vital that midwives are included in emergency preparedness and response planning (ICM 2014a, b). Professional midwives' associations can play an important part in lobbying for and contributing to national disaster planning and legislation, preparing midwives for their role in crisis situations and supporting those providing services (ICM 2014a, b). At programme level, it is also essential that communities themselves are directly involved in every stage of the disaster risk cycle (Sphere 2018).

Box 13.4. Suggestions for supporting midwives' wellbeing in emergency situations

- Take midwives' individual circumstances into consideration, especially those with additional support needs.
- Allow staff to raise concerns and find effective solutions.
- Ensure midwives have access to food and drink.
- Encourage midwives to take regular breaks.
- Give fair duty rosters.
- Provide psychological support.
- Give opportunity for peer support through video calls.
- Consider provision of temporary accommodation near health facilities (Hunter et al. 2020; Cuesta et al. 2018).

13.10 Rehabilitation and Recovery

After the immediate response to a crisis comes the rehabilitation phase, where basic services and life-lines are restored, even if on a temporary basis. The recovery phase is where reconstruction of infra-structure is carried out, along with restoration of livelihoods in affected populations (UNOOSA 2020). For maternal, newborn, adolescent, sexual and reproductive health, this means transition from the MISP to provision of comprehensive SRH services for the recovery phase or during chronic or protracted crisis situations (IAWG 2018a, b). Beek et al. (2019) report that the contribution of midwives to the rehabilitation and recovery after crises is largely missing from the literature. However, some encouraging papers do highlight the extraordinary work of midwives in post-conflict and crisis situations such as Afghanistan, Syria and Sierra Leone (Currie et al. 2007; Health Cluster/UNFPA 2018; O'Mally Floyd 2013).

13.11 Case Studies

Case Study 1: Rohingya Refugee Crisis, Bangladesh

In 2017, ethnic violence in Myanmar caused 742,000 Rohingya Muslims to flee to Cox's Bazar, Bangladesh, an already densely populated area. By 2020, this constituted the largest refugee site in the world (CRED 2020). Half of the refugees (51%) were women and girls of which 318,500 were of reproductive age and 31,200 were pregnant (UNFPA 2020). The Rohingya population have low levels of illiteracy and gender differences and traditional beliefs play important roles in their culture. Contraception is not widely accepted (CRED 2020).

The first direct-entry midwives in Bangladesh qualified in 2016, just before the Rohingya refugee crisis. Many of these midwives were deployed by UNFPA, or by non-governmental organisations such as Médecins Sans Frontières (MSF), to Cox's Bazaar; international midwives have also been deployed from within the region and further afield (UNFPA 2018a; UNV 2020; MSF 2020). Both local and international midwives faced many challenges: speaking a different language with their clients, caring for women who had faced trauma, assault and food shortages, working in muddy and overcrowded environments. Despite these difficulties, midwives have been providing comprehensive sexual and reproductive health services including antenatal care, 24/7 intrapartum care, postnatal and newborn care, counselling and health promotion, family planning services, menstrual regulation, post-abortion care and adolescent sexual and reproductive health services. In the camps, UNFPA set up women-friendly spaces, gender-based violence services and dignity kits for women including hygiene, sanitary and clothing items (UNFPA 2018b).

Case Study 2: Earthquake, Nepal

In April 2015, a huge earthquake (magnitude 7.8) shook Nepal. The epicentre of the earthquake was near the densely populated capital city, Kathmandu, causing enormous loss of life, injury and homelessness. UNFPA (2015) estimated that 126,000 pregnant women were affected by the earthquake. Despite structural damage to its office, the Midwifery Society of Nepal (MIDSON) launched an immediate response to the crisis, setting up a helpdesk for women at the national maternity hospital and conducting maternal, newborn, adolescent, sexual and reproductive health outreach clinics in earthquake-affected areas.

At the time, MIDSON was twinned with the Royal College of Midwives (RCM) in the UK. Through this partnership, funds were raised to deploy local nurse-midwives to work alongside remaining staff in badly affected rural sites, role-modelling high-quality maternity care and providing training in essential skills. MIDSON provided coaching, mentoring and support to health facility staff and, through partnerships with other organisations strengthened through the twinning project, were able to supply health centres and clinics with necessary equipment and supplies (Kemp et al. 2017). MIDSON's response during the crisis ensured that midwives had a seat at the policymaking table and gave them a higher profile with stakeholders for the future development of midwifery in Nepal going forward. In 2017, the Government of Nepal launched the first Bachelor in Midwifery programme.

13.12 Conclusion

Conflict and crises are increasing around the world. Women, newborns and adolescent girls are especially vulnerable in emergencies and midwives have a key role in protecting and promoting health at all stages of the disaster risk cycle. Women and their families have the right to quality midwifery care, even in crises; midwives also have rights to a safe working environment and protection from harm. Midwives may be affected by emergencies in many ways and need support for their own physical and emotional well-being during crises. Midwives and midwives' associations should familiarise themselves with the core documents for reproductive and sexual health in humanitarian situations and should position themselves at the decision-making table for disaster preparedness and mitigation, actively training midwives for emergency response. Pre-service and in-service midwifery curricula should prepare midwives for their role in humanitarian settings. Further research is needed to build an evidence-base for effective community-based approaches to maternal and newborn health in humanitarian settings and for the role of midwives during crises (IWAG 2019; Beek et al. 2019).

Key Messages
Principles

Women and newborns are especially vulnerable in crises. Midwives and midwives' associations have a key role in humanitarian emergencies and must be ready to respond.

Policy

Countries, donors, implementing organisations and global policymakers must ensure participation of midwives in all stages of crisis preparedness and response. Midwifery education must include the preparation of midwives to work in humanitarian crises. Policy makers must mobilise around three key actions: greater emphasis on maternal and newborn health in vulnerable communities including preparedness, the MISP, maternal and newborn life-saving interventions in crisis settings, and strengthening the role of communities in delivering maternal and newborn health interventions (IAWG 2019; UNFPA 2019a).

Practice

Midwives must ensure they have the competence to perform all signal functions of BEmONC and to provide respectful maternity care in all situations, including in crises when regular health systems may be fractured. To perform these competencies, midwives must work in an enabling environment and should engage with women and local communities in planning care and establishing a systematic feedback mechanism on their experience of care and recommendations for improvement (IAWG 2019).

Questions for Reflection or Review

1. Watch the short film 'War and Grace' (International Medical Corps 2020). What challenges does the film highlight for women giving birth in conflict settings? What is the difference that midwives can make in such situations? What barriers can you identify for midwifery education and practice in war-torn areas, especially with regard to the provision of respectful maternity care? https://www.youtube.com/watch?v=qr23J2M0WEM &feature=youtu.be&fbclid=IwAR2zAd e5n6MRxQqKsGePWofHZDNYthyJ_ izJnOwwLTzDmEKiVAfHaadFNxw

2. Familiarise yourself with the Minimum Initial Service Package (MISP) for Sexual and Reproductive Health (SRH) in crises situations. Reflect on how you would perform the signal BEmONC functions and provide respectful maternity care to women and their families were a crisis to occur in your locality.

3. Reflect on your education as a midwife, both pre-service and in-service, and whether it has (or has not) prepared you for working in emergencies. How can education for midwives be developed to reflect the growing number of global humanitarian crises?

Recommended Further Reading

Interagency working group (IAWG) on Reproductive Health in Crises (2018) Interagency field manual on reproductive health in humanitarian settings. https://resourcecentre.savethechildren.net/node/11145/pdf/iafm_on_reproductive_health_in_hs_2018.pdf. Accessed 6 May 2020

London School of Hygiene and Tropical Medicine (LSHTM) (2020) Health in humanitarian crises: a free Massive Open Online Course (MOOC). https://www.lshtm.ac.uk/study/courses/short-courses/free-online-courses/health-in-humanitarian-crises. Accessed 24 May 2020

Sphere (2018) Humanitarian standards. https://spherestandards.org/humanitarian-standards/. Accessed 6 May 2020

United Nations Office for Disaster Risk Reduction (2015) Sendai framework for disaster risk reduction. https://www.undrr.org/implementing-sendai-framework/what-sf. Accessed 17 May 2020

United Nations Children's Fund (UNICEF) (2018) Newborn health in humanitarian settings: a field guide. https://www.unicef.org/media/61561/file. Accessed 6 May 2020

References

Beek K, McFadden A, Dawson A (2019) The role and scope of practice of midwives in humanitarian settings: a systematic review and content analysis. Hum Resour Health 17(5). https://doi.org/10.1186/s12960-018-0341-5

Centre for Research on the Epidemiology of Disasters (CRED) (2019) Natural disasters 2018. https://www.cred.be/natural-disasters-2018. Accessed 23 Jul 2019

Centre for Research on the Epidemiology of Disasters (CRED) (2020) Refugee crisis in Bangladesh: a view from the field. CRED Crunch 57. https://www.emdat.be/publications. Accessed 18 May 2020

Cuesta J, van Loenhout J, de Lara-Banquesio M et al (2018) The impact of Typhoon Haiyan on health Staff: a qualitative study in two hospitals in Eastern Visayas, The Philippines. Front Public Health 6:208. https://doi.org/10.3389/fpubh.2018.00208

Currie S, Azfar A, Fowler R (2007) A bold new beginning for midwifery in Afghanistan. Midwifery 23:226–234

Direct Relief (2020) Direct Relief midwife kits: made for new life. https://www.directrelief.org/product/midwife-kit/. Accessed 29 May 2020

Enhancing Learning and Research for Humanitarian Assistance (ELRHA) (2014) Global survey on humanitarian professionalisation. https://www.humanitarianlibrary.org/sites/default/files/2014/02/global_humanitarian_professionalisation_survey.pdf. Accessed 31 May 2020

Flahault A, Wernli D, Zilberman P et al (2016) From global health security to global health solidarity, security and sustainability. Bull World Health Organ 94:863. https://doi.org/10.2471/BLT.16.171488. Accessed 17 May 2020

Fred M, Kernohan W (2015) Development of a framework to prepare midwives for relief work in West Africa. Afr J Midwif Womens Health 9(2):72–76

Guttermacher Institute (2020) Factsheet: Unintended Pregnancy and Abortion Worldwide. https://www.guttmacher.org/fact-sheet/induced-abortion-worldwide. Accessed 15 Nov 2020

Health Cluster/United Nations Population Fund (2018) Quality midwifery care in the midst of crisis: midwifery capacity building strategy for Northern Syria 2017–2021. https://reliefweb.int/report/syrian-arab-republic/quality-midwifery-care-midst-crisis-midwifery-capacity-building-strategy. Accessed 30 May 2020

Hobbs A, Moller AB, Kachikis A et al (2019) Scoping review to identify and map the health personnel considered skilled birth attendants in low-and-middle income countries from 2000–2015. PLoS One, 14(2): e0211576

Homer C, Friberg I, Dias M et al (2014) The projected scaling up of midwifery. Lancet 384(9948):1146–1157

Hunter B, Renfrew M, Downe S (2020) Supporting the emotional wellbeing of midwives in a pandemic: guidance for the Royal College of Midwives. https://www.rcm.org.uk/media/4095/rcm-supporting-the-emotional-wellbeing-of-midwives-during-a-pandemic-v1-submitted-to-rcm_mrd.pdf. Accessed 25 May 2020

INFORM (2020) Global risk index 2020. https://data.humdata.org/organization/inform. Accessed 22 May 2020

Inter-Agency Standing Committee (2015) Introduction to humanitarian action. https://interagencystandingcommittee.org/system/files/rc_guide_31_october_2015_webversion_final.pdf. Accessed 23 Jul 2019

Interagency Working Group (IAWG) on Reproductive Health in Crises (2018a) Interagency field manual on reproductive health in humanitarian settings. https://resourcecentre.savethechildren.net/node/11145/pdf/iafm_on_reproductive_health_in_hs_2018.pdf. Accessed 6 May 2020

Interagency Working Group (IAWG) on Reproductive Health in Crises (2018b) Newborn health in humanitarian settings. https://www.unicef.org/media/61561/file. Accessed 20 Aug 2020

Interagency Working Group (IAWG) on Reproductive Health in Crises (2018c) Manual: Newborn care supply kits for humanitarian settings. New York: UNICEF

Interagency Working Group (IAWG) on Reproductive Health in Crises (2019) Surviving day one: caring for mothers and newborns in humanitarian emergencies on the day of childbirth. https://www.healthynewbornnetwork.org/hnn-content/uploads/SavetheChildren-NBH-16Pager-ProductionV4.pdf. Accessed 27 May 2020

International Confederation of Midwives (2014a) Position statement: role of the midwife in disaster/emergency preparedness. https://www.nurse.or.jp/nursing/international/icm/basic/statement/pdf/Role_of_the_Midwife_in_DisasterEmergency_Preparedness_en.pdf. Accessed 23 Jul 2019

International Confederation of Midwives (2014b) Position statement: women, children and midwives in situations of war and civil unrest. https://www.internationalmidwives.org/assets/files/statement-files/2019/07/women-children-and-midwives-in-situations-of-war-and-civil-unrest-eng-july-1.pdf. Accessed 27 May 2020

International Confederation of Midwives (2017) Position statement: migrant and refugee women and their families. https://www.internationalmidwives.org/assets/files/statement-files/2019/06/eng-migrant_refugee_women-letterhead.pdf. Accessed 27 May 2020

International Confederation of Midwives (2018) Essential competencies for midwifery practice. https://www.internationalmidwives.org/assets/files/general-files/2019/02/icm-competencies_english_final_jan-2019-update_final-web_v1.0.pdf. Accessed 28 May 2020

International Confederation of Midwives (2020) Women's rights in childbirth must be upheld during the coronavirus pandemic: ICM official statement. https://www.internationalmidwives.org/assets/files/news-files/2020/03/icm-statement_upholding-womens-rights-during-covid19-5e83ae2ebfe59.pdf. Accessed 25 May 2020

International Federation of the Red Cross and Red Crescent Societies (2018) Information sheet: disaster risk reduction. https://media.ifrc.org/ifrc/document/disaster-risk-reduction-drr-information-sheet/. Accessed 31 May 2020

International Medical Corps (2020) War and Grace (short film). https://www.youtube.com/watch?v=qr23J2M0WEM&feature=youtu.be&fbclid=IwAR2zAde5n6MRxQqKsGePWofHZDNYthyJ_izJnOwwLTzDmE-KiVAfHaadFNxw. Accessed 20 May 2020

International Organization for Migration (2020) Who is a migrant? https://www.iom.int/who-is-a-migrant. Accessed 20 May 2020

IPPF (2015) How to talk about abortion: a rights-based messaging guide. https://www.ippf.org/sites/default/files/2018-08/ippf_abortion_messaging_guide_web_0.pdf. Accessed 15 Nov 2020

Kemp J, Shaw E, Bajracharya K (2017) Shaken into action. RCM midwives. Autumn 2017. https://www.rcm.org.uk/media/2690/midwives-magazine-autumn-2017.pdf. Accessed 18 May 2020

Kohrt B, Mistry A, Anand L et al (2019) Health research in humanitarian crises: an urgent global imperative. BMJ Glob Health 4:e001870. https://doi.org/10.1136/bmjgh-2019-001870

Manning A, Schaaf M (2018) Disrespect and abuse in childbirth and respectful maternity care. https://www.whiteribbonalliance.org/wp-content/uploads/2018/04/6422_RMC-Maternity-Care-Resources-PPG_English.pdf. Accessed 12 May 2020

Médecins Sans Frontières (2020) Midwife with MSF: care at every step. https://msf.org.au/article/stories-patients-staff/midwife-msf-care-every-step. Accessed 18 May 2020

Miyake S, Speakman E, Currie S et al (2017) Community midwifery initiatives in fragile and conflict-affected countries: a scoping review of approaches from recruitment to retention. Health Policy Plan 32:21–33. https://doi.org/10.1093/heapol/czw093

Mizutori M (2020) COVID-19 puts human rights of millions at risk: statement by the UN Secretary General's Special Representative for disaster risk reduction on the human rights dimensions of the COVID-19 pandemic. https://www.undrr.org/news/covid-19-puts-human-rights-millions-risk. Accessed 17 May 2020

Moxon S, Blencow H, Bailey P et al (2019) Categorising interventions to levels of inpatient care for small and sick newborns: Findings from a global survey. PLoS One, 14(7): e0218748

O'Mally Floyd B (2013) Lesson learned preparing volunteer midwives for service in Haiti: after the earthquake. J Midwifery Womens Health 58: 558–568

Office of the United Nations High Commissioner for Refugees (1991) Guidelines on the protection of refugee women. UNHCR, Geneva

OXFAM (2019) The Humanitarian-Development-Peace Nexus: what does it mean for multi-mandated organizations? https://reliefweb.int/report/world/humanitarian-development-peace-nexus-what-does-it-mean-multi-mandated-organizations. Accessed 22 May 2020

Partnership for Maternal, Newborn and Child Health (2019) Health and well-being of women. Children and adolescents on the move: knowledge Brief Series 1. https://www.who.int/pmnch/media/news/2019/new-knowledge-brief-series/en/. Accessed 17 May 2020

Prevention Web (2015) Poverty and inequality. https://www.preventionweb.net/risk/poverty-inequality. Accessed 22 May 2020

Relief Web (2008) Glossary of humanitarian terms. https://www.who.int/hac/about/reliefweb-aug2008.pdf?ua=1. Accessed 20 May 2020

Renfrew M, McFadden A, Bastos M et al (2014) Midwifery and quality care: findings from a new evidence-informed framework for maternal and newborn care. Lancet 384(9948):1129–1145

Renfrew M, Cheyne H, Craig J et al (2020) Sustaining quality midwifery care in a pandemic and beyond. Midwifery. Accessed 29 May 2020. https://doi.org/10.1016/j.midw.2020.102759

Safeguarding Health in Conflict Coalition (2020) Health workers at risk: violence against health care. Available at https://www.safeguardinghealth.org/sites/shcc/files/SHCC2020final.pdf. Accessed 15 Nov 2020

Save the Children, UNICEF, WHO and UNHCR (2019) Roadmap to Accelerate Progress for Every Newborn in Humanitarian Settings 2020 – 2025. Available at https://www.healthynewbornnetwork.org/hnn-content/uploads/Roadmap-to-Accelerate-Progress-for-Every-Newborn-in-Humanitarian-Settings-1-1.pdf. Accessed 15 Nov 2020

Schaaf M, Boydell V, Sheff MC, Kay C, Torabi F, Khosla R (2020) Accountability strategies for sexual and reproductive health and reproductive rights in humanitarian settings: a scoping review. Conflict and Health 14 (1)

Sphere (2018) Sphere handbook: the humanitarian charter and minimum standards in humanitarian response. https://handbook.spherestandards.org/en/sphere/#ch001. Accessed 05 May 2020

Steffens G (2018) Changing climate forces desperate Guatemalans to migrate. National Geographic. Available at https://www.nationalgeographic.com/environment/2018/10/drought-climate-change-force-guatemalans-migrate-to-us/. Accessed 10 Nov 2020

United Nations Children's Fund and Save the Children (2018) Newborn health in humanitarian settings: a field guide. https://www.healthynewbornnetwork.org/resource/newborn-health-humanitarian-settings-field-guide/. Accessed 26 May 2020

United Nations Office for the Coordination of Humanitarian Affairs (2017) A new way of working. https://www.unocha.org/es/themes/humanitarian-development-nexus. Accessed 22 May 2020

United Nations Office for the Coordination of Humanitarian Affairs (2020) Global humanitarian overview 2020. https://www.unocha.org/sites/unocha/files/GHO-2020_v9.1.pdf. Accessed 16 Nov 2020

United Nations Office for the Coordination of Humanitarian Affairs (2020a) How the private sector helps in emergencies. https://www.unocha.org/es/themes/engagement-private-sector/how-private-sector-helps-emergencies. Accessed 22 May 2020

United Nations Office for the Coordination of Humanitarian Affairs (2020b) Before and after: how COVID-19 is changing humanitarian operations. https://unocha.exposure.co/before-and-after. Accessed 22 May 2020

United Nations Office Human Rights Office of the High Commissioner (2019) Protecting rights in humanitarian crises. https://www.ohchr.org/EN/Issues/HumanitarianAction/Pages/Crises.aspx. Accessed 23 Jul 2019

United Nations Officer for Outer Space Affairs (2020) UN-Spider knowledge portal: disaster risk management. http://www.un-spider.org/risks-and-disasters/disaster-risk-management. Accessed 31 May 2020

United Nations Population Fund (2015) News on the earthquake in Nepal. https://www.unfpa.org/emergencies/earthquake-nepal. Accessed 18 May 2020

United Nations Population Fund (2018a) Sexual and reproductive health needs immense amongst Rohingya refugees. https://www.unfpa.org/news/sexual-and-reproductive-health-needs-immense-among-rohingya-refugees. Accessed 18 May 2020

United Nations Population Fund (2018b) Annual report 2018: progress and highlights. https://bangladesh.unfpa.org/sites/default/files/pub-pdf/UNFPA_Bangladesh_2018_annual_report-HR-MAY%2020.pdf. Accessed 18 May 2020

United Nations Population Fund (2019a) Humanitarian action 2019 overview. https://www.unfpa.org/sites/default/files/pub-pdf/UNFPA_HumanitAction_2019_PDF_Online_Version_16_Jan_2019.pdf. Accessed 5 May 2020

United Nations Population Fund (2019b) State of the world population report 2019: unfinished business, the pursuit of rights and choice for all. https://www.unfpa.org/sites/default/files/pub-pdf/UNFPA_PUB_2019_EN_State_of_World_Population.pdf. Accessed 20 May 2020

United Nations Population Fund (2020) UNFPA Bangladesh situation report: Rohingya humanitarian response programme, Cox's Bazaar Jan-Feb 2020. https://bangladesh.unfpa.org/sites/default/files/pub-pdf/External%20Sitrep_Jan-Feb_21Apr20.pdf. Accessed 18 May 2020

United Nations Refugee Agency (UNHCR) (2020) Refugee facts: what is a refugee? https://www.unrefugees.org/refugee-facts/what-is-a-refugee/. Accessed 20 May 2020

United Nations Volunteers (2020) UN Volunteer strengthens midwifery care in Bangladesh. https://www.unv.org/Success-stories/UN-Volunteer-strengthens-midwifery-care-Bangladesh. Accessed 18 May 2020

White Ribbon Alliance (2019) Respectful maternity care: the universal rights of women and newborns. https://www.whiteribbonalliance.org/wp-content/uploads/2019/10/WRA_RMC_Charter_FINAL.pdf Accessed 15 Nov 2020

Williams J (2020) Can resilience be taught in midwifery education? https://www.rcm.org.uk/news-views/rcm-opinion/2020/can-resilience-be-taught-in-midwifery-education/. Accessed 15 Nov 2020

World Health Organization (2009) Monitoring emergency obstetric care: a handbook. https://apps.who.int/iris/bitstream/handle/10665/44121/9789241547734_eng.pdf?sequence=1. Accessed 28 May 2020

World Health Organization (2010) What is a pandemic? https://www.who.int/csr/disease/swineflu/frequently_asked_questions/pandemic/en/. Accessed 20 May 2020

World Health Organization (2014) Early essential newborn care: clinical pocket book guide. WHO Western Pacific Region. WHO/9789290616856_eng%20(3).pdf. Accessed 20 Aug 2020

World Health Organization (2016) Global strategy on human resources for health: workforce 2030. https://www.who.int/hrh/resources/pub_globstrathrh-2030/en/. Accessed 16 Nov 2020

World Health Organization (2019a) Ten threats to global health. https://www.who.int/news-room/spotlight/ten-threats-to-global-health-in-2019. Accessed 16 Nov 2020

World Health Organization (2019b) Draft global action plan: promoting the health of refugees and migrants (2019–2023). https://www.who.int/migrants/GlobalActionPlan.pdf?ua=1. Accessed 23 Jul 2019

World Health Organization (2019c) Framework for action: strengthening quality midwifery education for universal health coverage 2030. https://www.who.int/maternal_child_adolescent/topics/quality-of-care/midwifery/strengthening-midwifery-education/en/. Accessed 28 May 2020

World Health Organization (2020) Humanitarian health action definitions: emergencies. https://www.who.int/hac/about/definitions/en/. Accessed 20 May 2020

Crossing Borders: International Consultancies and Student Electives

14

Expected Learning Outcomes

By the end of the chapter, the reader should be able to:

1. Reflect on the history of international exchange and the current practice of development co-operation.
2. Identify the key concepts associated with culture, consider the importance of cultural competence and how these impact on ethical norms and the qualities which contribute to acceptability in those who cross borders.
3. Describe how the processes of modernization and development affect countries at different levels on the Human Development Index and consider how these impact on health services.
4. Discuss issues surrounding the 'gaps' and 'shocks' which can be encountered when crossing international borders such as: 'epoch gap', 'quality gap' 'concept gap', 'perception gap', 'culture shock' and 'reverse culture shock'.
5. Consider the differing concepts of time in diverse cultures.
6. Discuss the variety of roles in which a consultant may be required to function and identify ways in which she/he can prepare for these.
7. Identify the important issues in considering student electives and explore the responsibilities of students, faculty staff and those hosting students in country.

14.1 Early Beginnings

From the earliest times, man has sought to establish international relationships, though the aim of these relationships appears to differ widely. It is possible to trace international exchange back through the last two millennia; however, the concept of development co-operation has been recognised as a 'relatively recent chapter in the history of mankind' (Juva 1994:19) with technological advances making this even more practicable as time proceeds. There has undoubtedly been an increasing mobilisation of personnel in recent centuries. International interaction through the ages can be related to various religious and political movements. Beyond the early mission journeys of the apostolic witnesses, there is evidence of Roman Catholic workers from the Portuguese colony of Goa travelling to the courts of the Mughal emperors in North India as early as 1579 (Alter and Singh 1966). Sardesi (1983) traces the path of Brahmin advisers to the royal courts of India through the early centuries of South East Asian history and in the Ottoman Empire following the fall of Constantinople in

© Springer Nature Switzerland AG 2021
J. Kemp et al., *Global Midwifery: Principles, Policy and Practice*,
https://doi.org/10.1007/978-3-030-46765-4_14

1453 a considerable number of foreign personnel with specific expertise were employed. These included specialists in politics, administration and military skills Goldhamer (1978). It is, however, distinctly apparent that the tremendous growth of scientific knowledge, technical advances, economic prosperity and social development which occurred in Europe from the early eighteenth until the mid-twentieth centuries was largely confined to the European continent (Juva 1994).

So, from this perspective, in the latter part of the twentieth century and into the twenty-first century, the exchange of technical assistance and professional expertise has become something of a new concept. It is into this environment that midwives and other experts have begun to cross international borders in order to assist development, provide technical assistance and share skills with the aim of meeting the most important needs of childbearing women and their families. Migration from north to south has been a regular feature of this kind of intercontinental exchange. However, more recently, south to south exchange has developed, and this concept is discussed in Chapter 15.

14.2   Custom and Culture

It is advantageous for those who cross international borders to acquire some knowledge of the history and geography of the region and to attempt to understand the political climate. But wherever consultants or other experts originate from, it is vital that the custom and culture of a country are observed and respected. In a doctoral study of the acceptability of short-term international consultants, Maclean (1998) identifies cultural offensiveness as being one of the most unacceptable qualities of consultants. She states that cultural sensitivity therefore is paramount in offering advice that will be crystallized in the recommendations, and this can in fact affect whether such counsel may be heeded and recommendations implemented. This is particularly relevant when consultants travel north-south or west-east, and it is important to realise that there

may be a considerable difference in what might work when ideas are transferred across cultural boundaries (Maclean 1998:337).

It has been emphasised that thoughtfulness and purposeful communication must lie at the heart of international consultancy. From this perspective, the consultant's attitude and advice need to be encapsulated in cultural sensitivity which is expressed through a mind-set of ethnic humility (Maclean 2011a). The latter has been defined as 'the extent to which advisers can overcome ethnocentrism and cultural arrogance, to become genuinely multicultural protean individuals' (Fry and Thurber 1989:84–5). This requires an ability and willingness to evaluate one's own culture with open eyes, recognising its faults and weaknesses (Maclean 2011a).

It is important to realise that professional ethics are also often embedded in cultural roots. Veatch (2000) in considering medical ethics from a cross-cultural perspective, asserts that in facing an ethical dilemma, an individual is inevitably working, implicitly if not explicitly, from within a certain framework. In respect of ethical issues, as with cultural preferences, expatriates cannot assume that their own stance is the norm and need to recognise their own position for what it is. It may be very different and seem 'the right thing to do', but it is not necessarily acceptable when crossing cultures.

Cultural competence is therefore a skill that needs to be acquired by the would-be international consultant. This has been described as adopting 'a set of congruent behaviours, attitudes, and policies' anticipating that these will mingle into a structure that would enable professionals to work effectively in cross-cultural situations (Cross et al. 1989:13). Lough (2011) asserts that in spite of numerous international voluntary agencies which send professionals overseas claiming that volunteering will increase intercultural competence; this learning will only take place in the presence of certain pre-conditions. These include cultural immersion, service duration and guided reflection. Lough explains that guided reflection tends to moderate the relationship between duration and intercultural competence. In a study by Monkhouse (2018:13), professionals returning to the United Kingdom after a global exchange experience reported a process of 'experiential learning, reflection and evolving cultural intelligence'. This emphasises the value of reflective practice for short-term professionals, especially if reflection is guided by a skilled and experienced mentor. It needs to be acknowledged too that culture shock can be a very real experience for anyone crossing borders, and this is discussed further below in the context of student electives.

Drawing from their experience of cross-cultural work, Humbert et al. (2011:301) have identified 'cultural awareness', 'complexity' and 'connectedness' as important insights when crossing borders. They claim that practitioners need to be able to integrate these layers of insight into their practice. Their definitions of these terms are summarised in Box 14.1.

Box 14.1. Defining the Terms Used to Describe Layers of Cultural Insight

'**Cultural awareness**' describes recognising a different culture and attempting to understand it

'**Complexity**' incorporates the idea that cultural differences are intricate, dynamic and multifaceted

'**Connectedness**' describes the formation of relationships during cross-cultural encounters

(Humbert et al. 2011:305)

Cultural awareness calls for an individual to compare the insights gained with their own culture and then respond appropriately to the differences. Recognising the complexity of the situation, it is essential to establish the all-important relationships borne out of connectedness. It is crucial for the cross-cultural visitor to infiltrate these layers of cross-cultural manners in order to attain that critical quality of cultural competence (Humbert et al. 2011:300). It has been stressed that a multidimensional learning process is essential to acquiring cultural or intercultural competence and that this cannot be obtained by just learning the cultural do's and don'ts. It is suggested that such a core competency surrounds the ability to manage change whilst remaining in control, and the ability to do this in situations of additional complexity when crossing cultures (Steixner 2011).

Even though the world is rapidly evolving into an ever smaller 'global village' identified decades ago by McLuhan (1962) people continue to perceive some essential issues from very different perspectives, often relating to whether they originate from the eastern or the western hemisphere, from the north or from the south. These perceptions can be considered in the context of culture though they are likely to relate to the degree of modernization and development of the nation which is discussed below. In the western world and in the northern hemisphere, 'big' has become 'beautiful', trade and business mergers are the order of the day and 'time is money'. These are some of the products of industrialization and secularism that can impact on various aspects of life, not least on health and health services (Maclean 1998:10), and these will affect the care which a woman can and often does expect to receive when giving birth.

The concept of time can sometimes be related to the level of modernization being experienced in a country. It may be argued that one's concept of time relates to personal priorities in that business or income-generating issues may take precedence over punctuality; but these vary considerably, and in order to understand, the matter calls for some insight in cross-cultural encounters. In this context, Hall (1973) introduced the concepts of monochronic and polychronic time which he dubbed 'the silent language'. If cross-cultural visitors fail to interpret this silent language, there is potential for misunderstanding at best and conflict at worst. People from northern and central Europe, Australia and North America tend to fall into the former category and may be described as 'M people' whilst those inhabiting South America, Africa, Asia and the Mediterranean region are known as 'P People'. Their attitudes to time vary considerably, and some of the main characteristics are summarised in the Table 14.1.

Table 14.1 Contrasting characteristics of monochronic and polychronic cultures

Monochronic cultures 'M people'	Polychronic chronic 'P People'
Define time as linear	Define time in terms of tasks
Time can be saved, spent, wasted, lost	Time is flexible due to the unpredictability of life
Events scheduled one at a time	Several events happen simultaneously
Schedule may take precedence over interpersonal relationships	People and their involvement take precedence over schedules
Emphasis on schedules, punctuality, preciseness	Subject to interruptions and can be distracted. Base the importance of promptness on the relationship
Value productivity and getting things done on time	Emphasis on completion of transactions rather than schedules and deadlines
Committed to the job	Committed to people and relationships
Adhere strictly to plans	Change plans easily, often
One task at a time appropriate	Multitasking valued
Everything is organized and dominated by a very rigid conception of time	Appointments can be changed and most projects can undergo important changes until the last minute
Meeting format: Agenda scheduled, only one person speaks at a time	Meeting format: May bounce from subject to subject as seems fit, more than one person may speak at a time
Uncomfortable with 'P' style meetings	Uncomfortable with 'M' style meetings

Sources: Hall (1973), Duranti and Di Prata (2009), and Brenner (2018)

Decades ago, Kluckhohn and Strodtbeck (1961) proposed that people adopt a time orientation derived from their culture but looked at it slightly differently from Hall (1973) cited above. This, they maintain, is acquired through a complex process of socialisation and can be described as a past or future orientation. The perceptions of Kluckhohn and Strodtbeck (1961) were reintroduced by Hofstede (2001) who regards 'long-term versus short-term orientation' as the fifth dimension of culture. The contrasting characteristics of long- and short-term orientation are summarised in Box 14.2 and bring out some additional issues to those cited above (Table 14.1). Countries that score highly in long-term orienta-

tion include China, Japan, South Korea and Brazil. Conversely the Philippines, Ghana, Nigeria and Sierra Leone do not have high long-term orientation scores.

Box 14.2. Contrasting Characteristics of Long- and Short-Term Orientation

Long-term orientation	Short-term orientation
*Emphasis on persistence	*Emphasis on quick results
*Relationships ordered by status	*Status not a major issue in relationships
*Personal adaptability important	*Personal steadfastness and stability important
*'Face' considerations common but seen as a weakness	*Protection of one's 'face' is important
*Leisure time not too important	*Leisure time important
*Save, be thrifty	*Spend
*Invest in real estate	*Invest in mutual funds
*Relationships and market position important	*Bottom line important
*Good or evil depends on circumstances	*Belief in absolutes about good and evil

Derived from Hofstede 2001:359

In addition to the orientations described above, Hofstede and Minkov (2010) have further identified a total of six cultural dimensions of relevance to the cross-cultural visitor, and these are listed in Box 14.3.

Box 14.3. The Six Dimensions of Culture

1. **Power distance index** defines the degree of inequality existing and accepted between people with and without power.

2. **Individualism versus collectivism** describes the strengths of the ties that people have to others in their community.

---

3. **Masculinity versus femininity** refers to the distribution of roles between men and women.
4. **Uncertainty avoidance index** describes how well people can cope with anxiety.
5. **Long-term versus short-term orientation** refers to the time horizon people in a society display.
6. **Indulgence versus restraint** indicates the degree to which gratification of people's own drives and emotions is allowed or encouraged (according to Hofstede and Minkov 2010).

Beugelsdijk and Welze (2018) have taken opposing paradigms presented by Hofstede and Inglehart and propose that younger generations have become 'more individualistic and joyous'. They acknowledge however that although economic development and generational replacement drive the cultural change, approximately half of the variation occurring in national cultural orientations is totally unique to each country. These are considered to arise from variation in the route in which development has taken and are rooted in historical forces (Beugelsdijk and Welze 2018:1469). Inglehart (1997) had proposed some controversial theories in the context of modernization and post-modernization, claiming that economic development and cultural and political change combine in logical and somewhat predictable patterns.

14.3 Modernization and Development

Ever-increasing dimensions of cultural norms and contrasts can be discovered by the dedicated cross-cultural visitor. However, an understanding of the concepts of modernization and development is another desirable asset for the international consultant. These concepts have been variously defined. Modernization is typically depicted as a transition from a traditional rural society to an urban, secular, industrial civilisation (Encyclopaedia Britannica 2016). Modern societies are predominantly individualistic by contrast with those described as collectivist. Hofstede (1991:261) describes the former as:

> ...societies in which ties between individuals are loose: everyone is expected to look after himself or herself and his or her immediate family.

Collectivism, on the other hand, is described as the opposite of individualism pertaining to:

> ...societies in which people from birth onwards are integrated into strong, cohesive groups, which throughout people's lifetime continue to protect in exchange for unquestioning loyalty. (Hofstede 1991:260)

It stands to reason therefore that a person who may be described as 'modern' is almost inevitably individualistic or is likely to be moving in that direction. Smith and Bond (1993) suggest that in fact individualism may be another name for modernity.

Beyond modernity, postmodernism is described as 'a late 20th-century movement characterized by broad scepticism, subjectivism, or relativism; a general suspicion of reason; and an acute sensitivity to the role of ideology in asserting and maintaining political and economic power' (Online Encyclopaedia Britannica 2019). It is from a post-modern world that most international consultants and advisors travel in order to share expertise with colleagues who may be in a totally different place along the road to post-modernity and holding a contrasting worldview. It can be useful to consider some of the concepts that influence thinking and action as societies move through different stages of modernization and development (Table 14.2). These inevitably need to be taken into account when sharing expertise and ideas. The conceptual level of a society and its individuals by comparison with that of the visiting consultant or advisor will inevitably influence the degree of congruence which can exist between them. The difference may be considered a 'concept gap'. The usefulness and acceptability of an international exchange may well be determined by how well this gap can be bridged or minimised. This matter could account for why south to south and north to

Table 14.2 The transition of concepts held in diverse societies

Concept	Traditional society	Modern society	Postmodern society
Community and individuals	Society is like an organism, existing as a 'whole'; individuals are like organs of that whole and cannot exist if separated	People are independent, self-reliant, having an individualistic orientation towards others	People are separate, coherent individuals thinking and acting independently
Identity and purpose	Society dictates the place and function of the individual	Individuals possess cognitive and behavioural flexibility; they are highly motivated to achieve	Identity is not fixed, but in process; multiple identities are required to achieve a successful life
Beliefs	Observes and influenced by traditional religion or philosophy	Secularization in religious belief	Relativism—All truth is relative
Attitude of mind	Fatalistic	Anti-fatalistic	Anti-fatalistic

Sources: Yang (1988), The Science Forum (2009), NZCER (2017) and Zevada (2019)

north cooperations are increasingly developing in an ever-changing world. These systems of international cooperation are discussed in Chapter 15.

In a comparison of the various worldviews, Burnett claims that it was the mechanical model of man proposed in the secular worldview that ultimately led to the individualistic concept of human populations (Burnett 1990:43). This contrasts with the worldview of most traditional societies where the stress lies on the community or society as a whole rather than on the individual. This has relevance in attempting to promote woman-centred care in a collectivist environment, especially where masculinity takes precedence over femininity (see Box 14.3:3). Additionally, this directs the power distance index (Box 14.3:1) to the disadvantage of women and Hofstede and Minkov's (2010) sixth dimension of culture (Box 14.3:6) may tend to discourage the physical and emotional needs of a birthing woman from being satisfied.

Development has traditionally been associated with the achievement of economic and social progress. The World Bank (2019a) maintains that empirical evidence and operational experience demonstrate that social development promotes economic growth leading to better interventions and a higher quality of life. However, Barder (2012) maintains that 'development consists of more than improvements in the well-being of citizens, even broadly defined: it also conveys something about the capacity of economic, political and social systems to provide the circumstances for that well-being on a sustainable, long-term basis'. Sustainability is the issue that has been at the heart of the 2030 Agenda (United Nations 2015) which enshrines the Sustainable Development Goals (SDGs) (United Nations 2019), and these issues are discussed in Chapter 1.

Currently, countries are designated into four groups: high, upper middle, lower middle and low-income countries, according to their relative economic level which is reviewed annually (World Bank 2019b).

Through its development programme, the United Nations uses human development indicators to analyse regional and national trends in development. The Human Development Index (HDI) was created to emphasise that people and their capabilities should be the ultimate criteria for assessing the development of a country, not economic growth alone (United Nations Development Programme 2019). This concurs with the sentiment of Barder (2012) cited above. In considering achievements in health, education and income there is a considerable disparity confronting people living in contrasting conditions at the higher and lower ends of the HDI. By comparing the latest maternal mortality ratios (MMR) from these countries, it is clear that there is a vast difference in the relative risk to women giving birth living at either end of this index (Box 14.4).

(Box 14.5).

Box 14.4. The Highest and Lowest Ranking Countries in the 2018 Human Development Index (HDI)

Highest ranking 5 countries	Lowest ranking 5 countries
1. Norway (**5**)	185. Burundi (**712**)
2. Switzerland (**5**)	186. Chad (**856**)
3. Australia (**6**)	187. South Sudan (**789**)
4. Ireland (**8**)	188. Central African Republic (**882**)
5. Germany (**6**)	189. Niger (**553**)

(Derived from 189 countries and territories indexed by United Nations Development Programme 2018)
(The bold numbers in brackets indicate the latest available MMRs* according to WHO 2015)
MMRs are cited per 100,000 births
*MMR maternal mortality ratio

numerous skills. Indeed, a technical adviser or consultant who crosses borders may encounter the need to function in a multiplicity of roles (Box 14.5).

Box 14.5. The Multiplicity of Roles Played by Consultants

• Adviser	• Advocate	• Capacity builder
• Change agent	• Colleague	• Diplomat
• Educator	• Evaluator	• Expert
• Friend	• Interpreter	• Networker
• Practitioner	• Researcher	• Writer

Sources: Bingham (1954), Bruner (1975), Goldhamer (1978), Craig (1980), Fry and Thurber (1989), Forss et al. (2006) and Maclean (2013)

Maclean (1998:11) identifies an 'epoch gap' that can be encountered when travelling between countries that are at inconsistent levels of modernisation and development. A person travelling from a high-income country into one with a lower-income or one that is lower on the HDI scale may well encounter situations that were customary in their country of origin decades or even centuries ago. This may affect numerous issues including for example the availability of clean, running water and reliable electricity supplies upon which modern life is very dependent. The short-term visitor will only be exposed to such inconveniences temporarily, but it is important that a consultant is aware of the situation in which women habitually give birth and colleagues live and work and not allow the living environment of an international standard hotel, if that is the hospitality offered, to cloud the real picture. Any recommendations need to be relevant to reality in a country that is less modernised or developed, or where the HDI is comparatively low.

14.4   Essential Attributes in Cross-Cultural Exchange

An international consultant may be required to undertake various assignments that call for

Little wonder therefore that Fry and Thurber (1989:85) cited earlier stress that those who cross international borders must become 'genuinely multicultural protean individuals'. Cultural competence and sensitivity have been outlined above, and the necessity of gaining insight into the historical, geographical and political situations is reiterated. The need to take cognizance of the current level of human development and the place of women in society and to consider the path of development the country has and is taking is a valuable exercise prior to undertaking an assignment and certainly before offering advice and making recommendations for the way ahead. Political awareness and correctness and an insight into the accepted ethics in a country are all basic requirements of those who would cross borders.

Whether or not a cross-cultural visitor, professional consultant, volunteer or student on an elective study will be acceptable or will not depend on a multitude of issues. The concept of the undesirable is described in Maclean's 'nightmare consultant' derived from a synthesis of respondent opinions expressed in a major study (Box 14.6), and very similar criticisms have continued to be echoed more recently (Box 14.7). Those who aspire to cross borders would do well to take note!

Box 14.6. 'The Nightmare Consultant'

A 'nightmare consultant' is critical and bossy. She fails to establish a good relationship with us and does not discuss her decisions with us. She tries to tell us what to do and her usual approach in advising us is to say: 'You must...' She is emotional and sometimes she fights with us.

Culturally insensitive, she dresses improperly and carries too much baggage. She neither understands our culture nor our problems. She does not obtain our views. She fails to understand our problems and is totally unaware of our needs. She identifies 'problems' which are not problems to us. She ignores the 'grassroots workers.' She is incompetent in the very area we require expertise and is unskilled clinically.

In writing her report, she makes criticisms based on her own inaccurate observations. She is impractical and inflexible. She is unable to work independently and therefore demands too much of our time. She talks a lot but we see no action. We call them 'NATO' consultants—No Action, Talking Only!

Derived from: Maclean (1998:301, 302).

Box 14.7. Unsatisfactory Volunteers in Global Health Exchange

Unacceptable volunteers demonstrate.

> Lack of cultural understanding.

> Insufficient cultural sensitivity and awareness.

> Attitudes of superiority.

> Disrespect of local customs and practices.

> Imposition of own methods and opinions inappropriate to the practice environment.

> Inexperience so that they are ill prepared to work in low-income countries.

> Difficulties with cultural and language barriers.

> Differences in norms and values.

> Lack of understanding about local health practices and challenges.

> Limited skill sets.

> Inadequate training to work in the new environment.

> Undervaluing of local staff knowledge.

> Unwillingness to support the public health system.

> Lack of understanding of their role.

> Lack of communication on the terms of reference or job description.

> Differing expectations.

Laleman et al. 2007, Green et al. 2009, Kraeker and Chandler 2013, Kung et al. 2016, Lasker 2016.

Before undertaking an international assignment, it behoves a consultant to prepare herself/himself in the areas of professional policy and practice, evidence-based practice and to ensure she/he has the requisite clinical skills and experience appropriate to the assignment. Some of the most essential topics needful in consultant preparation are summarised in Box 14.8 and offer a personal checklist.

Organizations could strengthen their efforts considerably in promoting more effective and valuable interventions in partner communities.

Box 14.8. A Personal Checklist for Consultant Preparation

• Do I have 'cultural competence' and a cultural sensitivity?

• Am I politically aware and do I aim to be politically correct?

• Am I aware of my personal professional ethics and stance?

• Am I aware of the historical, geographical and political issues shaping the country I am visiting?

- Do I know where the country is placed on the 'Human Development Index'?
- Do I have a linguistic ability or at least recognise my limitations?
- Do I possess good interpersonal communication skills?
- Am I aware of the cultural differences in educational approaches?
- Am I aware of the traditional approaches to birth and medicine in the region?
- Am I cognizant with the tropical or climatic conditions and the health issues relevant in the area?
- Am I up to date with evidence-based practice?
- Do I have an adequate level of clinical practice skills?
- Am I conscious of gender issues and attitudes and how these may impact birthing experiences and my approaches to offering counsel?
- Can I be described as non-discriminatory in my approach, being respectful to others whatever their ethnicity, culture, religion, educational or social standing?
- Am I familiar with rights-based approaches?
- Am I knowledgeable about capacity building?
- Do I have monitoring and evaluation skills?
- Am I aware of the 'pathways of power' through which I will need to work and how to use 'evidence-based advocacy' to the best advantage?
- Am I familiar with current reports and strategies, e.g. the Sustainable Development Goals and 2030 Agenda?
- Am I a team worker but capable of working alone when required?
- Am I knowledgeable about 'terms of reference', contracting, report writing and making recommendations?
- Am I able to write reports of good quality?

- Am I prepared to discuss possible recommendations with the implementers before finalising them?
- Do I know to whom I am accountable during and after the assignment?

Derived from: Fry and Thurber 1989; Maclean 1998, 2011a, 2013; Nanda et al. 2005; Forss et al. 2006; Lough et al. 2018.

In considering the most appropriate practices in cross-cultural exchange from the partner organisation point of view, Lough et al. (2018:9) maintain that the important issues centre around 'service duration, volunteer skill-level, language capacity, and training in the local community'. They conclude that evidence-based practices need to be integrated into programmes, in this way. In addition, those who cross borders, cross cultures and cross timelines need to be aware of personal safety and health issues. These include an awareness of risk and how to minimise it. An ability to counteract jet lag and culture shock can make a difference to the quality of consultancy offered and hence help determine whether long term partnerships can be established.

Partnership and co-presence are key concepts in current international development cooperation. Consultancy therefore needs to encapsulate the aspirations and objectives of both the consultant and the clients. Bellman (1990:238) summarises an ideal professional partnership almost as an equation which has remained accurate through several decades:

> …the client's investment in the consultant's unique combination of abilities equals the consultant's investment in the client's unique combination of opportunities.

A successful partnership is dependent on equity and on a reciprocated esteem. It needs to encompass a shared vision that incorporates mutual respect and meaningful communication which lead to reciprocal insight (Fig. 14.1). Without these elements, there is a high risk of a 'perception

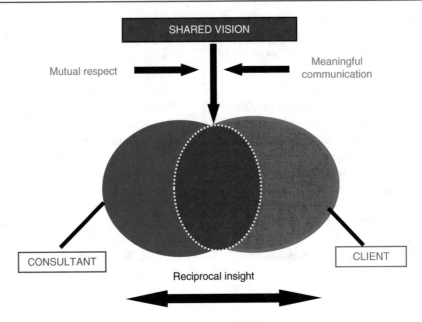

Fig. 14.1 The importance of attaining a shared vision (Maclean 1998, 2011) (reproduced with permission from the British Journal of Midwifery)

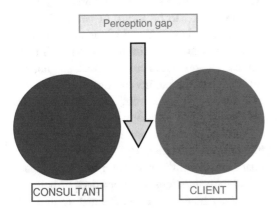

Fig. 14.2 Where there is no shared vision (Maclean 1998, 2011) (reproduced with permission from the British Journal of Midwifery)

gap' (Fig. 14.2) with the possibility of considerable misunderstanding and even distress (Maclean 1998:97–99, 2011b:389).

It has been claimed that the principle of 'co-presence' lies at the heart of a sustainable volunteering project. It has been applauded as 'an indicator of the quality of relationships established between professional volunteers and their...mentors and peers' (Ackers and Ackers-Johnson 2014:2). In this context, it could feasibly be applied to the principles of consultancy since co-presence has been identified as 'working together to share knowledge and ideas'. Co-presence recognizes that 'different types of knowledge and skills can move between different health workers in multiple directions', and therefore, it can be noted that 'skills transfer is not a one-way process' (Ackers and Ackers-Johnson 2014:1). In a study examining the impact of health partnership schemes, it is reported that 74% of UK volunteers believed that they brought back 'new approaches and techniques which can improve their practice in the UK'. Furthermore, it discovered that '765 participating institutions in low and middle-income countries are demonstrating a higher quality of specified health services' (THET 2019:1). The principles and practice of partnership are further discussed in Chapter 16.

Any consultant who considers that she/he has nothing to learn from national colleagues is under a considerable misconception and is unlikely to be able to offer much in wise counsel.

Maclean (2011b) warns those who are crossing borders that they are usually entering a world that is very different from that with which they are most familiar. Often consultants hail from the affluent West and as indicated above, in order to cross boundaries effectively and offer relevant counsel, consultants need special preparation and 'a commitment that will endure in the adversity of the unknown that lies ahead' (Maclean 2011b:391). The International Confederation of Midwives (International Confederation of Midwives 2019) offers a consultancy service which includes preparation for this role, and this is described in Chapter 6.

14.5   Student Electives

Anyone, who aspires to cross borders, whatever their purpose or status, faces similar challenges in respect of culture and custom and modernization and development, and these have been discussed above. Students can avail themselves of unique opportunities that may be offered during an elective placement. However, like anyone else, students can experience culture shock during international assignments. This is more likely if she/he is an inexperienced traveller or has not adequately prepared for the transition between countries and cultures (UKCISA 2018). In a seminal work, Furnham and Bochner (1986:31) maintain that culture shock arises from a range of different situations including the degree of difference between the new culture and that of the country of origin, previous experience of crossing cultures and adapting to them, the preparation made for the change, individual psychological characteristics and the social support networks that exist. Winkelman (1994) recommends that culture shock can be minimised by 'preparing for problems and using resources that will promote coping and adjustment' (Winkelman 1994:123), suggesting that 'all atypical problems encountered during cross-cultural adaptation are caused by or exacerbated by cultural shock', and this will have the effect of increasing typical negative reactions. Therefore, it is suggested that problems need to be reframed

in such a way that greater tolerance is fostered and problem resolution strategies implemented. Essentially therefore universities need to take cognizance of these issues and adequately prepare elective students.

Some students may choose an elective in a country that seems similar in many respects to their country of origin, but culture shock can still occur, the unexpected taking the visitor sometimes by surprise. If travelling to a country that is considerably dissimilar along the HDI described above, has a different climate or contrasting environment, this will call for more adaptability. The university or school in the new environment may lack many of the familiar resources. The library may not offer up to date textbooks and journals and even the electricity or internet connection for the previously 'essential' technology and study may not be available or may be unreliable. Another contrast in such a different setting can occur in clinical practice. The student might observe contrasting standards of care compared to that with which s/he is familiar. In travelling to a lower income country essential supplies may be limited or scarcely existent at all. The woman's needs may not be considered and she may be denied an informed choice. The reactions which an elective student may experience here can range between disbelief and disgust, between pity and anger, a determination to 'change the world' or a feeling of hopelessness and despair. This experience, described as a 'quality gap', exists where the working environment and the standards of available care differ considerably from that to which the visitor is accustomed and can be comprised of numerous issues which are summarised in Fig. 14.3 (Maclean 1998, 2013).

Since an elective period forms part of an undergraduate curriculum, it is important for students to identify personal learning targets during the assignment giving due regard as to how these will help in overall personal professional development. Talking with a student or new graduate who has undertaken an elective that involved international travel can prove helpful, particularly if that person has studied or worked in an area similar to the planned elective location. It is

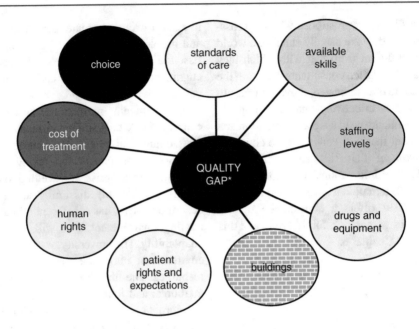

Fig. 14.3 Examples of issues contributing to a 'quality gap' in available health care between countries at different levels of modernisation and development (Maclean 2013) (reproduced with permission from Quay Books, MA Healthcare)

important also for students in consultation with their tutors or supervisors to discover lines of support. An identified member of staff on site in the visiting country who is able to offer this can be greatly advantageous. It is also essential to identify a faculty member at the university where the student is normally based who can advise about preparation, where practicable provide a guided mentorship during the elective and offer debriefing on return. Keeping a reflective diary is invaluable during an elective period of study, but its value is limited if that element of guided mentorship by an experienced member of staff either on site or back at base is not available (Lough 2011; Maclean 2013).

Ethical viewpoints that may be at variance when cultures are crossed have been mentioned above. Udokang (2014) acknowledges the influence of Western colonisation in Africa and concludes that it is impossible to make a complete and total reversal of the impacts that were made on traditional ethics. However, he proposes that 'a healthy integration of the positive elements of the Western and traditional values is imperative'. Udokang suggests that:

> the challenges and opportunities presented by globalization and international interdependence should be explored in charting a new culture and cultural policies for modern Africa. (Udokang 2014:269)

However, Pinker (2011) and Flynn (2012) concur that people in post-industrial societies are accustomed to dealing with complex situations; they cope with abstract ideas and exist amidst social diversity. Therefore, their capacity to reason about ethical issues increases and their empathy increases. Nevertheless, change needs to come from within an organisation, and Gentile (2016) stresses that discovering 'creative ways to reframe issues' may be appropriate, but genuine commendable qualities of the culture need to be acknowledged and respected. Some countries do not have a historical experience of Western colonisation and traditional ethical norms will be rooted elsewhere. Box 14.9 displays some of the principles fundamental to East Asian ethics and provides an example of a mindset that may be at variance with a western approach. It can be useful for students and their supervisors to reflect on these in practical situations and compare them with the sort of ethical decision that would most likely prevail in their country of origin and usual place of practice. Again, considering the issue of woman centred care within such a framework could render certain challenges. Each culture or region is likely to have their own set of ethical principles and discovering them can prove both educational and have practical application for the student on a clinical elective placement.

Box 14.9. Six Principles of East Asian Ethics
- Interdependence over independence.
- Hierarchy over equality.
- Obligations over rights.
- Others over self.
- Harmony over confrontation, resignation over protest.
- Stability of form over change.

(Derived from Becker 1997:1089–1091)

From the point of view of the sending university, it is necessary that sites for elective study are inspected and approved for the purpose. There needs to be adequate experience and supervision available on site, but in the real world, by nature of the situation, the ideal may not prove practicable and the student may find that she/he lacks the supervision and support experienced back home. In addition, clinical conditions never previously observed will almost inevitably be encountered in a country that is lower on the HDI scale. If the conditions have been seen, it is likely that the severity of the problem exceeds the student's previous experience. The student, for example, may have observed a woman experiencing a prolonged labour, but it would likely be unfamiliar to encounter obstructed labour, rup-

tured uterus or vesico-vaginal fistulae, the sequelae of prolonged labour. These occur where recognition is not prompt, access to emergency obstetric services limited or unavailable or referral and transfer of patients to the appropriate level of care may be beyond the reach of many of the population (Indra et al. 2017).

Culture shock may well be expected, and every effort is made to minimise it, but reverse culture shock has been recognised as a very real issue that confronts students, professional workers, business people and others crossing borders (Jordan 1992; Pascoe 2000; Knell 2006; Presbitero 2016). Adequate preparation is again a good precautionary measure and provision for debriefing on return can be beneficial for students and all kinds of travellers. Raschio (1987) in a small study of elective students after returning home asserts that reverse culture shock most usually surrounds comparisons made between lifestyles and societies. Students recognised that changes personally experienced and those they perceived in others gave rise to a sense of personal conflict. Respondents had experienced adjustments in their interactions with peers and in their friendships. However, students reported personal growth in respect of greater independence. They had also acquired a changing global perspective and had increased their language skills. An increased quality of patience and the ability to be more objective were claimed as assets after their overseas electives. Students had habitually required support from their family and friends to help them adjust back to their home environment, but Raschio (1987) recommends that institutional support systems should exist through which students can be helped with this process of re-entry into their own culture. Storti (2001) suggests that the negative feelings of loneliness, unpleasantness and frustration of returnees can frequently become precursors of personal growth and insight and proffers:

> …re-entry is an experience to be reckoned with, but when the reckoning is done and the accounts are cleared you are likely to find that the price you paid for your overseas sojourn was the bargain of a lifetime. (Storti 2001: xxi)

14.6 Finally…

It is apparent therefore that those who would cross borders need to be carefully selected, adequately prepared and appropriately debriefed. Although evaluating the success of a consultancy or any international sojourn for that matter has been recognised for decades as notoriously difficult (Alexander 1966; Chambers 1981; Fry and Thurber 1989; Laleman et al. 2007; Motamedi 2015), maybe Storti's conclusion is one that should reflect the conclusion of a returned consultant or elective student.

Fry and Thurber (1989:130) conclude that *'exemplary consultants'* can be described as *'inners and outers'* as they make the transition between academic and practice areas with ease; they are adaptable and able to communicate with both 'peasants' and 'princes'. However, they warn that the best consultants are never available, because they are always in demand!

Questions for Reflection or Review

1. Consider the characteristics of long- and short-term orientation described by Hofstede (Box 14.2); identify your own position and then that of a country you have visited, reflect on ways of achieving cultural competence in crossing such a border.
2. Discuss the importance of consultant and client acquiring a shared vision.
3. Consider the different ethical perspectives that could impact on clinical decision making and on how teams work together. Identify your own ethical framework and reflect on areas where there may be differences or conflict of opinion in providing woman centred midwifery care.

Key Messages

Principles

Cross-cultural exchange should be nurtured within an enabling philosophy that aims to provide mutual benefits to both parties and be framed within an atmosphere of reciprocal respect.

Policy

There needs to be a strategy in place to guide selection and ensure appropriate preparation and debriefing for all who cross borders, whether professionals or students, in order to facilitate maximum effectiveness and minimal disruption.

Practice

The safety, health and well-being of women and babies within a human rights framework should be a priority whether in clinical, academic or consultancy practice.

Additional Resources for Reflection and Further Study

Consider Hofstede's six dimensions of culture, see: https://www.mindtools.com/pages/article/newLDR_66.htm- Explore these in respect of your own country and a country in which you are working or visiting. How should these insights affect your approach to cross-cultural cooperation or collaboration and influence any recommendations you may propose?

Using the principles of partnership described by the Tropical Health and Education Trust (THET), compile a checklist that can be used to assess the quality and effectiveness of a cross-cultural project with which you are familiar: https://www.thet.org/principles-of-partnership/

How many of the 'gaps' identified in this chapter exist between you and the partnership you have experienced and evaluated?

Lough BJ, Tiessen R, Lasker JN (2018) Effective practices of international volunteering for health: perspectives from partner organizations. Glob Health 14:11 https://globalizationandhealth.biomedcentral.com/articles/10.1186/s12992-018-0329-x

Maclean GD (2013) Electives and international midwifery consultancy: a resource for students, midwives and other health professionals. Tiger Stripes and Tears. Quay Books, London

UKCISA (2018) Facing Culture Shock. UK Council for International Student Affairs. https://www.ukcisa.org.uk/Information%2D%2DAdvice/Preparation-and-Arrival/Facing-culture-shock

References

Ackers L, Ackers-Johnson J (2014) Policy report: understanding co-presence. Sustainable volunteering project. University of Salford, England

Alexander Y (1966) International technical assistance experts: a case study of the UN experience. Praeger, New York

Alter JP, Singh HJ (1966) The church in Delhi. Part a in Hayward VEW. The church as Christian community. Lutterworth Press, London

Barder O (2012) What is development? Center for Global Development, Washington, DC. https://www.cgdev.org/blog/what-development. Accessed 7 May 2019

Becker CB (1997) Social ethics in East Asia. Drug Inf J 31:1089–1096

Beugelsdijk S and Welze C (2018) Dimensions and Dynamics of National Culture: Synthesizing Hofstede With Inglehart. Journal of Cross-Cultural Psychology. 9(10):1469–1505. Article first published online: October 2, 2018; Issue published: November 1, 2018 [last accessed 10.11.2020]

Bingham J (1954) Shirtsleeve diplomacy. Point 4 in action. John Day, New York

Brenner R (2018) Polychronic Meetings. Point Lookout 18:1

Bruner J (1975) The role of the researcher as an adviser to the educational policy maker. Oxf Rev Educ 1(83):183

Burnett D (1990) Clash of worlds. MARC, Monarch Publications, Eastbourne

Chambers R (1981) Rural poverty unperceived: problems and remedies. World Dev 9:1–19

Craig J (1980) Culture shock! What not to do in Malaysia and Singapore, how and why not to do it. Times Books International, Singapore

Cross T et al (1989) Towards a culturally competent system of care, vol 1. CASSP Technical Assistance Center, Georgetown University Child Development Center, Washington, DC

Duranti G, Di Prata O (2009) Everything is about time: does it have the same meaning all over the world? Paper presented at PMI® global congress 2009—EMEA, Amsterdam, North Holland, the Netherlands. Project Management Institute, Newtown Square, PA

Encyclopaedia Britannica (2016) Modernization. Encyclopaedia Britannica Inc. https://www.britannica.com/topic/modernization. Accessed 15 May 2019

Encyclopaedia Britannica (2019) Postmodernism. https://www.britannica.com/topic/postmodernism-philosophy. Accessed 12 Jul 2019

Flynn R (2012) Are we getting smarter? Rising IQ in the twenty-first century. Cambridge University Press, New York

Forss K, Carlsen J, Frojland E et al (2006) Can evaluations be trusted? An enquiry into the quality of Sida's evaluation reports. Sida, Stockholm, Sweden

Fry and Thurber (1989) The international education of the development consultant: communicating with peasants and princes. Pergammon Press, Oxford

Furnham A, Bochner S (1986) Culture shock, Methuen, London. In: For thoroughly updated version see: Ward CA (2001) psychology of culture shock, 2nd edn. Routledge, Hove, East Sussex

Gentile MC (2016) Talking about ethics across cultures. Harv Bus Rev. https://hbr.org/2016/12/talking-about-ethics-across-cultures. Accessed 10 Jul 2019

Goldhamer H (1978) The adviser. Elsevier, New York

Green T, Green H, Scandlyn J et al (2009) Perceptions of short-term medical volunteer work: a qualitative study in Guatemala. Globalization and Health 5:4. https://globalizationandhealth.biomedcentral.com/articles/10.1186/1744-8603-5-4 [last accessed 10.11.2020]

Hall ET (1973) The silent language. Anchor Books, New York

Hofstede G (1991) Cultures and organizations: software of the mind. McGraw-Hill Book, London

Hofstede G (2001) Cultures consequences: comparing values, behaviors, institutions and organizations across nations, 2nd edn. Sage, London and New Delhi

Hofstede GJ, Minkov M (2010) Cultures and organizations, software of the mind, 3rd revised edn. McGraw Hill, London. ISBN 0-07-166418-1

Humbert TK, Burket A, Deveney R et al (2011) Occupational therapy practitioners' perspectives regarding international cross cultural work. Aust Occup Ther J 58(4):300–309

Indra, Usharani N, Bendigeri M (2017) A study on clinical outcome of obstructed labour. Int J Reprod Contracept Obstet Gynecol 6(2):439–442

Inglehart R (1997) Modernization and post-modernization: cultural, economic and political change in 43 societies. Princeton University Press, Princeton, NJ

International Confederation of Midwives (2019) ICM consultancy service. International Confederation of Midwives, The Hague. https://www.internationalmidwives.org/icm-publications/icm-consultancy-service.html. Accessed 25 Feb 2019

Jordan P (1992) Re-entry: making the transition from missions to life at home. YWAM Publishing, Seattle

Juva M (1994) The roots of development cooperation. Chapter 3. In: Lankinenen KS et al (eds) Health and disease in developing countries. Macmillan Press, London

Kluckhohn F, Strodtbeck FL (1961) Variations in value orientations. Row, Peterson, Evanston IL

Knell M (2006) Burn up or splash down: surviving the culture shock of re-entry. Authentic Publishing, Milton Keynes

Kraeker C, Chandler C (2013) "We learn from them, they learn from us": global health experiences and host perceptions of visiting health care professionals. Academic Medicine 88:483–7. https://journals.lww.com/academicmedicine/Fulltext/2013/04000/_We_Learn_From_Them,_They_Learn_From_Us____Global.20.aspx [last accessed 10.11.2020]

Kung TH, Richardson ET, Mabud TS et al (2016) Host community perspectives on trainees participating in short-term experiences in global health. Medical Education; 50:1122–30. Wiley Online Library https://doi.org/10.1111/medu.13106 [last accessed 10.11.2020]

Laleman G, Kegels G, Marchal B et al (2007) The contribution of international health volunteers to the health workforce in sub-Saharan Africa. Hum Resour Health 5(1):19

Lasker JN (2016) Global health volunteering; understanding organizational goals. International Journal of Voluntary and Nonprofit Organizations. 27:574–94. Springer

Lough BJ (2011) International volunteers' perceptions of intercultural competence. Int J Intercult Relat 35(4):452–464

Lough BJ, Xiang X, Kang S (2018) Effective practices of international volunteering for health: perspectives from partner organizations. Glob Health 14:11. Accessed 23 May 2019. https://doi.org/10.1186/s12992-018-0329-x

Maclean GD (1998) An examination of the characteristics of short-term international midwifery consultants. PhD thesis. University of Surrey, Guildford

Maclean GD (2011) Short term international midwifery consultancy: Preparing and promising. British Journal of Midwifery 19(9):594–99. https://doi.org/10.12968/bjom.2011.19.9.594

Maclean GD (2011a) Short term international midwifery consultancy: evaluating practice. Br J Midwifery 19(12):814–819

Maclean GD (2011b) Short term international midwifery consultancy: discussing the need. Br J Midwifery 19(6):594–599

Maclean GD (2013) Electives and international midwifery consultancy: a resource for students, midwives and other health professionals. Tiger Stripes and Tears. Quay Books, London

McLuhan M (1962) The Glutenberg galaxy, the making of typographic man. University of Toronto Press, Canada

Monkhouse A (2018) The improving global health fellowship: a qualitative analysis of innovative leadership development for NHS professionals. Glob Health 14:69. Accessed 23 May 2019. https://doi.org/10.1186/s12992-018-0384-3

Motamedi K (2015) A framework to evaluate consulting efforts: evaluation research and consulting agreements. Grazadio Business Rep 18(1)

Nanda G, Switlick K, Lule E (2005) Accelerating progress towards achieving the MDG to improve maternal health: a collection of promising approaches. In: Health, Nutrition & Population Discussion Paper. The International Bank for Reconstruction and Development/The World Bank, Washington, DC, p 20433

New Zealand Council of Education Research (2017) Shifting to 21st century thinking in education and learning. New Zealand Council for Educational Research http://www.shiftingthinking.org/?page_id=61. Accessed 13 Jul 2019

Pascoe R (2000) Homeward bound. Expatriates' Press, Vancouver

Pinker S (2011) The better angels of our nature. Allen Lane, London, England

Presbitero A (2016) Culture shock and reverse culture shock: the moderating role of cultural intelligence in international students' adaptation. Int J Intercult Relat 53:28–38

Raschio RA (1987) College students perceptions of reverse culture shock and re-entry adjustments. J Coll Stud Pers 28(2):156–162

Sardesi DR (1983) South East Asia past and present. Vikas, Delhi

Smith PB, Bond MH (1993) Social psychology across cultures: analysis and perspectives. Harvester Wheatsheaf, Hemel Hempstead

Steixner M (2011) Intercultural competence: describing a developmental process—methods and processes of intercultural development in training and coaching. Gr Organ 42(3):237–251

Storti C (2001) The art of coming home. Intercultural Press, Yarmouth, ME

The Science Forum (2009) What is traditional thinking? http://www.thescienceforum.com/philosophy/13976-what-traditional-thinking.html. Accessed 13 Jul 2019

Tropical Health Education Trust (2019) Health partnership schemes. Impact report: 2011–2019. Relationships for Global Health, Tropical Health and Education Trust, London

Udokang EJ (2014) Traditional ethics and social order: a study in African philosophy. Cross Cult Commun Canada 10(6):266–270

United Kingdom Council of International Student Affairs (2018) Facing culture shock. UK Council for International Student Affairs. https://www.ukcisa.org.uk/Information%2D%2DAdvice/Preparation-and-Arrival/Facing-culture-shock. Accessed 10 Jul 2019

United Nations (2015) Transforming our world: the 2030 agenda for sustainable development. United Nations General Assembly, 4th Plenary Meeting, 70/1. United Nations, New York

United Nations (2019) About the sustainable development goals. United Nations, New York. https://www.un.org/sustainabledevelopment/sustainable-development-goals/. Accessed 29 Apr 2019

United Nations Development Programme (2018) Human development indices and indicators: 2018 statistical update. United Nations Development Programme, New York. http://hdr.undp.org/sites/default/files/2018_summary_human_development_statistical_update_en.pdf. Accessed 7 May 2019

United Nations Development Programme (2019) Human development reports: human development index. United Nations Development Programme, New York. http://hdr.undp.org/en/content/human-development-index-hdi. Accessed 7 May 2019

Veatch RM (2000) Cross cultural perspectives in medical ethics, 2nd edn. Jones and Bartlett Publishers International, London

Winkelman MJ (1994) Cultural shock and adaptation. J Couns Dev 73(2):121–126

World Bank (2019a) Social development. Updated 09 April 2019. https://www.worldbank.org/en/topic/socialdevelopment/overview. Accessed 31 May 2019

World Bank (2019b) New country classifications by income level: 2018–2019. https://blogs.worldbank.org/opendata/new-country-classifications-income-level-2018-2019. Accessed 7 May 2019

World Health Orgnization (2015) Trends in Maternal Mortality 1990–2015. World Health Organization, Geneva. https://apps.who.int/iris/bitstream/handle/10665/194254/9789241565141_eng.pdf;jsessionid=3B3C058496BBF7ECE88C0C9C048620C9?sequence=1. Accessed 15 May 2019

Yang KS (1988) Profile of a modern person in: Smith PB and Bond MH (1993) Social psychology across cultures analysis and perspectives. Harvester Wheatsheaf, Hemel Hempstead

Zevada J (2019) What is postmodernism in religion? https://www.learnreligions.com/what-is-postmodernism-700692. Accessed 13 Jul 2019

Global Midwifery Partnerships

15

15.1 An Introduction to Midwifery Partnerships

In recent years, global health partnerships have been increasingly promoted as a way of accelerating progress towards the Sustainable Development Goals (SDGs) (The Global Goals 2020; Jones 2016; THET 2019). At the highest of levels, there is recognition of the need for partnership in maternal, newborn and child health, as demonstrated by the Partnership for Maternal, Newborn and Child Health (PMNCH), an alliance of more than 1000 organisations across 192 countries which believes that working together allows organisations to deliver more than they would working alone (WHO 2020a).

Midwifery is a profession based on partnership, most importantly the partnership between a midwife and the woman and her family (ICM 2017). Midwives also work in partnership with each other, with other health professionals and with wider communities. However, this chapter focuses specifically on global midwifery partnerships, where midwives or midwifery organisations come together formally for mutual learning and strengthening.

15.2 The Purpose of Global Midwifery Partnerships

WHO (2020a) describes a partnership as:

> a collaborative relationship between two or more parties based on trust, equality and mutual understanding for the achievement of a specified goal. Partnerships involve risks as well as benefits, making shared accountability critical.

The aim of global midwifery partnerships is to build midwifery capacity (Dawson et al. 2015), improving the quality of maternity care resulting in better maternal and newborn health outcomes and contributing to Universal Health Coverage and the Sustainable Development Goals. Global midwifery partnerships may be formed for a variety of reasons such as developments in midwifery education and regulation, quality

© Springer Nature Switzerland AG 2021
J. Kemp et al., *Global Midwifery: Principles, Policy and Practice*,
https://doi.org/10.1007/978-3-030-46765-4_15

improvement for midwifery practice, uplifting and expanding the profession of midwifery or for strengthening the organisational capacity of each partner (Spies et al. 2017). In female dominated professions, such as midwifery, partnerships can lead to women's empowerment and leadership opportunities (Ireland et al. 2015). Historically the flow of knowledge, capacity building and service delivery of international health partnerships has been almost exclusively unidirectional; however, the landscape is changing and such partnerships can cultivate 'reverse innovation' (see Chapter 9) and bi-directional learning (Kulasabanathan et al. 2017).

15.3 Types of Midwifery Partnerships

Global midwifery partnerships may be strategic, prudent or ill-advised. Strategic partnerships will help an individual partner to achieve their goals, to raise their profile and to enhance and extend midwives' influence at a policy level. Prudent partnerships are those where a failure to work together will mean that midwives lose their professional space, perhaps to others such as nurses or obstetricians, especially in countries where midwifery is not yet well-established. Ill-advised partnerships are those where the relationship will be detrimental either to midwives, and/or to women, their newborns and families. For example, partnerships with infant formula milk companies who do not uphold the international code of marketing of breastmilk substitutes (IBFAN 2018) would be ill-advised, as this could prove detrimental to newborn health.

15.3.1 Twinning Partnerships

Since 2008, twinning partnerships between professional midwives' associations in different countries have been promoted by the International Confederation of Midwives for mutual support and capacity building (ICM 2014). Therefore, the literature about global

midwifery partnerships largely focuses on twinning. Cadée et al. (2018) suggest that twinning differs from other forms of partnership because of its explicit emphasis on the core value of reciprocity; giving and receiving, learning with and from each other. Twinning has many potential benefits, for example exchange of best practice, relationship building, networking and solidarity (ICM 2014). In countries where midwifery is relatively new or marginalised (such as Bangladesh and Canada), twinning partnerships can raise the profile of the profession and provide a platform for advocacy (Kemp and Moran 2018; Sandwell et al. 2018). Twinning can also increase midwives' power to be change agents in their communities and to make a substantial contribution to global development, challenging the conventional aid-driven top-down models of international development and contesting traditional hierarchies (Cadée et al. 2018; Sandwell et al. 2018). Twinning is one way in which midwives can be 'midwifed' themselves. This leads to empowerment and enables midwives to provide competent, compassionate care for women and their families around the world (Brodie 2013).

15.3.1.1 Twinning at an Individual Level

Partnerships may be formed between individual midwives (such as those in Sierra Leone, Morocco and the Netherlands or the UK and Uganda) (Cadée et al. 2013, 2020; Kemp et al. 2018a). Twins collaborate to share knowledge and skills and to debate challenges. Twinning fosters personal and professional growth and engenders creative solutions through shared perspectives and problem solving (Twintowin 2019). Midwives from the UK and Uganda, twinned through the MOMENTUM project (Kemp et al. 2018a, b), explain the benefit of twinning:

> My UK twin and I observed the practice in our clinic together and made a plan to improve the learning environment. Now we are more organised and systematic, and teaching has become a core activity' (Ugandan Twin).

I have learned so much from Uganda. I see my own situation with different eyes and see things that I didn't see before. This experience has inspired me to return to university and study for a Master's degree (UK Twin).

Participating in a successful twinning partnership can prepare midwives for other strategic partnerships with non-midwives.

15.3.1.2 Twinning at an Organisational Level

Twinning partnerships may be established between different groups or organisations such as professional midwives' associations, universities or training institutions, professional networks, hospitals and clinics, non-governmental organisations or Ministries of Health (Dawson et al. 2015). Midwifery partnerships may also be local, regional, or global. For example, in the UK, university student midwifery societies are affiliating with local professional midwives' association branches for mutual benefit (RCM 2020a); in Europe, a regional twinning partnership has been formed between the Dutch and Icelandic midwives' associations to enhance midwifery leadership development (Codina 2018); globally, the Canadian Midwives Association is twinned with the Tanzania Midwives Association (Sandwell et al. 2018). Partnerships may also be between organisations in countries where the context and access to resources is similar (global north to north or south to south) or between differently resourced contexts (global south to north).

15.3.2 Partnership with United Nations (UN) Agencies, Multilateral and Bilateral Agencies

Multilateral agencies are international organisations that include several nations acting together (e.g. the World Health Organization). A bilateral organisation is a government agency that receives funding from its home country's government for assistance to a developing country (Borgen Project 2017), for example SIDA, the Swedish International Development Cooperation Agency. The World Health Organization (WHO) and the United Nations Population Fund (UNFPA) are multilateral organisations and UN agencies with a mandate to strengthen midwifery (WHO 2020b; UNFPA 2020). These agencies work in partnership with other international organisations, such as the International Confederation of Midwives (ICM 2018) and with smaller organisations such as individual professional midwives' associations, to strengthen midwifery through collaborative, time-bound projects. Strong professional midwives' associations have the competencies that multinational organisations need to fulfil their objectives in strengthening midwifery, so such partnerships are complementary. These initiatives can be useful sources of resource and support, but caution is required before entering into any partnership where one partner is a huge organisation with financial power; the less powerful organisation/s may feel themselves being pushed in a direction in which they did not wish to travel, engaged in activities which derail midwives from a focus on midwifery, swallowed up to the point at which their lose their identity, or are bullied.

15.3.3 Partnerships with Other Healthcare Professional Associations

A midwives' association will not achieve its vision without strategic collaborations with other relevant professional associations that share a common goal in improving maternal and newborn health outcomes (Moyo and Renard 2016). Partnerships between healthcare professional associations can enable co-learning and interprofessional education, strengthen advocacy efforts and promote leadership development. They also enable healthcare professionals to present a united front to policymakers. In some countries, professional associations come together in formal partnerships such as a Perinatal Society or other partnership. An example is shared in Box 15.1.

Box 15.1. The One Voice Partnership

In the UK, health professional associations representing midwives, obstetricians and gynaecologists, paediatricians and health visitors have joined together in the 'One Voice' initiative with a leading parents' charity and a network of baby loss charities. The aim of this partnership is to have one voice and common purpose to improve the safety of maternity care in the UK and the experience of women and families using services. Together, the partnership holds parliamentary events and issues joint press statements on key issues. The policy and communications teams from each organisation have developed strong working relationships, and this has led to a stronger, more influential voice and more constructive management of the news media (RCM 2020b).

15.3.4 Partnerships with Local and International Non-governmental Organisations

Non-governmental organisations (NGOs) have a long history of programmes and partnerships to strengthen maternal and newborn health. Some NGOs are very large and work across the globe (e.g. Save the Children and Jhpiego); others are very small, working in just one community. Many NGOs work on specific projects funded by overseas development aid or from corporate social responsibility sources. Some NGOs act as grant managers for overseas development aid; for example, THET coordinated the UK-Aid Health Partnerships Scheme, supporting 191 partnerships between the NHS and UK institutions and developing countries' health systems (THET 2019). The Global Midwifery Twinning Project between midwives' associations in Cambodia, Nepal and Uganda with the UK (RCM 2015) was facilitated by THET.

15.3.5 Partnerships with For-Profit Organisations

Some corporate organisations provide opportunity for partnerships with midwives, for example Laerdal Global Health and Johnson and Johnson. Engagement with health professionals enables companies to have greater access to populations, either to sell their products or to contribute goods or activities philanthropically. Commercial partnerships should be developed with caution; there may be hidden agendas or ethical conflicts which would make such partnerships ill-advised. Commercial partners should only be chosen if they are like-minded organisations, sharing similar values, goals and ethics.

15.3.6 Educational Partnerships

Partnerships between educational institutions, for example through the Erasmus exchange scheme in Europe, can contribute to upscaling midwifery, can enhance students' personal and professional development, prepare them to address global health concerns and promote change at a global level (Marshall 2017).

15.4 Characteristics of Strong Partnerships

The New Zealand College of Midwives (2019) suggests that midwifery partnerships are based on trust, shared decision-making and responsibility, negotiation and shared understanding. THET (2015) puts forward eight principles of partnership, drawn from experience of facilitating more than 180 global health partnerships. These principles are illustrated in Fig. 15.1. Evaluation of THET's Health Partnerships Scheme (THET 2019) found that health workers participating in the scheme had learned new skills, developed in their leadership and become more adaptable; as a result, health systems in the UK and in partner countries had been strengthened.

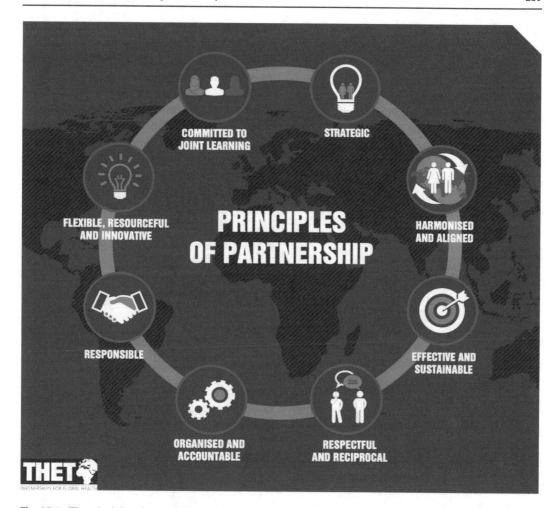

Fig. 15.1   The principles of partnerships

Cadée et al. (2018) research, which gathered the views of experts in midwifery twinning from around the world, outlined 25 critical success factors for midwifery twinning projects. Most of these critical success factors depend upon power-sharing and equity; they highlight the importance of shared values and commitment, good management and clear communication to successful partnerships. Reciprocity is an important aspect of twinning projects; this means a two-way mutually beneficial partnership that is started on an equal footing (ICM 2014). Donor-funded projects may be short-term, but ICM suggests that partners should enter twinning partnerships with a long-term commitment to one another. An example of the key steps in twinning is provided in Box 15.2.

> **Box 15.2. Key Steps in Twinning Between Canada and Tanzania**
> - Twinning relationship between Canadian and Tanzanian midwives' associations facilitated by the International Confederation of Midwives.
> - Donor funding secured for set-up phase.
> - Partnership agreement signed and joint strategic plan developed.
> - Organisational development outcomes identified and achieved for both partners.
> - First phase evaluated and future plans developed.
> - Further external funding secured for follow-on project (Sandwell et al. 2018).

15.5   The Partnership Cycle

Tennyson (2013) suggests that there are four phases in the partnering cycle: scoping and building, managing and maintaining, reviewing and revising, and sustaining outcomes (Fig. 15.2). Each of these phases contains several steps; every step is important and should not be neglected if the partnership is to move forward and achieve its goals.

Literature on midwifery twinning goes further, proposing 10 (Cadée et al. 2018) or 12 (ICM 2014) steps to twinning partnerships.

15.5.1 Choosing a Partner Organisation

Choosing the right partner is vitally important for success. ICM (2014) suggests drawing up a shortlist of three potential partners and talking with each in turn to find the right 'fit'. It is important that the decision to enter a partnership is supported by the leadership of each organisation, that there is genuine interest in learning from each other and an openness to change. Several midwifery twinning partnerships have been formed between midwifery associations in high-resource settings wishing to make a difference to their sis-

ters in low-resource settings where maternal and newborn health outcomes are poor (Cadée et al. 2013; Sandwell et al. 2018; RCM 2015). However, this can be challenging when trying to achieve the equity and power sharing which are critical to the success of such partnerships. Barriers of distance, different time zones, languages and expectations of partnership have all been reported. Conversely, organisations can find much in common despite being far-removed geographically. For example, in Canada and Tanzania, both midwifery associations were new and mainly run by volunteers; both had few members spread across large distances and shared an interest in supporting midwives in remote and rural settings. A twinning partnership led to significant transformation for both partners (Sandwell et al. 2018).

15.5.2 Starting a Global Midwifery Partnership

Most of the literature on global health partnerships recommends a scoping phase prior to the start of a formal partnership. This may include in-country visits to either or both partners to develop an understanding of the different contexts in which midwives live and work. During

Fig. 15.2 The partnering cycle (Tennyson 2013). (Copyright © The Partnering Initiative 2020, reproduced with permission)

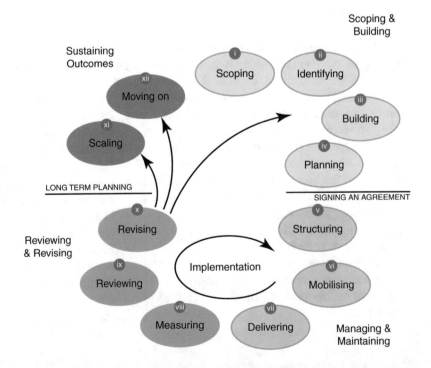

this phase, it is important that partners are honest with each other and that expectations are managed as, sometimes, a scoping visit may result in a decision not to start a partnership. Whilst virtual connection is becoming the norm for many international partnerships, in-country face-to-face contact is invaluable before launching a new partnership. Additionally, access to internet, power and virtual conferencing software may not be equally available to both partners.

Various tools can be helpful during the scoping phase, such as a SWOT or PESTLE analysis (Symonds 2011; French 2017). Where possible, both partners should undertake such exercises together so that a joint understanding of the context is achieved. Appreciative Inquiry (AI) and Appreciative Dialogue are also useful frameworks for identifying mutual strengths and opportunities for change; these methodologies can help to create a safe, positive environment in which to develop new ideas (Sharp et al. 2017; Hung 2017).

It may be helpful, where possible, for the scoping phase to be facilitated by a third party. For example, the International Confederation of Midwives facilitated the early stages of the twinning partnership between the Canadian and Tanzanian Midwifery Associations. Once the scoping stage is complete, signing agreement/s such as memoranda of understanding and terms of reference mark the formal start of the partnership (ICM 2014; Tennyson et al. 2009). Involving key stakeholders, such as the Ministry of Health, in the scoping phase and ensuring that the partnership is legal in both countries may help to avoid future problems.

15.5.3 Funding for Global Midwifery Partnerships

Raising funds for the partnership is a joint responsibility. If one or both partners is located in a low-resource setting, overseas aid funding may be available. For example, the midwifery twinning project between Bangladesh and the UK is funded by the governments of the UK, Sweden and Canada through the United Nations Population Fund (UNFPA) (Kemp and Moran 2018). However, Cadée et al. (2013) suggests that

development aid is often a 'one-way process', with top-down support from high- to low-income countries; this can compromise the critical success factors of equity and power-sharing and is also not sustained beyond the end of the funding period. Therefore, where possible both partners should engage in fundraising, ring-fencing their membership funds for core organisation business (ICM 2014). Resourcefulness, innovation and sustainability are key to the principles of partnership (THET 2015). Some suggestions for accessing resources for funding are listed in Box 15.3.

15.6 Facilitating Factors in Implementing a Global Midwifery Partnership

---

Box 15.3. Potential Funding Sources for Global Midwifery Partnerships
- Overseas development aid.
- Non-governmental organisations.
- Commercial partners (ensure ethical 'fit').
- Fundraising events and sales.
- Crowd-funding.
- Engaging with members to raise local funds.

15.6.1 Taking Baseline Measurements

For organisational development partnerships a joint assessment of organisational capacity will provide a baseline from which to measure change and can inform the development of a strategic plan for the partnership (ICM 2014). Most midwifery twinning projects will start with using the ICM's Member Association Capacity Assessment Tool (MACAT) (ICM 2011); this is preferably facilitated by an objective external consultant and takes place over several days. A revised version of the MACAT is currently being piloted. However, other capacity assessment tools are available (Moyo 2016). For midwifery education partnerships, the Midwifery Assessment Tool for

Education (MATE) (Hunter 2019) can provide a helpful baseline. A stakeholder analysis and mapping exercise will also identify those persons or bodies important to the success (or failure) of the project, as well as providing a baseline for measuring growth in the partnership's networks and visibility. Another important step is to conduct a joint risk assessment, especially if midwives will be travelling to countries with security challenges.

15.6.2 Shared Vision, Goals and Outcomes

A shared vision, mission and core principles are the foundations of a strong partnership (Girls Not Brides 2019). If the partnership is implementing an externally funded project, donors will usually require a robust project plan using a logical framework or similar tool with identified goals, objectives and outcomes with and an accompanying monitoring and evaluation plan. However, it is also important to articulate a shared vision and to set goals and outcomes for the partnership itself (THET 2015).

15.6.3 Theoretical Underpinning

Midwifery partnerships have reported the use of various theoretical frameworks. For example, the 'Twin2twin' project between the Netherlands and Sierra Leone midwives' associations used a feminist methodology of mutual exchange (Cadée et al. 2013). The MOMENTUM project (Kemp et al. 2018a, b) used Action Research, Appreciative Inquiry and work-based learning to improve the quality of clinical learning for student midwives in Uganda.

15.6.4 Human Resources

Most global midwifery partnerships will require dedicated paid staff in each country who can manage the systems and coordinate activities. This is especially important for those projects funded by external donors who will require regular reporting and careful management of funds. Where possible, both partners should be involved in recruitment and appointment of project staff, and relevant organisational policies should be developed, for example finance and human resource policies.

15.6.5 Shared Governance and Management Structures

A governing body or steering committee with representatives from both partners should be established for the partnership or project, and this should meet regularly, with minutes being taken and shared with appropriate stakeholders. With advances in technology, such meetings can take place online, though opportunities to meet in person should be taken when they arise, for example when making exchange visits or attending international conferences together. An example of a twinning project structure is outlined in Box 15.4.

Box 15.4. Example of a Twinning Project Structure (Kemp et al. 2018b)

Category	UK actors	Ugandan actors
Project management team	UK project lead UK project officer Support staff in UK: Finance officer, communications, HR and marketing personnel Executive support and governance	Ugandan project coordinator Ugandan monitoring and evaluation officer Ugandan support staff: Driver, secretary, finance officer, caretaker/guard executive support and governance
Twinned units	11 UK midwives	11 Ugandan midwives

15.6.6 Effective Communication

Communication is a critical success factor for midwifery partnerships (Cadée et al. 2018). Therefore, setting up an effective communication strategy and an action plan is imperative. Different organisations have different preferred ways of communicating, so this needs careful exploration. Participants may need the provision of a smartphone, tablet or laptop and sufficient airtime or Wi-Fi connectivity to enable effective communication. Some users may be older and/or unfamiliar with such technology so will need training and support with this. The MOMENTUM twining project between midwives in Uganda and the UK was effective because it created a powerful community of practice that was enabling, fulfilling and transformative. Communication in this project was achieved through email and WhatsApp messages/calls, supported by intermittent workshops that brought participants face-to-face and hands-on quality improvement work together in clinical sites. Project participants received smartphones, training in how to use them and support when problems arose (Kemp et al. 2018b).

15.6.7 Celebration of Success

Celebration of success, however small, is another important activity of twinning (Cadée et al. 2013; Kemp et al. 2018b). Such celebrations are empowering, boost morale and encourage continuation of the partnership. They can also generate media interest.

15.7 Management of Cross-Cultural Exchange Placements in Partnership Projects

Until the COVID-19 pandemic, most global midwifery partnership projects included the use of cross-cultural exchange placements, with midwives spending some time in the partner country for exposure and learning or to contribute specific skills. The number and length of such placements varied between partnerships. However, they shared common features; identification of a placement opportunity, developing a role descriptor for the visiting midwife, making necessary preparations in-country including arrangements for accommodation and transport, recruiting, interviewing and briefing the midwife or volunteer, cross-cultural preparation, deploying the midwife individually or in a group with others, in-country orientation and support, safeguarding, problem solving, debriefing, supporting re-entry to the home country and finally facilitating reflection, reporting and dissemination.

COVID-19 has changed the landscape of cross-cultural exchange, with very few opportunities available for international travel and strict quarantine requirements in place. However, whilst posing challenges for partnerships and limiting scope for in-person cultural exchange, many partnerships have embraced creativity and found new ways to communicate and to provide mutual support, harnessing technologies such as Zoom and Skype to host online meetings and events. Opportunities to participate in 'virtual volunteering' have been created where volunteers can share knowledge to meet partners' priority needs, with a focus on remote mentorship and capacity development (THET 2020). This may contribute to redressing the previous imbalance of power where, in partnerships between differently resourced contexts, opportunities for exchange visits may have favoured midwives from high-resource settings, compounding inequalities. Whether or not cross-cultural exchange placements continue in the future to the same extent, going forward effort must be made to afford equal opportunity to midwives from each partner organisation. Aside from global pandemics, concerns about the environmental impact of international travel is likely to reduce such exchange visits in the future.

Global health competencies for midwives have been developed to identify the breadth of global expertise that may be required for midwives to care for clients, or to work with colleagues, from different cultures or to participate in global exchange placements. These competencies provide structure for evaluating such opportunities (ACNM 2018) and are outlined in

Table 15.1 Global health competencies for midwives (ACNM 2018)

Areas of competence	Skills include
Global understanding	Past, present, and anticipated future of global maternal, newborn and reproductive (MNR) health
Clinical practice	Safe and appropriate clinical practice based on knowledge of maternal, perinatal, and under five health and illnesses in resource-constrained settings
Health equity and justice	Application of the principles of health equity and justice in the provision of global MNR health
Professionalism / ethics	Self-awareness, respect of and sensitivity towards others, flexibility, and ability to address ethical/professional issues in global MNR health experiences
Communication	Effective, appropriate, and adaptive communication skills in a variety of global health settings
Leadership, organisation, and programme management	Leadership and organisation skills to develop programmes that improve global MNR health
Teaching and learning	Expertise in teaching, learning, and evaluation in low resource settings
Research/quality improvement (QI)	Utilises internationally accepted research and QI approaches to improve global MNR health
Health systems strengthening	Co-develops solutions to health systems challenges using local health systems knowledge and leadership

Table 15.1. Others suggest additional global health competencies; for example, cultural competence, political awareness/correctness, gender issues, capacity development and sustainable development (Maclean 2013). However, few pre-service curricula offer any education in global health competence (Al-Sharkarchi et al. 2018; Wilson et al. 2012).

Embracing the principle of 'co-presence' (Ackers and Ackers-Johnson 2014) can be helpful for midwives participating in cross-cultural exchange placements. Put simply, visiting midwives should always be working alongside national counterparts. Co-presence has many benefits; firstly, it minimises risk by avoiding lone working; secondly, it allows for co-creation of knowledge and skills-sharing; thirdly, it facilitates reciprocity and cultural exchange.

Cross-cultural exchange visits and virtual volunteering can have many benefits, but partnerships must be aware of the amount of work and the potential risks involved. Despite these risks and challenges, many partnership projects report successful exchange visits/programmes and significant resulting changes in participants, projects and partner organisations. Where possible, midwives experienced in cross-cultural work can travel or work with and support those newer to the field.

Lasker et al. (2018) suggest six core principles for effective and ethical intercultural exchange placements/programmes: appropriate recruitment, preparation and supervision of visitors/virtual volunteers; a host partner that defines the programme, including the needs to be addressed and the role of the host community/organisation in directing and teaching the visitors/virtual volunteers; sustainability and continuity of programmes; respect for governance and legal and ethical standards; regular evaluation of programmes for impact and, finally, mutuality of learning and respect for local health professionals. Cross-cultural exchange is explored in more detail in Chapter 14 of this book.

15.8   Challenges to Global Midwifery Partnerships

Challenges can arise at any stage of the partnership cycle. Tennyson (2013) suggests that there are three core challenges that have recurred time and again in partnerships: power imbalance, hidden agendas and the desire to win at any cost. All published global midwifery partnerships have described obstacles as well as successes. These can arise from outside or within the partnership. External obstacles may include a difficult political or economic context, inflated expectations from outsiders and bureaucracy (Tennyson 2013). Challenges within the partnership include communication difficulties; these may stem from differences in language and culture, poor internet connectivity, different time zones, unwillingness or inability to embrace new technologies or lack of time to commit to the partnership (Kemp et al. 2018b; RCM 2015; Sandwell et al. 2018). Differences in organisational cultures may cause tension; for example, expected behaviours of presidents and senior officers of professional associations. Leaders of the partnership on either side may have personal limitations or lack certain skills. Either partner organisation may face staff changes or abrupt reduction or cessation of funds. Potential obstacles to exchange visits and placements include political unrest or geographical disasters in the destination country, global pandemics such as COVID-19, problems with obtaining visas or permission to travel or difficulties in being released from home or work to undertake the placement. Partners may not engage with, or commit time to, the midwife during the visit. Travelling midwives will require robust travel and health insurance; flexible travel arrangements are advised. For short-term placements, it is often not possible for midwives to arrange professional registration in the host country; therefore, they will be limited to observation of practice only which may cause frustration.

All of these challenges can be addressed by the guiding principles of equity, transparency and mutual benefit which must be discussed and agreed at the start of the partnership (Tennyson 2013).

15.9   Reciprocal Benefits of Global Midwifery Partnerships

Benefits of twinning partnerships can be numerous. Growth in organisational capacity for either partner can include an increase to core staffing, development of organisational policies, new skills in strategic planning, improved financial systems and skills, improved member engagement and development of services for members, increased networks and linkages with key stakeholders, improved connection with maternity service users and women's organisations, better communication systems, more effective advocacy for midwives, for the midwifery profession and for and maternity service users and broader engagement with the news media (Cadée 2013; Sandwell 2018; Kemp et al. 2018a, b; Brodie 2013).

Global north to global south partnerships often report on outcomes and impact in the low-

Table 15.2 Reciprocal benefits of health exchange placements in international health partnership projects

Reciprocal benefits to health systems	Reciprocal benefits to individuals
• Productivity increase for 24–41% for each returned volunteer (Zamora et al. 2019) • System learning • Capacity building • Enhanced recruitment and retention • Professional development of the workforce • Improved patient/client experience • Reputational development	• Leadership and management development • Improved communication and teamwork • Improved clinical skills • Enhanced policy awareness and experience • Enhanced academic skills • Improved understanding of the patient experience and need for dignity • Strengthened resilience, satisfaction and interest

resource partner country but do not elucidate any reciprocal benefit. However, this is changing. As a result of their twinning partnership, the Canadian and Tanzanian midwives' associations reported capacity building of both partners (Sandwell et al. 2018). The Netherlands and Sierra Leone twinning partnership (Cadée et al. 2013) reported several shared outputs and products of benefit to each country; for example, increased membership and engagement of members, a film, leaflets, and teaching resources. The partnership may also enable better care for the diaspora community in the partner country; for example, the twinning partnership between the UK and Bangladesh is enabling better engagement with Bangladeshi midwives in the UK and hopes in turn to improve care for diaspora maternity service users. Basu et al. (2017) cite improvements in innovation and client-centred care, environmental responsibility and making wiser healthcare choices as examples of the reciprocal benefits of health partnerships. Recent publications (Zamora et al. 2019; Fergusson and McKirdy 2017) have focused on learning and reverse innovation to health services in high-income countries, where health professionals have participated in exchange placements as part of an international health partnership project. These are outlined in Table 15.2.

In some cases, partnerships themselves spawn new partnerships; for example, the Global Midwifery Twinning Project (RCM 2015) provided the building blocks for the MOMENTUM project in Uganda and the SUSTAIN project in Nepal (RCM 2015).

15.10 Monitoring and Evaluation of Global Midwifery Partnerships

There has been a lack of evidence about the impact and effectiveness of global midwifery partnerships (Dawson et al. 2015). Many partnerships start on an ad hoc basis and grow in a haphazard fashion, making it difficult to start the partnership with a robust monitoring and evalua-

Table 15.3 Examples of tools for evaluating global midwifery partnership projects

Example of tool, framework or methodology	Aspects of the tool or framework
Critical Success Factors for midwifery twinning partnerships (Cadée et al. 2018)	Includes setting goals together, having an M&E plan and adapting goals if circumstances change
Partnership Health Check (THET 2017)	Based on the principles of partnership (Box 15.1)
Partnership baseline matrix and monitoring tool (World Wildlife Fund undated)	Includes a spider diagram for mapping progress towards agreed goals
Realist evaluation	Appropriate for evaluating programmes of change set within complex social organisations, such as health services, and can help to understand variations in outcomes and experiences (McInnes et al. 2018)

tion (M&E) plan. However, being committed to joint learning, including M&E and reflection, is one of the principles of partnership (THET 2015). It is important to be clear about the purpose of M&E. What is being measured: the partnership or a project being implemented by the partners? Are the partners themselves being evaluated, or the partnership—or perhaps both? For example, are the objectives which led to the partnership being met? Is the partnership bringing the expected outcomes to midwives? Is the partnership having an impact on the quality of midwifery care for women and their families? Co-creation is important in a partnership and that includes the co-creation of any M&E. Therefore, when developing a M&E framework or plan, collecting M&E data, developing terms of reference for an evaluation, or selecting an evaluation team, the principles of equity and shared power must be followed. Pasanen (2016) advises partners to define a hypothesis for the partnership early on and to set up monitoring and evaluation systems to test it.

Different tools are available for evaluating partnerships, examples of which are shown in Table 15.3. Many of these are self-assessment tools; however, Pasanen (2016) advises that such self-perception data may be subjective and should be triangulated with more objective indicators such as whether all partners are represented in major decision-making bodies, or whether the decisions made reflect the views of all of the partners or just one. Global midwifery partnerships can be complex with far more actors than originally envisaged and with a network of individuals and organisations involved. Deciding what and who to evaluate is not straightforward. Alternatively, certain aspects of the partnership may be evaluated separately, for example a process evaluation. Cadée et al. (2013) recommend setting evaluation moments throughout a partnership and considering the reliability of cross-cultural evaluation; for example, how hierarchies may limit participants' ability to speak out in a self-assessment exercise, how freely participants may criticise a partnership funded by a donor agency or how effective a written evaluation may be within an oral culture?

15.11 Sustainability of Midwifery Partnerships

Sustaining outcomes is the final section of the partnering cycle (Fig. 15.2) and includes scaling up/down and moving on. ICM (2014) recommends that midwifery twinning partnerships should be long-term.

However, those funded by donor agencies are almost always time-bound, and there is a risk that the partnership may not be formally sustained beyond the length of any funded project or that partnerships may be quiet or even dormant between projects. Staff may be funded through a project grant and may not be retained afterwards, thus reducing organisational capacity once more. Partnerships that span a wide geographical divide may struggle to continue without regular in-country visits and contact; however, these can be costly and unaffordable long-term. It is therefore important that sustainability is planned for at the start of any partnership. This means ensuring that the right stakeholders are involved at the start of the partnership.

If wider stakeholders are involved in building the partnership and assessing the need prior to any intervention, inputs are more likely to be sustained. For example, the MOMENTUM project in Uganda was requested by the Ugandan Nurses and Midwives Council and the Ugandan Ministries of Health and Education and Sports. Representatives from each body attended the project inception workshop and every subsequent event and were included in the project management team. This ensured that project outputs were taken up by these bodies and continued after the project ended (Kemp et al. 2018b).

15.12 The Future of Global Midwifery Partnerships

Advances in technology and innovation are already changing midwifery partnerships. Social media, virtual meeting software and messaging Apps allow partners to connect instantly across the globe, to form online communities and to access information instantly. The 2020 COVID-19 pandemic has shown how quickly the context of international work can change and the role of technology in allowing work and relationships to continue. These issues are discussed further in Chapter 17. Environmental concerns are likely to reduce the amount of international travel within midwifery partnerships. The landscape of donor funding has changed, and significant grants will be given only to those organisations that can demonstrate partnership working and a long-term commitment. Professional boundaries also change, requiring midwives and midwife educators to form strategic interprofessional partnerships to improve multidisciplinary care and teamwork (Luyben et al. 2018).

However, despite the challenges, there has never been a more favourable policy context for midwives. With ample evidence building for the role of midwives in helping countries to achieve the Sustainable Development Goals (Lancet 2014; WHO 2019) the time is ripe for midwives to partner across the world and develop new ways of working together to ensure that every woman and her family have access to high-quality maternity care from a midwife.

Key Messages

Principles

Successful midwifery partnerships depend upon power-sharing and equity; they need shared vision, values and commitment, good management and clear communication.

Policy

Midwifery partnerships can enhance the capacity of professional midwives' associations to improve the quality of maternity care and are worthy of support by policymakers.

Practice

Participating in a global midwifery partnership can foster personal and professional benefit to individuals, having an impact on the organisations in which midwives work. Managing a partnership takes commitment from both partners and will benefit from dedicated staff and resources.

Questions for Reflection or Review

1. Face-to-face in-country contact helps to facilitate global midwifery partnerships. However, international travel can be harmful to planetary health and is not always possible. How can global health actors support cross-cultural partnerships in the future?

2. Equity and power-sharing can be difficult where one partner has access to more resources than another. How can this be mitigated?

3. With reference to the toolkit in the additional resources section, consider how health professionals participating in global midwifery partnerships can assimilate cross-cultural experiences and bring back benefit to their own health systems.

Additional Resources for Reflection and Further Study

Foster D, Newton M, McLachaln H et al (2011) Exploring implementation and sustainability of models of care: can theory help? BMC Public Health 11(Supplement 5):S8

The Health Professional Association Strengthening Project. http://www.strongprofassoc.org/

Twintowin. http://twintowin.com

The Principles of Partnership. https://www.thet.org/principles-of-partnership/

Toolkit for the collection of evidence of knowledge and skills gained through participation in an international health project. https://www.hee.nhs.uk/sites/default/files/documents/2312-HEE%20Toolkit%20for%20evidence%20Interactive%20v4.pdf

References

Ackers L, Ackers-Johnson J (2014) Understanding 'Co-presence' in the Sustainable Volunteering Project: University of Salford Policy Report. tinyurl.com/co-presence. Accessed 5 Feb 2019

Al-Sharkarchi N, Obolensky L, Walpole S et al (2018) Global health competencies in UK postgraduate medical training: a scoping review and curricular content analysis. BMJ Open 9:e027577. Accessed 2 Apr 2020. https://doi.org/10.1136/bmjopen-2018-027577

American College of Nurse Midwives (2018) Global health competencies and skills. https://www.midwife.org/acnm/files/cclibraryfiles/filename/000000007496/Global%20Health%20Competencies.pdf. Accessed 2 Apr 2019

Basu L, Pronovost P, Edwards N et al (2017) The role of south-north partnerships in promoting shared learning and knowledge transfer. Glob Health 13:64

Borgen Project (2017) What is a bilateral organisation? https://borgenproject.org/bilateral-organization/. Accessed 5 Apr 2020

Brodie (2013) Midwifing the midwives. Midwifery 29:1075–1076

Cadée F, Perdok H, Sam B et al (2013) Twin2twin' an innovative method of empowering midwives to strengthen their professional midwifery organisations. Midwifery 29:1145–1150

Cadée F, Nieuwenhuijze M, Largo-Janssen A et al (2018) From equity to power: critical success factors for twinning between midwives, a Delphi study. J Adv Nurs 74:1573–1582

Cadée F, Nieuwenhuijze M, Largo-Janssen A et al. (2020) Paving the way for successful twinning: using grounded theory to understand the contribution of twin pairs in twinning collaborations. Women and Birth. Accessed 5 Apr 2020. https://doi.org/10.1016/j.wombi.2020.01.013

Codina M (2018) Twinning up North! https://share-netinternational.org/new-twinning-project-royal-dutch-organisation-midwives-knov/. Accessed 31 Mar 2020

Dawson A, Brodie P, Copeland F et al (2015) Collaborative approaches towards building midwifery capacity in low income countries: a review of experiences. Midwifery 30(4):391–402

Fergusson S, McKirdy M (2017) Global citizenship in the Scottish health service: the value of international volunteering. Royal College of Physicians and Surgeons of Glasgow. https://rcpsg.ac.uk/documents/publications/global-citizenship-report/204-global-citizenship-in-the-scottish-health-service/file. Accessed 4 May 2018

French J (2017) Social marketing planning. In Social marketing and public health: theory and practice (2nd ed.). Oxford: OUP, 27–44

Girls Not Brides (2019) Partnering for success: a step-by-step guide to addressing your most common partnering challenges. https://ams3.digitaloceanspaces.com/girlsnotbridesorg/ https://www.documents/National-Partnership-Toolkit_FINAL.pdf. Accessed 16 Nov 2020

Hung L (2017) Using appreciative inquiry to research practice development. Int Pract Dev J 7(1):1–7. https://doi.org/10.19043/ipdj.71.005

Hunter B (2019) Collaborating to Improve Midwifery Education in Eastern Europe: Developing the WHO Midwifery Assessment Tool for Education (MATE). Presentation to IME Expo, Nov 2019

International Baby Food Action Network (IBFAN) (2018) International Code of Marketing of Breastmilk Substitutes. https://www.ibfan.org/international-code/. Accessed 16 Nov 2020

International Confederation of Midwives (2011) Member Association Capacity Assessment Tool. https://www.internationalmidwives.org/assets/files/association-files/2018/04/macat-eng.pdf. Accessed 1 Apr 2020

International Confederation of Midwives (2014) Twinning as a tool for strengthening midwives associations. https://www.healthynewbornnetwork.org/hnn-content/uploads/140419-Twinning-ICM-V04.pdf. Accessed 19 May 2019

International Confederation of Midwives (2017) Position statement: partnership between women and midwives. https://www.internationalmidwives.org/assets/files/statement-files/2018/04/eng-partnership-between-women-and-midwives1.pdf. Accessed 18 May 2019

International Confederation of Midwives (2018) Partners and projects. https://www.internationalmidwives.org/icm-projects/. Accessed 5 Apr 2020

Ireland J, van Teijlingen E, Kemp J (2015) Twinning in Nepal: the Royal College of Midwives UK and the Midwifery Society of Nepal working in partnership. J Asian Midwives 2(1):26–33

Jones A (2016) Envisioning a global health partnership movement. Global Health 12:1. Accessed 19 May 2019. https://doi.org/10.1186/s12992-015-0138-4

Kemp J, Moran C (2018) A world of difference. In: RCM Midwives Magazine, Spring edn, pp 61–65

Kemp J, Shaw E, Musoke M (2018a) Developing a model of midwifery mentorship for Uganda: the MOMENTUM project 2015–2017. Midwifery 59:127–129

Kemp J, Shaw E, Nanjego S et al (2018b) Improving student midwives' practice learning in Uganda through action research: the MOMENTUM project. Int Pract Dev J 8(1):7

Kulasabanathan K, Issa H, Bhatti Y et al (2017) Do International health partnerships contribute to reverse innovation? A mixed methods study of THET-supported partnerships in the UK. Glob Health 13:25

Lancet (2014) Midwifery Series: Executive Summary. Available at http://www.thelancet.com/series/midwifery. Accessed 14 Dec 2017

Lasker J, Aldrink M, Balasubramaniam R et al (2018) Guidelines for responsible short-term global health activities: developing common principles. Glob Health 14:18

Luyben A, Barger M, Avery M et al (2018) What is next? Midwifery education building partnerships for tomorrow's maternal and neonatal health care. Midwifery 64:132–135

Maclean G (2013) Tiger stripes and tears: electives and international midwifery consultancy: a resource for students, midwives and other healthcare professionals. Quay Books, Salisbury, p 17

Marshall JE (2017) Experiences of student midwives learning and working abroad in Europe: The value of an Erasmus undergraduate midwifery education programme. Midwifery 44:7–13

McInnes R, Martin C, McArthur J (2018) Midwifery continuity of carer: developing a realist evaluation framework to evaluate the implementation of strategic change in Scotland. Midwifery 66:103–110

Moyo NT(2016) Module 9: the health, growth and development of a professional association. The Health Professional Association Strengthening Project. http://www.strongprofassoc.org/wp-content/uploads/2016/05/PAS-Module-9-May2016.pdf. Accessed 1 Jan 2020

Moyo NT, Renard C (2016) Module 4: functions of a professional association. The Health Professional Association Strengthening Project. http://www.strongprofassoc.org/wp-content/uploads/2016/05/PAS-Module-4-May2016.pdf. Accessed 6 Apr 2020

New Zealand College of Midwives (2019) Midwifery: a partnership model. https://www.midwife.org.nz/midwives/midwifery-in-new-zealand/. Accessed 18 May 2019

Pasanen T (2016) How can we assess the value of working in partnerships? Better evaluation. https://www.betterevaluation.org/en/blog/assessing_partnerships. Accessed 6 Apr 2020

Royal College of Midwives (2015) The Global Midwifery Twinning Project. https://www.rcm.org.uk/promoting/global/projects/global-midwifery-twinning-project/. Accessed 31 Mar 2020

Royal College of Midwives (2020a) Student midwifery societies. https://www.rcm.org.uk/influencing/activists/student-midwifery-societies/. Accessed 31 Mar 2020

Royal College of Midwives (2020b) Who we work with. https://www.rcm.org.uk/about-us/who-we-work-with/. Accessed 19 Apr 2019

Sandwell R, Bonser D, Hebert E et al (2018) Stronger together: midwifery twinning between Tanzania and Canada. Global Health 14:123. Accessed 19 May 2019. https://doi.org/10.1186/s12992-018-0442-x

Sharp C, Dewar B, Barrie K et al (2017) How being appreciative creates change. Action Res 16(2):223–243

Spies L, Garner S, Faucher M et al (2017) A model of upscaling global partnerships and building nurse and midwifery capacity. International Nursing Review. 64:331–344

Symonds M (2011) SWOT analysis in project management. Available at https://www.projectsmart.co.uk/swot-analysis-in-project-management.php. .Accessed 14 Apr 2020

Tennyson R (2013) The partnering toolbook. https://thepartneringinitiative.org/publications/toolbook-series/the-partnering-toolbook/. Accessed 31 Mar 2020

Tennyson R, Huq N, Pyres J (2009) Partnering step by step. https://thepartneringinitiative.org/wp-content/uploads/2014/08/partneringstepbystep.pdf. Accessed 19 May 2019

The Global Goals (2020) Goal 17: partnership for the goals. https://www.globalgoals.org/17-partnerships-for-the-goals. Accessed 16 Nov 2020

Tropical Health Education Trust (2015) Principles of partnership. https://www.thet.org/principles-of-partnership/. Accessed 18 May 2019

Tropical Health Education Trust (2017) Partnership Health Check. https://www.thet.org/resources/partnership-health-check-tools/. Accessed 6 Apr 2020

Tropical Health Education Trust (2019) Health partnership scheme impact report 2011–2019. https://www.thet.org/resources/impact-report-hps-2011-2019/. Accessed 19 May 2019

Tropical Heath Education Trust (THET) (2020) Global Health Virtual Volunteering Opportunities. https://www.thet.org/get-involved/volunteering-with-thet/. Accessed 16 Nov 2020

Twintowin (2019) What is twinning? http://twintowin.com/#twinning. Accessed 5 Apr 2020

United Nations Population Fund (2020) Midwifery. https://www.unfpa.org/midwifery. Accessed 5 Apr 2020

Wilson L, Faan D, Harper C et al (2012) Global health competencies for nurses in the Americas. Prof Nurse 28:213–222

World Health Organization (2019) About the partnership for maternal, newborn and child health. https://www.who.int/pmnch/about/en/. Accessed 19 May 2019

World Health Organization (2020a) Twinning partnerships for improvement. https://www.who.int/service-deliverysafety/twinning-partnerships/en/. Accessed 19 Aug 2020

World Health Organization (2020b) Nursing and midwifery resource centre. https://www.who.int/nursing-midwifery-resources/en/. Accessed 5 Apr 2020

World Wide Fund for Nature (undated) Partnership Toolbox. http://assets.wwf.org.uk/downloads/wwf_parthershiptoolboxartweb.pdf. Accessed 6 Apr 2020

Zamora B, Gurupira M, Rodes Sanchez M et al (2019) The value of international volunteers' experience to the NHS. Glob Health 15:31. Accessed 19 May 2019

Part VI

Looking Ahead

Harmonising Midwifery: Creating a Common Philosophy and Professional Identity

16

Expected Learning Outcomes

After reading this chapter, the reader should be able to:

1. Define harmonisation, common philosophy and professional identity and why these are important in midwifery.
2. Explain why midwifery needs harmonisation.
3. Outline the advantages and challenges of harmonisation.
4. Discuss some approaches to harmonisation including how these have been implemented in different parts of the world.
5. Suggest a way forward for the benefit of women, newborn and midwives.

16.1 Definition of Harmonisation, Common Philosophy and Professional Identity

16.1.1 Harmonisation

The European Union defines harmonisation as the process of minimising redundant or conflicting standards which may have evolved independently. According to World Health Organisation European Region (2009), it is a term used in European Union law where the process of harmonisation sets a threshold which national legislation must meet. Harmonisation is similar to but not the same as standardisation. The main difference between harmonisation and standardisation lies in the degree of strictness of the standards. Harmonisation involves reduction of variations whilst standardisation entails moving towards eradication of any variation (Quora.com 2020).

Standardising midwifery on a global scale would be difficult if not impossible. Harmonisation on the other hand is most relevant given the variety or lack of standards used in midwifery education, regulation and practice globally (WHO 2016, 2018, 2019; Castro-Lopes et al. 2016).

16.1.2 Common Philosophy

Amongst the series of definitions that can be explored, the general concepts that came through were that a philosophy is a theory or attitude that acts as a guiding principle to behaviour. It is a set of ideals, standards and beliefs used to describe behaviour and thought, a way of thinking about the world, the universe and society (YourDictionary 2020). The ideas in a philosophy are usually general and abstract and consist of self-generated guidelines and perspective-shaping action, reaction and meditated response to life events (Quora.com 2020).

© Springer Nature Switzerland AG 2021
J. Kemp et al., *Global Midwifery: Principles, Policy and Practice*,
https://doi.org/10.1007/978-3-030-46765-4_16

Having a common philosophy ensures that professionals share a common view of the world, a way of thinking and how things should be. It unites the individuals in their perspectives and principles of behaviour. According to Hughes et al. (2018), a common philosophy encourages people to think critically about the world and forms the foundation of critical thinking and problem solving.

These qualities are must-haves for any profession, especially in midwifery where the concept of midwifery itself differs even amongst midwives (Renfrew et al. 2014; Steenbruggen et al. 2011). If harmonisation contributes to the development of a common philosophy, then it is urgent to start the process to ensure that midwifery takes its rightful place in the many global initiatives whose achievement depends on the effective contribution of quality midwifery services.

16.1.3 Professional Identity

Another concept demanding urgent harmonisation of midwifery is professional identity. A number of authors have defined the concept of professional identity (Ibarra 1999; Schein 1978; Tsakissiris 2015; Olckers 2017). The underpinning thoughts are that professional identity is associated with how one perceives oneself, one's self-concept in relation to the profession and one's membership of it. Professional identity is created through one's attributes, attitudes, beliefs, values, motives and experiences through which one defines oneself. Tsakissiris (2015) further stated that professional identity has typically been associated with expectations that professions have of how the professionals perform their roles, with professionalism being the ultimate aim of developing that identity (Olckers 2017). White and Ewan (1997:190) went further to state that professional identity gives a sense of 'personal adequacy and satisfaction and autonomy in the interpretation of performance of the expected role'. They further argued that identities based on group membership generate internal controls which enhance the individuals' desire to conform to the standardised identity. This self-identification addresses various self-related needs and is associated with a variety of individual and organisational outcomes. A strong, positive, self-selected professional identity has been shown to influence an individual's professional success and satisfaction (Skorikov and Vondracek 2011). Cowin et al. (2013) observed that nurses who had formed a strong professional identity were more productive and committed to the healthcare industry, and this was beneficial to other healthcare workers and patients. This is what midwifery needs. But it can only happen when individuals carrying the title 'midwife' share a common identity and a common philosophy, have gone through an education programme similar to that undertaken by colleagues carrying the same title and are regulated and practicing in a similar manner, hence the need for harmonisation.

Putting together these three concepts—harmonisation, professional identity and common philosophy—it becomes clear that for midwifery to be recognised by other healthcare professionals as an autonomous profession, it is mandatory for it to display minimum variations in the education, regulation and practice of its members. The members should perceive themselves as belonging to the profession and develop self-generated guidelines and a perspective that shapes their actions. The viewpoint should also display similar attributes, attitudes, values, motives and beliefs which become hallmarks of the profession. Joynes (2018) goes further to state that there is a clear relationship between professional identity and interprofessional responsibility, and these have an implication on the education of healthcare professionals. Professional identity amongst midwives is further discussed in Chapter 10.

The intricate relationship between harmonisation, common philosophy and professional identity cannot be addressed in detail here, but literature demonstrates that harmonisation constitutes the first step to the acquisition of the other two concepts. This is because it is the first step towards consolidating the uniqueness and unity amongst the professionals and the oneness of the profession (Tsakissiris 2015). Harmonisation leads to enhancing similarities in education, regulation and practice. Individuals display similar attributes, attitudes, values and motives and start developing a similar perspective of the world and of themselves, thus becoming a unified profession with an identity. Individuals who belong to the profession develop a sense of self interest and self-concept which enhances the development of self-generated guidelines on how they expect themselves to behave as professionals (Tsakissiris 2015).

16.2 Why Midwifery Needs Harmonisation

16.2.1 The State of Midwifery Globally

As demonstrated in the previous chapters of this book, midwifery is developing at different paces and has different positions in healthcare systems. In some countries, midwifery does not exist. In some, it is only beginning to develop. In others, though it has been there for a while, because of lack of leadership and status, investment in its development is limited. The education of midwives can be weak. There are varied education pathways in different parts of the world without recognisable alignment to the global standards for midwifery education. In some countries, midwives do not have all the relevant competencies expected of a qualified midwife and other individuals also carry the title 'midwife' despite their not having been educated as such (WHO 2016, 2017, 2018, 2019; Castro-Lopes et al. 2016; UNFPA 2011, 2014; Renfrew et al. 2014). In some settings, there are so many titles used for different grades of midwives and others providing maternity care that it is confusing to women and their families. Such variations pose a problem for individual midwives to develop any professional identity. Multiple titles exist for midwives, and these titles create ambiguity and confusion for women, their families and employers (Kennedy et al. 2018; Grundy-Bowers et al. 2018). These titles have been listed in Chapter 2: Box 2.4.

The same applies to regulatory processes and frameworks. Very few countries have regulatory bodies specific for midwifery (UNFPA 2014). The scopes of practice differ from country to country. In some countries, regulation is missing. In others, just like in education, regulation is weak and occasionally even inhibitive of some care provision (WHO European Region 2009; Kennedy et al. 2018).

Practice is no different. Individuals in most professions do pretty much the same thing no matter where they live. The protocols and expectations do not vary much. Not so with midwifery. Midwives do different things in different countries with different permissions, protocols and expectations (Chen 2017; Kennedy et al. 2018). The issue of shortages of staff in low- and middle-income countries has widened these differences as countries embarked on task shifting as a way of addressing staff shortages, thus further expanding the role of the midwife (WHO European Region 2009). Hence, a midwife in one country is not necessarily a midwife in another.

Lack of harmonisation inhibits free movement of midwives in an age where health care and workforce are considered as commodities (WHO 2016). This presents a major obstacle to the freedom of movement of midwives in general, though movement could be a double-edged sword in relation to migration of midwives from poor countries to richer countries.

The lack of professional autonomy and identity for midwifery contributes to the need for harmonisation. Because of small numbers of midwives compared to numbers of nurses, many major health organisations and governments find it more cost-effective to address midwifery together with nursing (Kennedy et al. 2018). This poses problems for professional identity and autonomy of midwifery. In some countries, midwifery is perceived as a specialisation of nursing, making it difficult to separate the two professions (Katende and Nabirye 2015; Browne and Kambo 2016). Harmonisation of midwifery would contribute to some uniformity and alignment of midwifery education and practice, producing a distinctness that would facilitate creating a whole mindset in organisations and governments about the identity and autonomy of midwifery.

The achievement of global health initiatives in maternal, newborn and child health demands effective midwifery services provision. The value of midwifery in maternal and newborn health is no longer under discussion (Renfrew et al. 2014). Harmonising the profession will contribute to supporting governments and agencies willing to invest in strengthening midwifery by providing them with areas of focus and definite, undisputed outcomes and returns for their investments (UNFPA 2014).

16.2.2 Relationship with Other Healthcare Professions

Throughout history, midwifery has had to contend with opposition and pressure from other healthcare professionals. These issues have been discussed in some detail in Chapters. 4 and 10. In the United States of America, doctors wanted midwives to be called 'obstetric nurses' (Hellman 1971). In a large part of Southern Africa, midwifery is perceived as a specialisation of nursing. In some countries, nursing is perceived as superior or more attractive than midwifery as midwives are perceived as not highly educated (Burst 2005; Luyben et al. 2017). In a considerable number of countries, because of this perception that midwives are not highly educated, midwives are educated by doctors and nurses and not by midwives (Fullerton et al. 2011). Additionally, some care providers who also work with women and their families, who, however, are not themselves educated as midwives, have designated titles that contain the word 'midwife'. This adds to the confusion, making harmonisation more than needed for the survival of midwifery (Hobbs 2019; Stones and Arulkumaran 2014).

16.3 Advantages of Harmonisation

Harmonisation will strengthen midwifery by improving the initial education and access to higher education. Harmonisation calls for the establishment of necessary legislative and regulatory frameworks in each country. The role and function of various bodies relevant to mid-

wifery services would be clarified, taking into account local factors in each country and applying general principles to make a consistent framework (Keighley 2009). Harmonisation gives a common vision to all those who carry the title 'midwife' and creates common public expectations from midwives. The European Union Directives are one example where the education of healthcare providers was harmonised (Keighley 2009).

Harmonisation can be employed as part of a midwifery development package which incorporates all the global tools and strategies available for the development of midwifery education, guidance on the utilisation of the midwifery workforce, recommendations on strengthening midwifery practice and the use of the global standards for midwifery education and regulation (WHO Europen Region 2009, 2016, 2018, 2019; ICM 2013a, 2019). Chapters 4 and 5 address the issues relating to education and regulation, and Chapter 10 considers the influence of higher education.

Harmonisation facilitates free movement of midwives from country to country and can result in the development of globally accepted, mutually recognised processes to facilitate the acceptance of education and training and qualifications acquired in another country, a system similar to the European Union (EU) Directives (EU 1977, 1980, 2005; WHO European Region 2009). Harmonisation thus aids quality assurance in education and practice (Steenbruggen et al. 2011).

16.3.1 Professional Identity

Harmonisation provides a foundation for professional identity and a sense of self-interest and respect which enhances individuals' desire to do the right thing. Professional identity unifies individuals through a common philosophy and a common view of the world and how things should be done. As described earlier, professional identity binds midwives through self-generated guidelines for quality, thus creating a self-reinforcing quality assurance mechanism within the profession and amongst professionals.

Additionally, movement of midwives across regions will be less costly by avoiding lengthy bridging courses and administrative processes and easier for both governments and midwives.

16.3.2 Raised Profile and Status

Harmonisation of midwifery implies adherence to a minimum set of general standards and protocols and therefore enhances the possibility of adherence to and commitment to best practices, sharing of approaches and expertise and prevents duplication (Keighley 2009). This raises the profile of the profession and of individual midwives as the meaning and the concept of *midwife* will be the same globally, fulfilling the maxim 'a midwife, is a midwife is a midwife'. This will enable the population served to approach midwives with knowledge and understanding of who these care providers are and what they can do (WHO 2019). This knowledge is likely to strengthen women's respect and support for midwives. A strong partnership between women and midwives is a powerful advocacy tool for improving maternal and newborn health services (Dixon et al. 2018).

16.3.3 Aspects to Be Harmonised

The major areas to be harmonised are midwifery education, midwifery regulation, midwifery governance and leadership and midwifery practice. Most of the elements of each aspect are diagrammatically presented in Fig. 16.1.

16.4 Challenges to Harmonisation of Midwifery

The gaps in different aspects of midwifery demonstrated above are already known. Global surveys have been conducted by WHO through the global consultations conducted between 2016 and 2018 of how to strengthen midwifery education. The ICM has conducted gap analysis workshops in upward of 75 countries on the status of midwifery in those countries culminating

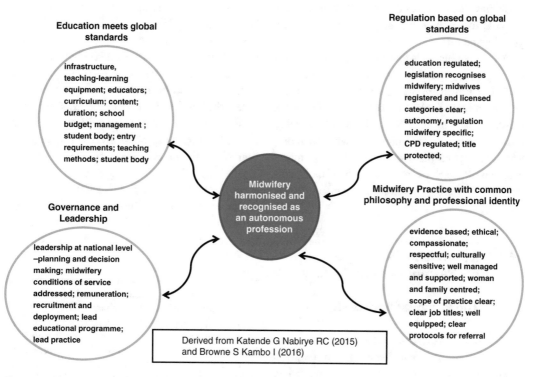

Fig. 16.1 Harmonised midwifery showing most of the aspects to be reviewed. (Derived from Katende and Nabirye (2015) and Browne and Kambo (2016))

in the creation of the ICM Midwifery Services Framework which attempts to place midwifery into the heath system (ICM 2015). The UNFPA has overseen the coordination and resourcing of the State of the World Midwifery Reports (UNFPA 2011, 2014) and other projects, and most of the areas of variation have been identified (UNFPA 2011, 2014; WHO 2016, 2019; ICM 2013a). Midwife experts have conducted studies on the state of midwifery education, regulation and association in 73 countries (Castro-Lopes et al. 2016). This will be extended to more countries in the 2021 State of the World's Midwifery Report. All these activities revealed the discrepancies in midwifery as a profession. Each of these groups provided recommendations and possible strategies; however, challenges exist. For the variations to be addressed, there is need for political will to invest in midwifery. This is not available in many countries (WHO 2019). Addressing the variations requires resources—a considerable amount of resources and expertise. Not every country is able to provide such resources. The WHO (2019) reported that even the 3-year duration for midwifery education is not achievable in some countries because they are not able to resource a programme which meets global standards.

A final challenge is that the needs of countries differ greatly, and the countries cannot do anything but utilise midwives to do more and ask non-midwives to take on some midwifery work (Castro-Lopes et al. 2016). There is a possible risk that some of the midwives who do more, which is beyond the scope of midwifery, might perceive themselves as better than their colleagues, rendering harmonisation efforts quite challenging.

16.5 Approaches/Strategies for Harmonising Midwifery

16.5.1 The Regional Approach

16.5.1.1   The European Union
In the European Union, healthcare professions, specifically midwifery, nursing and medicine, were required to create advisory committees that agreed on the minimum standards for the profession concerned. This was regarding the nature, minimum content and length of education and training programmes required to obtain qualifications that were mutually recognised by all member states. Directives were created based on this agreement. Certain bodies, recognised by law to administer the directives called 'competent authorities' were established in each member state. These bodies were responsible for handling the applications for recognition of qualifications, education and training in another EU country. Relevant directives were instituted for the recognition of diplomas, certificates and other evidence of the formal qualifications of professionals (Directive 80/154/EEC and Directive 80/155/EEC).

In 1999 the Bologna Declaration put in motion a series of reforms that created a common degree-level system for undergraduates, graduates and doctoral degrees across all sectors including health. This improved recognition of degrees and academic qualifications in every field across 46 countries (Keighley 2009). National centres for the recognition of qualifications were created.

The process was progressively refined until 2005 when 15 directives were replaced by one, based on the three concepts and processes of mutuality,[1] harmonisation and recognition. This meant that a professional recognised in one state could also be recognised in another provided the profession concerned was regulated in both member states. General directives were created to cover diplomas awarded on completion of a higher education course of at least 3 years duration, following general education equivalent to A-Level / Baccalaureate; and diplomas gained on completion of professional education and training of less than 3 years duration in higher education. Common platforms[2]

---

[1]Mutuality is the process by which decisions reached in one member state are honoured in another, unless there are clear grounds for doubt (Keighley 2009).

[2]A common platform is a set of criteria which make it possible to compensate for the widest range of substantial differences which have been identified between the education requirements in at least two thirds of the member states including all member states which regulate that profession (Keighley 2009).

were created to lead to an extension of automatic recognition within the general system. Administrative cooperation was required, meaning that competent authorities of the host member state and the home member state were required to work in close collaboration. Contact points and committees on the recognition of professional qualifications were put in place in each member state (Keighley 2009). All these principles also applied to midwifery. Some applications were addressed on a case-by-case basis. This involved the recognition of midwives who entered the profession via a field of practice that was not related to health and midwives who had taken a specialist training. This incorporated practitioners who wished to be recognised in their specialist field in another member state, particularly where the receiving member state did not have that particular field of practice. Harmonisation introduced greater flexibility with solutions found through either a period of compensatory training and supervised practice or the applicant being required to take an examination (Keighley 2009).

Of equal importance within the harmonisation system was the recognition of professional development and vocational studies. The Commission recommended the creation of a common reference framework which served as a translation device between different qualifications systems and their levels, whether for general and higher education or for vocational education and training (Keighley 2009).

16.5.1.2 The South Eastern European Countries

Gosic and Tomak (2019) explored the possibility of harmonising midwifery in six countries in the South Eastern European region, namely Bosnia and Herzegovina, Croatia, Montenegro, North Macedonia, Slovenia and Serbia. They started with a study to determine the state of midwifery in these countries. This included professional standards, legal and ethical norms that oblige midwives to provide quality midwifery care and the activities of the professional associations. They found that, though all the countries were following the Bologna Declaration of 1999, there were differences in the way midwives were educated, their titles, and the definitions of a midwife.

Midwives were educated at higher education level in all countries except Montenegro. Midwifery education was taking place in different departments of universities, some in medical schools and others in non-medical departments or in health departments. Those who were educated at higher education level were awarded different qualifications on completion of the programme even though all programmes were 3 years duration. Some received a bachelor's degree in midwifery but others could also qualify as a midwife. For those who entered the programmes after secondary school, involving 4 years education after elementary school, some completed the programme to become midwives, some to become nurse-midwives and others midwife assistants. In some countries, continuing professional development is mandatory. In some, it is needed for specialisation though it remained as a right and obligation. In others, it was desirable but not obligated. The definitions and scopes of practice differed in these countries (Gosic and Tomak 2019:4).

These findings were used as a basis for advocacy for the mobilisation of financial support to enable students to enter midwifery at graduate level in line with the Bologna Declaration. This resulted in the creation of a regional education centre for midwifery educators and researchers. It also led to harmonisation of the standards and laws impacting midwifery across these countries and the design and implementation of joint teaching projects for midwifery education at both levels, namely secondary and higher education.

This study demonstrates what could be considered on a global level.

16.5.1.3 The East African Countries

Six East African countries (Burundi, Kenya, Rwanda, Uganda, mainland Tanzania and the state of Zanzibar), in collaboration with Partner States and various International Development Partners and stakeholders, undertook to harmonise midwifery and nursing in the region, in 2015. The purpose of the exercise was to strengthen regional and national policies, laws, regulation, human resources, institutional and infrastructure capacity for the provision of high-quality nursing and midwifery services. The first step was to determine the status of midwifery in the aspects to be harmonised. Midwifery was addressed together with nursing.

A series of meetings was held with Ministries of Health, chief nursing and midwifery officers, regulatory bodies and professional associations in each country/state, after which a consultancy was commissioned to develop harmonisation guidelines.

The objectives of the process were, firstly, to review the existing midwifery education programmes (this incorporated curricula and guidelines, standards and procedures, admission criteria, regulation, certification, internship, registration, practice, inspection, accreditation and mutual recognition in the East African Community Partner States); secondly, to review the midwifery governance structure in all East African States.

The findings revealed variations in all aspects according to the desires of each state. There were different curricula, guidelines, policies and accreditation processes where they existed. Entry requirements for different levels varied and the qualifications awarded at the end of each programme were diverse with different titles at different levels of the profession. The study recommended the establishment of task forces to synchronise education, regulation and practice of the professions based on international criteria developed by the International Confederation of Midwives, International Council of Nurses and the World Health Organization (Katende and Nabirye 2015; Browne and Kambo 2016).

16.5.1.4   The South East Asian Nations

The Association of South East Asian Nations (ASEAN) established an Asian Economic Community (AEC), a single market to compete in the global economy (Law et al. 2019). The ASEAN Vision 2020 perceived equitable development and the free flow of trade in services and

skilled labour across the ten nations[3] as critical to the AEC.

Processes to facilitate mobility, information exchange on standards and qualifications, promotion of best practices and opportunities for capacity building and professional education of seven key occupations including nursing and midwifery were initiated (Law et al. 2019:6). In most of the countries, midwifery is included in nursing (Law et al. 2019).

Regional structures were established. These included the Mutual Recognition Arrangements (MRA) and Joint Coordinating Committees for each discipline. The key areas considered were the quality of education and standards including clinical exposure, registration and mobility of practitioners. Governance of each discipline remained in the member states.

Because of the great diversity amongst countries, implementation was inconsistent. Some countries feared the depletion of already strained human resources. Others saw an opportunity for nurses migrating from countries with surplus to those with shortages. Hence, whilst the values implicit in the MRAs were shared, specific mechanisms appeared driven by internal needs and commitment to improve standards rather than regional reform. For example, in Cambodia, the Khmer Rouge war in the 1970s had decimated the health workforce. In the following few years, non-governmental organisations (NGOs) trained a range of healthcare providers in refugee/displaced persons camps along Cambodia's border. At the end of the conflict, demobilised military health staff were integrated into the health system. The result was a bloated workforce of uncertain quality. This impacted the country's response to MRA (Law et al. 2019). Regionally, despite severe sanctions for failure to meet registration requirements (Amaro 2016; Ven 2016), enforcement mechanisms were inadequately resourced. Continuing professional development for nurses and midwives was difficult because of low incomes and lack of financial support.

---

[3]The ten nations are Brunei Darussalam, Cambodia, Indonesia, Lao PDR, Malaysia, Myanmar, Philippines, Singapore, Thailand and Viet Nam (Law et al. 2019).

Solutions were developed. Concerns over clinical standards at registration led to the introduction of mandatory entry and exit examinations. A mandatory foundation year was introduced for all health professional students to address the uneven secondary schooling and establish a common platform for the health workforce. Because of high maternal and neonatal mortality rates, Cambodia introduced the associate degree in midwifery (Annear et al. 2015) and unlike the rest of the region, midwifery and nursing have discrete preservice education and two separate professional councils (Law et al. 2019).

16.6   Lessons from Regulation

Efforts have been made in harmonising some aspects of midwifery. The most visible efforts have been in the harmonisation of midwifery regulation and education (see Chapters. 4 and 5). The Eastern Mediterranean Region started in 2002 to harmonise regulation (WHO EMRO 2002). There were a variety of weak or missing regulatory processes in each of the six[4] EMRO countries. The conclusion was that nursing and midwifery would be of better quality if there was harmonisation across countries. In the United States of America, the development of a consensus document in 2015 by the United States Midwifery Education Regulation and Association (US MERA) provided clarity and guidelines for policymakers in relation to midwifery regulation. The variety of regulatory processes across the 50 states were said to have been causing confusion amongst care providers, policymakers, women and their children and in some cases the inhibition of access to certain types of care for women and their families (Kennedy et al. 2018). The Regulatory Collaboratives across 17 countries in East and Central Africa (McCarthy et al. 2013; Gross et al. 2015) achieved the same objective during the time of HIV and AIDS and facilitated task shifting in this region.

The World Health Organization conducted a series of global consultations between 2016 and 2018 as a first step towards strengthening and harmonisation of midwifery education and came up with a number of strategies to be implemented for this purpose (WHO 2019). The same approaches employed for regulation and education could be used for the harmonisation of other aspects of the profession until variations are reduced to a minimum globally.

16.6.1   Harmonisation Levels

Midwifery can be harmonised at national level, amongst a group of hospitals (NHS Foundation Trust 2015) or at facility level (Grundy-Bowers et al. (2018). Harmonisation can also be achieved in only one aspect of the profession for example in regulation which was discussed in Chapter 5; education including curricula, duration of programmes and the quality of educators which were discussed in Chapter 4, as well as job titles (Grundy-Bowers et al. 2018). The process is the same. It is a question of scale and resources.

16.6.2   Tools Available

The tools for the harmonisation of midwifery were already in place at the time of writing. These are presented in Box 16.1.

Box 16.1. Tools Available for Harmonisation of Midwifery
- Global Standards for Midwifery Education (ICM 2013a).
- Global Standards for Midwifery Regulation and the Regulation Toolkit (ICM 2013b).
- Essential Competencies for Basic Midwifery Practice (ICM 2019).
- Model curricula for the education of midwives, including a curriculum concordance (ICM 2013c).

---

[4]ASEAN countries: Cambodia, China, Lao People's Democratic Republic, Papua New Guinea, Solomon Islands, Viet Nam.

- Midwifery Education Accreditation Programme (ICM 2018).
- WHO Midwifery Educator Competencies (WHO 2014).
- WHO Global Strategy for Strengthening Midwifery 2016–2020 (WHO 2015).
- WHO Global Advocacy Strategy for Strengthening Midwifery (WHO 2018).
- WHO Seven-step Plan for Strengthening Midwifery (WHO 2018).

16.6.3 Pre-Requisites for Harmonisation

For successful harmonisation of midwifery, there is need for resources and expertise to address the issue on a global level. The fact that harmonisation has been achieved in other aspects of the profession and in some regions demonstrates that the expertise is available. There is need for strong leadership and advocacy for the process and for the mobilisation of resources (WHO 2018). The EU established what was referred to as the Copenhagen criteria (European Council 1993). These are presented in Box 16.2.

Box 16.2 The Copenhagen Criteria for Harmonisation

- Stable institutions that guarantee democracy, the rule of law, human rights and respect for and protection of minorities.
- A functioning market economy, as well as the ability to cope with pressure of competition and the market forces at work inside the union.
- The ability to assume the obligations of membership, in particular, adherence to the objectives of political, economic and monetary union.

Source: Keighley (2009).

Some level of these criteria would be relevant and adapted to the global level. Quality management systems would be required similar to the competent authorities, common platforms, contact points and mutuality of the European Union.

Democracy, rule of law and respect for human rights are greatly desirable globally. At the same time, these are not easily achievable in settings of population upheaval and civil unrest which has been experienced everywhere during the third decade of the twenty-first century. Neither can market economies function in some of these settings. On a global scale, some countries have no competitive economic strength against larger global economies, and their midwifery workforce finds it more appealing to emigrate to the larger economies. In low- and middle-income countries, one of the biggest challenges to midwifery has been the lack of investment in the profession largely due to lack of political will and lack of financial resources (Renfrew et al. 2014). Were harmonisation of midwifery to be attempted at a global scale, these are issues which would require to be addressed and strategies devised to circumvent them or to reduce their impact on the processes. Be that as it may, the EU approach offers a lot in terms of a possible framework for the harmonisation of midwifery globally.

16.7 Conclusion

16.7.1 Where Are We Now in Harmonising Midwifery; Are Any Landmarks Visible?

The need for harmonisation of midwifery has been acknowledged across the world. Regions have taken steps to harmonise midwifery. The objectives for harmonisation are shared, and the demands of the harmonisation process is understood.

A lot has already been done. Global surveys on the state of midwifery have been conducted especially in low- and middle-income countries (UNFPA 2011, 2014; Castro-Lopes et al. 2015, 2016; Lancet Series on Midwifery 2016). The areas requiring urgent harmonisation were identified through these surveys and the gap analysis activities conducted by the International Confederation of Midwives 2008–2013 (ICM 2014). The next steps would be to collate the work that has been done and carry out the harmonisation process on a global scale and thus reduce variations in midwifery education, regulation, governance and practice.

16.7.2 What Else Has to be Done and by Whom with What Results?

The way forward therefore is a strong advocacy campaign for the strengthening of midwifery globally. With all the tools and the regional efforts in the early part of the twenty-first century, the ground was fertile for the implementation of the WHO Seven-Step Plan (WHO 2019), and the Global advocacy strategy for the strengthening of midwifery. Models have become available from which elements can be identified to develop implementation and monitoring mechanisms for any agreed processes. The EU model offers most of the elements that would be desirable for this purpose, for example the competent authorities, the common platforms, contact points, and the qualification recognition centres to establish mutuality. The creation and implementation of such systems would go a long way in making midwifery distinct, visible and autonomous. This would make it possible to extract midwifery from nursing without damaging the collegial relationship between the two professions that is both desirable and beneficial for women and their families.

The world could also borrow from the processes put in place to strengthen midwifery education globally. According to the WHO (2019) report on strengthening quality midwifery education, it is important to establish strategic priorities, be innovative and radical in thinking, establish methods of measuring progress and quality management in all settings including conflict and humanitarian settings. The latter is discussed in Chapter 13.

Making it happen, just like in midwifery education, will require the involvement of all stakeholders. Governments, parliamentarians, decision-makers and policymakers would need to make quality midwifery services a political priority, strengthening midwifery leadership and aligning partners, including in humanitarian and fragile settings, and providing funding. They would need to embed midwifery within the health system and to be accountable for resources and rights to quality midwifery services in cities and rural areas and adverse humanitarian settings. Enabling legislation would need to be put in place. In addition, laws, policies and regulations are needed. These should enhance effective midwifery service provision and protect women, midwives and other female health workers from gender-based or other discrimination in seeking, accessing or providing midwifery care.

The United Nations and other multilateral and bilateral organisations and global health initiatives would be required to increase numerous efforts. These include mobilising resources at global, regional and country level to invest in midwifery. Provision of technical support to countries is also needful, through innovative financing and other support mechanisms. Healthcare professional associations (HCPAs), midwifery associations, midwifery educators and practitioners, together with managers of educational and service institutions, civil society, academic and research institutions, even the business community and the media, would all need to take part (WHO 2019).

Harmonisation would go a long way in enabling midwifery to stand shoulder to shoulder with other healthcare professions and receive the respect that it deserves.

- **Principles**
- Principles of harmonisation that have been used in different regions and countries and at different levels of the profession can be adapted and used to harmonise

midwifery globally. Harmonisation, unlike standardisation, is flexible enough to allow individual country needs to be taken into account without compromising the quality of midwifery and its alignment with global standards.

- **Policy**
- Political commitment and advocacy are critical components for harmonisation. Despite harmonisation being a big ask, if the evidence about midwives' contribution to achieving the SGDs is to be believed, governments and other key stakeholders must be willing to tackle the process.
- **Practice**
- Harmonisation enhances the provision of quality midwifery services as individual professionals will share a common philosophy and a common professional identity which will compel them to provide care according to agreed professional standards.

Questions for Reflection

1. In many low and middle-income countries of Africa and in parts of Asia, midwifery is perceived as a part of nursing and sometimes as a post basic qualification to nursing. If global harmonisation of midwifery were to take place, what impact do you think this will have on midwifery service provision in these countries? Should midwifery be separated from nursing where there are extreme staff shortages?

2. The text argued that harmonisation will raise the profile of midwifery. Do you agree? What will be the challenges to harmonisation and how can these be addressed?

Additional Resources for Reflection and Further Study

Borrelli SE, Spiby H, Walsh D (2016) The kaleidoscopic midwife: A conceptual metaphor illustrating first-time mothers' perspectives of a good midwife during childbirth. A grounded theory study Midwifery 2016 Midwifery. May 2016. https://www.kennispoort-verloskunde.nl/wp-content/uploads/2016/12/11.-KALEIDOSCOPIC-MIDWIFE-Midwifery-2016.pdf. Accessed 8 Mar 2020

European Midwives Association: European Midwives Association (EMA) position on the proposal for a Directive of the European Parliament and of the Council amending Directive 2005/36/EC on the recognition of professional qualifications and regulation on administrative cooperation through the Internal Market Information System (COM (2011) 883). http://www.european-midwives.com/upload/filemanager/content-images/novice/ema_response_to_the_professional_qualifications_directive_proposal.pdf. Accessed 8 Mar 2020

European Commission Directive 2005/36/EC of the European Pariament and the Council of 7 September 2005 on the recognition of professional qualifications. Offical Journal of the European Union, 2005, L 255:22-142

European Commission (2020) The Siengle Market. Regulated professions database. https://ec.europa.eu/growth/tools-databases/regprof/index.cfm?action=regprof&id_regprof=8011. Accessed 8 Mar 2020

International Confederation of Midwives (2013) Global Standards for midwifery education. https://internationalmidwives.org/education. Accessed 8 Mar 2020

World Health Organisation (2008) Task shifting: global recommendations and guidelines. World Health Organisation, Geneva. https://www.who.int/healthsystems/TTR-TaskShifting.pdf?. Accessed Oct 2019

References

Amaro Y (2016) Enforcement a concern as health law moves forward. Phnom Penh. The Phnom Penh Post. http://www.phnompenhpost.com/national/enforcement-concern-health-law-moves-forward. Accessed 10 Apr 2020

Annear PL, Grundy J, Ir P et al (2015) The Kingdom of Cambodia health system review. Health in transition policy note 5(2). World Health Organization, Regional Office for the Western Pacific, Manila, p 2015

Browne S, Kambo I (2016) Harmonising nursing and midwifery education, regulation and licensure and practice across East Africa. Conference paper September 2016. ResearchGate. Accessed 15 Mar 2020

Burst HV (2005) The history of nurse-midwifery/midwifery education. J Midwifery Womens Health 50(2):129–137

Castro-Lopes S, Ten Hoope-Bender P, Bokosi M et al. (2015) The involvement of midwives' associations in policy planning about the midwifery workforce: a global survey. Midwifery 1096–1103

Castro-Lopes S, Nove A, Ten Hoope-Bender P et al (2016) A descriptive analysis of midwifery education, regulation and association in 73 countries: the baseline for a post-2015 pathway. Hum Resour Health 14. https://doi.org/10.1186/s12960-016-0134-7

Chen J (2017) Midwifery around the world: a glimpse at midwifery around the world. https://www.thebump.com/a/midwifery-around-the-world. Accessed 15 Mar 2020

Cowin LS, Johnson M, Wilson I et al (2013) The psychometric properties of five professional identity measures in a sample of nursing students. Nurse Educ Today 33(6):608–613

Dixon L, Neely E, Martis R (2018) Editorial: consumer representation on the editorial board. NZ Coll Midwives J 54:4

European Commission (2005) Directive 2005/36/EC of the European Pariament and the Council of 7 September 2005 on the recognition of professional qualifications. Offical Journal of the European Union L 255:22–142

European Council (1993) The Copenhagen accession criteria. European Council in Copenhagen 21–22 June 1993. https://eurlex.europa.eu/summary/glossary/accession_criteria_copenhague.html

European Union Council (1977) Directive 77/452/EEC of 27 June 1977 concerning the mutual recognition of diplomas, certificates, and other evidence of the formal qualifications of nurses responsible for general care, including measures to facilitate the effective exercise of this right of establishment of freedom to provide services. Official Journal of the European Union L 176:1–7

European Union Council (1980) Directive 80/154/EEC of 21 January 1980 concerning the mutual recognition of diplomas, certificates and other evidence of the formal qualifications in midwifery and including measures to facilitate the effective exercise of the right of establsihment and freedom to provide services. Official Journal of the European Union L 033:1–7

Fullerton JT, Johnson PG, Thompson JB et al (2011) Quality considerations in midwifery pre-service education: exemplars from Africa. Midwifery 27(3):308–315

Gosic N, Tomak T (2019) Professional and normative standards in midwifery in six south east European countries: a policy case study. Eur J Midwifery 3

Gross JM, Kelly M, McCarthy CF (2015) A model for advancing professional nursing regulation: the African health profession regulatory collaborative. J Nurs Regul 6(3):29–33

Grundy-Bowers M, O'Brien S, Harmer V (2018) Harmonising nursing and midwifery titles in an acute hospital. Nurs Times 114(1):36–39

Hellman LM (1971) Nurse midwifery: fifteen years bulletin of the American College of Nurse. Midwives 16(3):1542–2011

Hobbs AJ (2019) Scoping review to identify and map the health personnel considered skilled birth attendants in low-and-middle income countries from 2000–2015. PLoS One 14(2):e0211576

Hughes M, Rigtering C, Covin JG et al (2018) Innovative behaviour, trust and perceived workplace performance. Br J Manag 29(4):29(4). Accessed March 2020. https://doi.org/10.1111/1467-8551.12305

Ibarra H (1999) Provisional selves: experimenting with image and identity in professional adaptation. Adm Sci Q 44(4):764–791

International Confederation of Midwives (2013) Global Standards for midwifery education. https://www.internationalmidwives.org/education

International Confederation of Midwives (2013a) Global standards for midwifery education. https://www.internationalmidwives.org. Accessed 9 Mar 2020

International Confederation of Midwives (2013b) Global standards for Midwifery regulation. https://www.internationalmidwifery.org/regulation-resources/. Accessed 10 Mar 2020

International Confederation of Midwives (2013c) Essential competencies for basic midwifery practice. https://www.internationalmidwives.org/education

International Confederation of Midwives (2013c) Model curricula for the education of midwives. https://www.internationalmidwives.org/education

International Confederation of Midwives (2014) Gap analysis for the assemsnet of midwifery services in a country. https://www.internationalmidwives.org/projects

International Confederation of Midwives (2014) The regulation toolkit. https://www.internationalmidwives.org/regulation

International Confederation of Midwives (2015) The Midwifery Services Framework for developing and strengthening sexual reproductive maternal and newborn health. https://www.internationalmidwives.org/msf

International Confederation of Midwives (2018) The Global Midwifery Education Assessment Programme. https://www.internationalmidwives.org/education

International Confederation of Midwives (2019) Essential competencies for basic midwifery practice. www.internationalmidwives.org/competencies. Accessed 15 Nov 2019

Joynes VCT (2018) Defining and understanding the relationship between professional identity and interprofessional responsibility: implications for educating health and social care students. Adv Health Sci Educ 23:133–149

Katende G, Nabirye RC (2015) Development of regional guidelines for the harmonisation of nursing and midwifery for recognition in EAC Partner states. ResearchGate. Accessed Mar 2020. https://doi.org/10.13140/RG.2.1.1433.9043

Keighley T (2009) European Union standards of nursing and midwifery: information for accession countries, 2nd edn. World Health Organisation, Geneva

Kennedy HP, Myers-Cieko JA, Camacho Carr K et al (2018) United States model of midwifery legislation and regulation: development of consensus document. J Midwifery Women Health 63:652–659

Law KMH, Te V, Holl PS (2019) Cambodia's health professionals and the ASEAN mutual recognition arrangements: registration, education and mobility. Hum Resour Health 17:14. https://doi.org/10.1186/s12960-019-0349-5

Luyben A, Barger M, Avery M et al (2017) Exploring global recognition of quality midwifery education: vision or fiction? Women Birth 30:184–192

McCarthy FC, Voss J, Verani AR et al (2013) Nursing and midwifery regulation and HIV scale up: establishing a baseline in east, central and southern Africa. J Int AIDS Soc 2013(16):18051

Olckers C (2017) Measuring psychological ownership: a critical review. In: Olckers L, van Zyl L, van der Vaart C (eds) Theoretical orientations and practical applications of psychological ownership. Springer, Berlin, pp 61–78

Quora.com (2020) What is philosophy used for? Accessed 20 Mar 2020

Renfrew MJ, McFadden A, Bastos MH et al (2014) Midwifery and quality care: findings from a new evidence-informed framework for maternal and newborn care. Lancet 384(9948):1129–1145

Royal United Hospitals Bath NHS Foundation Trust (2015) Safer staffing Midwifery Six-monthly Report: November 2015. https://www.ruh.nhs.uk/about/trust-board/2015_11/documents/10a.1.pdf. Accessed 16 May 2020

Schein EH (1978) Career dynamics: matching individual and organizational needs. Addison-Wesley, Reading, MA

Skorikov VB, Vondracek FW (2011) Occupational identity handbook of identity theory and research. Springer, New York, pp 693–714

Steenbruggen I, Mitchell T, Severin P et al (2011) Harmonising spirometry education with HERMES: training a new generation of qualified spirometry practitioners across Europe. Eur Respir J 37: 479–481

Stones W, Arulkumaran S (2014) Health-care professionals in midwifery care. Lancet 384(9949):1169–1170

The Lancet (2016) Executive summary. Maternal health series. www.thelancet.com. Accessed 9 Oct 2019

Tsakissiris J (2015) The role of professional identity and self interest in career choices in the emerging ICT workforce. Thesis, School of Management, Faculty of Business, Queensland University of Technology Australia

United Nations Population Fund (2011) State of the World's midwifery. Delivering health, saving lives. United Nations Population Fund, New York

United Nations Population Fund (2014) State of the World's Midwifery Report. A universal pathway, a woman's right to health. UNFPA 2014 New York

Ven R (2016) Health professionals face registration reform. Phnom Penh: Khmer Times 2016. http://www.khmertimeskh.com/news/32694/health-professionals-face-registration-reform/. Accessed April 2020

White R, Ewan CE (1997) Clinical teaching in nursing, 2nd revised edn. Nelson Thornes, Cheltenham

World Health Organisation (2008) Task shifting: global recommendations and guidelines. World Health Organisation, Geneva. https://www.who.int/healthsystems/TTR-TaskShifting.pdf?ua-1 Accessed October 2019

World Health Organisation (2014) Midwifery educator competencies. World Health Organisation, Geneva

World Health Organisation (2015) Skilled attendants: management systems and other logistics need to be addressed. World Health Organisation. Geneva

World Health Organization (2016) Global strategy for human resources for health: Workforce 2030. WHO, Geneva

World Health Organization (2017) Strengthening quality midwifery education. WHO Meeting report July 25–26, 2016. In support of Global Strategy for Women's, Children's and Adolescents' Health 2016–30. WHO, Geneva

World Health Organization (2018) Definition of skilled health personnel providing care during childbirth. The 2018 Joint statement by WHO, UNFPA, UNICEF, ICM, ICN, FIGO, IPA

World Health Organization (2019) Strengthening quality midwifery education for universal health coverage 2030: Framework for action. ISBN 978-92-4-151584-9

World Health Organisation Europe Region (2009) Nurses and Midwices: a force for health. Survey on the situation of nursing and midwifery in the member states of the European Region of the World Health Organisation 2009. WHO Regional Office of Europe. Copenhagen, Denmark

World Health Organisation Regional Office of the Eastern Mediterranean: Regional Office for Europe Cairo (2002) Nursing and Midwifery: A guide to professional regulation. WHO Technical publication series:27. https://apps.who.int/bookorders/anglais/detart1.jsp?codlan=1&codcol=25&codcch=27

YourDictionary (2020) Definition and usage of philosophy. Accessed 10 Mar 2020

The Principles, Policy and Practice of Global Midwifery: 2030 and Beyond

17

Expected Learning Outcomes
By the end of the chapter, the reader should be able to:

1. Reflect on issues relating to the principles, policy and practice of global midwifery across the globe and consider the key issues in looking forward to 2030 and beyond.
2. Identify the political and economic factors that influence the provision of high-quality, respectful maternity care by midwives and the fiscal benefits to a nation where this is provided.
3. Discuss the socio-cultural issues that influence maternal and neonatal health and the importance of the midwife's role in understanding and addressing these.
4. Evaluate the influence of new technologies on midwifery education and practice and their impact on childbearing women/people and their families.
5. Identify the legal frameworks required to protect women during pregnancy and birth and to regulate the profession so that only midwives competent to global standards are licensed to practise midwifery.
6. Discuss environmental factors that may influence the lives of women and their families, midwives' practice and efforts to strengthen midwifery globally.
7. Evaluate the final recommendations offered in this book and consider how these may be prioritised, progressed and implemented to the maximum benefit of every woman, newborn and midwife across the globe.

17.1 Introduction

This book set out to be an authoritative, in-depth publication about global midwifery, exploring the available evidence for the contribution of skilled, professional midwives to the provision of high-quality, respectful maternity care and to the achievement of the 2030 Sustainable Development Goals through partnership with women and their families, enabling them to 'survive, thrive and transform' (Every Woman Every Child 2015).

This final chapter uses two well-known tools, PESTLE (Political, Economic, Social, Technological, Legal and Economic) and SWOT (Strengths, Weaknesses, Opportunities and Threats) analyses, to draw out from the detailed exploration in the previous chapters of this book,

© Springer Nature Switzerland AG 2021
J. Kemp et al., *Global Midwifery: Principles, Policy and Practice*,
https://doi.org/10.1007/978-3-030-46765-4_17

factors that have influenced the past and the present of global midwifery and those that will continue to have influence for the future. Drawing together the findings of these analyses, a detailed synthesis of the principles, policy and practice of global midwifery is then presented before offering recommendations for consideration by those who would attempt to continue to build a safer, more acceptable world for every woman and newborn on the planet at that crucial and costly time that surrounds birth.

17.2　The PESTLE Model

PESTLE analysis is a marketing and business model useful for identifying and addressing challenges that may affect the planning and implementation of a new strategy or project (Professional Academy 2020). It can also be a used in the health sector to view complex issues from a wide perspective (Edwards and Seda 2016; Ralph et al. 2014). PESTLE is an acronym that stands for Political, Economic, Social, Technological, Legal and Environmental factors. These factors are tackled in turn below.

17.2.1　Political Factors

Midwifery is political (Medway and Digance 2017), and this book has charted the struggle that midwives have faced in recent centuries for autonomy and political power. Midwifery is also closely linked to the politics of gender and patriarchy (Walsh 2016); women's lives can be saved, but only if their lives are considered worth saving (Chapter 2) (Fathalla 2006). Such a statement moves the ball firmly into the political arena.

Chapters 1–4 showed that the value of midwifery to the survival of women and newborns was recognised in 1987 with the launch of the Safe Motherhood Initiative (UN 1986, 2020a, 2015, 2016, 2019). However, the subsequent drive to meet globally agreed targets such as the Millennium Development Goals led to the blurring of midwives' identity. Different cadres and initiatives (such as skilled birth attendants) were introduced to produce more 'midwifery personnel', to substitute for midwives and to provide short-term solutions to human resource shortages. In some situations, these short-term solutions became long-term solutions. As a result, midwifery education suffered, policymakers became confused about what midwifery actually is and does, and further disparities in midwifery practice emerged in low-, middle- and high-income countries (WHO 2008, 2013, 2017, 2018a; Gherrisi et al. 2016; Luyben et al. 2017).

With an indistinct identity and a variety of education programmes of differing quality, midwifery has struggled to make itself visible and to be acknowledged as a separate profession. Since the 1950s, midwifery has often been conflated[1] with nursing; this has compromised women's sexual and reproductive health right to have care from a midwife, as the appropriate care giver, and means that midwifery, as a smaller profession, has often been overlooked (Cadée and Wikund 2020). Midwives have not always been involved in decision-making at national, regional and global levels. Weak health systems where the need for midwifery was greatest meant that midwifery was not supported to achieve at its best; nor were midwives able to perform the full scope of practice for which they had been educated, nor to meet the needs of women, babies and their families.

Because midwives lack political power, in many countries, the midwifery workforce strategy is developed in the absence of midwives. As a result, midwifery is not prioritised. Political and civil unrest, wars and massive population movements have also hampered, and continue to hamper, the development of midwifery globally. The COVID-19 pandemic overwhelmed demands on healthcare systems globally, further delaying progress. The initial lack of recognition of midwives as key service providers during the pandemic, or appreciation of the risk of COVID-19 transmission to midwives due to the very nature of midwifery services, demonstrates the need for effective advocacy for political commitment to midwifery (ICM 2020).

---

[1] Combining or confusing two separate things as one.

There are examples from different continents where political commitment has improved outcomes from women and their families and increased access to care (Chapters 1 and 2). These include Sweden, having educated and appointed midwives in remote and rural areas from the mid-eighteenth century (Högberg 2004) and, during the early twentieth century, countries including Thailand, Malaysia and Sri Lanka and later Egypt, Cuba, Honduras and Tunisia (Meléndez et al. 1999; Koblinsky 1999, 2003; Pathmanathan et al. 2003; Shiffman 2007; Shiffman and Smith 2007). However, the lack of political leadership and advocacy at national and regional levels have slowed down the growth of midwifery and recognition of midwives in other countries, which have therefore not gained maximum benefits from their investment.

In the second decade of the twenty-first century, the Sustainable Development Goals, with the accompanying concept of Universal Health Coverage and the global agenda of 'leaving no one behind' (World Health Assembly 2013), catapulted midwifery back into the limelight and created a more positive political environment for midwives. Evidence from the State of the World's Midwifery Reports (UNFPA 2011, 2014) and The Lancet Midwifery Series of papers (The Lancet 2014) provided vital evidence for the contribution of midwives, prompted a seminal shift from fragmented to women- and newborn-centred care services and showed policymakers that midwifery and midwives are crucial to the achievement of national and international goals and targets in reproductive, maternal, newborn and child health (ten Hoope-Bender et al. 2014). Global policies were developed including the 'Midwifery Pathway: the 2030 agenda' and 'Survive, Strive Thrive and Transform' (WHO 2018b) which emphasised improving health outcomes and quality of life for women, newborns and their families rather than just preventing deaths and disabilities. Countries moved closer to talking about midwives instead of the other cadres and titles which had led to confusion. Political strategies adopted by many countries, such as 'Road Maps' for sexual, reproductive, maternal, newborn and child health, enabled midwifery to continue to rise

(WHO and World Bank 2017). A growing emphasis on human rights-based approaches also compelled governments to strive to meet global standards for developments in midwifery in education and regulation (Chapters 4 and 5); a difference began to appear between political rhetoric and political action (Chapter 16).

Undoubtedly, global leadership by the International Confederation of Midwives (ICM) and UN Agencies, including the United Nations Population Fund (UNFPA) and the World Health Organization (WHO), contributed to this shift in policy. Chapter 6 described the role of the International Confederation of Midwives (ICM), in championing midwifery on the global political stage and in strengthening regional and national midwives associations to be the political voice of midwives and midwifery, promoting autonomous, well-educated, regulated and supported midwives, working in an enabling environment, as the most appropriate caregivers for childbearing women (Jerie 2014).

Moving forward, global midwifery will be further strengthened if there is political will to support different models of midwifery practice (Chapter 7), to keep centre-stage the rights of women/childbearing people and their families to high-quality, respectful maternity care, to develop ambitious midwifery workforce strategies that promote gender-equity and social inclusion (Chapter 8) and to find responsible, innovative approaches (Chapter 9) to working together at policy level, ensuring that no one is left behind, especially those in fragile stages and conflict-affected populations (Chapter 14). Political support is welcomed for global midwifery partnerships (Chapter 15) as a way to accelerate progress. Political commitment and advocacy are also critical for the harmonisation of midwifery in order to develop a common philosophy and identify (Chapter 16).

17.2.2 Economic Factors

Health and economic wealth are closely linked. Poverty has a significant negative impact on health, especially for women and girls (WHO

2020b). In return, health also impacts economies, as evidenced by the global economic downturn resulting from the COVID-19 pandemic. The economics and distribution of wealth in a country have also influenced the development of midwifery. A mapping of midwifery across the globe (Chapter 3) revealed that in some situations, availability of wealth led to medicalisation of maternity care, especially in high-income countries, thus reducing the number of women who benefit from high-quality maternity care from midwives (Kennedy et al. 2018; Camacho et al. 2015).

This book has demonstrated that investing in midwives is cost-effective and efficient when they are educated to international standards, regulated, supported and organised by well-led and well-managed professional associations and are working in an enabling environment (World Health Organization 2019). Midwives can bring a 16-fold return on investment and an additional 50 positive health outcomes, besides the reduction of deaths and disability (UNFPA 2014; WHO 2019). However, some governments cannot afford, or are unwilling, to educate midwives according to global standards, especially for the 3-year direct entry programme (Nathe 2017; WHO 2018b, 2019) and continue to engage in the production of different cadres as substitutes for midwives, that do not bring the same returns in investment. In some situations, this is unwittingly propagated by donors who fund these programmes either to fulfil their own agendas or genuinely do not understand the reality of the value of well-educated midwives. E-learning, increasing in popularity, is more affordable but varies in quality.

Around the world, there are different models of maternity care (Chapters 7 and 8) and different remuneration packages for midwives. Many do not receive a salary sufficient to support their families' basic needs for survival (Chapter 3) (WHO 2016a, b). As a result, some midwives resort to holding two jobs or engage in unscrupulous practices such as asking for 'under the table' payments from women and their families for care (Mannava et al. 2015). Midwives can also be exposed to economic exploitation if they choose to migrate to higher-income countries, where

they believe they will be able to earn a living wage (Anderson and Isaacs 2007). Unfortunately, in this quest, they are sometimes trafficked and sexually and/or economically exploited. In settings where health professionals compete for wealth, some have made it difficult for midwives to work in private practice, as they are perceived as a challenge to other care providers.

To safeguard women's and newborn's health and the global economy for the future, midwives, their leaders, supporters and communities must advocate to governments and health policymakers about the value of investing in midwives educated to global standards. Midwives should be paid a living wage (Chapter 16), enabling them to support their families and to avoid migration to higher-resource settings. Countries should maximise the potential of educating indigenous women to serve their own communities; promising attempts have been initiated in some countries including, in the past, Sweden and more recently Indonesia and the Maldives (WHO: SEARO 2020). Midwives should be supported to practise privately in rural areas where many other healthcare professionals are not willing to work. Innovation by and for midwives has the potential to improve efficiency, effectiveness and affordability of midwifery care (Chapter 9).

17.2.3 Social Factors

Society is constantly changing and midwives must continue to examine and understand the social and cultural context in which they provide care to women (ICM 2014b). However, midwives also have the power to change society themselves (Chapter 8) and to act as change agents within the society of midwifery itself (Chapters 6, 9, 11, 12 and 15; van Teijlingen 2015). When maternity care services are provided in a dignified, respectful manner, women emerge at the end of the birthing process empowered, confident and able to look after their own health and that of their families (Alonso 2019).

Numerous societal issues have been explored throughout this book, and also the role of the midwife in caring for women and birthing people in many different circumstances. At the heart of these are the capabilities of a woman to make decisions both for herself and for both her unborn baby and her child and to take control of her life as a human being; midwifery strengthens women to do that (WHO 2020a; Alonso 2019). The midwifery model of care (International Confederation of Midwives 2014a), discussed in Chapter 7, has the concept of 'woman-centred' care at its core.

Gender inequity has been a key thread throughout almost all chapters. Readers will have understood that although Sustainable Development Goal (SDG) 3 promotes gender equity, midwives have thus far been unable to take their rightful place in many societies (Chapters 1 and 3) where midwives face cultural and societal prejudice and are held in low regard because of their gender. Male midwives also share in this experience because midwifery, as a female-dominated profession, is affected by gender-inequity as a whole (WHO 2016a, b). The impact of gender inequity on midwifery education (Chapter 4) and the professionalisation of midwifery (Chapter 10) have been explored. Effective quality midwifery care (Chapter 8) enables governments and health systems to focus on the SDGs' demands for gender-mainstreaming of programmes, women's empowerment, addressing gender-based violence and reduction or even abolition of infanticide. However, midwives report that, although they know the solutions to providing high-quality midwifery care, their ability to do so is seriously compromised by their lack of voice or seniority within the broader political arena (WHO 2016a, b).

Violence against women has also been discussed by the authors. This takes several forms whether it be domestic violence, violence as a result of war or migration, obstetric violence (Chapter 7) or female genital mutilation (FGM), an inhumane and unacceptable act of abuse. Since 2012 there has been an annual day promoting zero tolerance of FGM and, in 2020, the United Nations focused on 'unleashing the power of youth' in order to help eradicate harmful socio-cultural practices including FGM (UN 2020b). The book has also highlighted violence against midwives themselves, other female health workers and the systems in which they work (Chapter 13; Nathe 2017). Midwives have the right to a safe and respectful working environment, free from discrimination, coercion and violence (Chapter 13).

Discrimination in its many forms within midwifery has also been explored. Women and midwives both face race discrimination in maternity services; for example, in United Kingdom, women from black ethnic backgrounds are five times more likely to die in childbirth and are at greater risk from other adverse pregnancy outcomes; midwives and maternity support workers are more likely to experience bullying at work, to face disciplinary processes and less likely to advance in their careers (MBRRACE-UK 2019; RCM 2020a). LGBTI people have historically been marginalised within healthcare and the maternity services (ICM 2017; Lai-Boyd 2020), and many still experience discrimination and harassment (House of Commons 2019). Midwives themselves are diverse in sexual orientation; midwifery is strengthened and enriched by having a diversity of practitioners that reflects the communities they serve (ICM 2017). Younger midwives can also face discrimination; midwifery has been called an ageing profession (RCM 2017; Callender et al. 2020). In many parts of the world, young or newly qualified midwives are posted to hard-to-reach areas where health facilities have poor access to essential amenities such as running water, electricity and security. Midwives in such situations are often the only care provider, are separated from their families and receive minimal or non-existent support with no access to continuing professional development. To retain and develop young people in the profession, it is important that they are supported and nurtured; yet they must be offered significantly challenging responsibilities to develop as midwife leaders (Nathe 2017) who are prepared to lead services with diverse populations and midwifery practitioners from differing backgrounds and cultures (Chapter 11). Midwives must provide inclusive care to all clients with respect to human rights and without discrimination (ICM 2014b).

This book calls for the formation of creative, collaborative partnerships (Chapter 15) amongst midwives, women and other healthcare professionals in order to maximise efforts and ensure women's access to high-quality midwifery care and to work towards equity and equal respect for all healthcare workers including midwives. This demands a concerted effort for women's and midwives' empowerment.

17.2.4 Technological Factors

The role of technology in advancing midwifery globally has been highlighted by the book's authors, in particular in Chapters 4 and 9. Technology can facilitate monitoring of progress, identification of potential problems and access to treatment; it can also enable reporting of outbreaks before there is a risk to life. Improvements in communication technologies make it possible for midwives to receive remote support and guidance on care issues. Chapter 9 highlighted technologies that aid decision-making, provide solar power to health facilities in remote areas and give midwives easy access to evidence-based information.

Technology has also made health-related information more accessible to women and their families; this increased knowledge has encouraged women to demand high-quality care and to retain control of their bodies, their own care and that of their newborns, as well as to retain their right to make choices. This behoves midwives to be open minded, to remain current in their knowledge and practice and to include women in decision-making about their care.

Technology has transformed midwifery education (Chapter 4), making it possible for student midwives to study their curriculum's theoretical components remotely, in their homes or workplaces, through technologies including virtual reality. It has also enhanced clinical practice as practitioners can conduct research and learn from each other without being in the same physical space. Clients can participate in health education through technological applications without needing to attend a health facility (Chapters 4 and 9).

As a result of the COVID-19 pandemic, there was a significant expansion in the use of technology in midwifery to provide virtual consultations to clients, to offer antenatal education and to continue the delivery of midwifery education (Chapter 9). However, the RCM (2020b) cautions that virtual consultations must adhere to the same standards of care that would be provided during in-person consultations and that discussing sensitive issues is better managed in-person.

To utilise new technologies, midwives must be digitally literate. As midwifery is an ageing profession, this can pose challenges to older midwives who may need support with digital access. Additionally, the amount of digital information available can become overwhelming for midwives and their clients; in the COVID-19 pandemic, this was described as an 'infodemic', an overabundance of information, both online and offline, that undermined the global response and jeopardised measures to control the pandemic (WHO 2020c). In some countries, new career opportunities are being developed for 'digital midwives', harnessing the power of technology to improve maternity care and supporting colleagues in new ways of working.

Unfortunately, technology has also contributed to an increase in inequality, widening the gap between populations of different economic means. However, Chapter 9 explored how some companies are developing appropriate technology, such as the low-fidelity models developed by Laerdal Global Health in collaboration with its partners, making learning technologies accessible for midwives in low-resource countries.

The International Confederation of Midwives produced tools such as the Midwifery Services framework, to support governments who wish to enhance the quality of their midwifery services to engage in a consultative and collaborative approach to planning and developing the services. Other tools like the Health System Building Blocks have been produced by the World Health Organization. All these tools support governments to stay abreast of developments in technology.

17.2.5 Legal Factors

Chapter 5 demonstrated the legal struggles that have been faced by midwifery globally. These include lack of recognition by governments and other healthcare providers, lack of professional identity as the word 'midwife' is not always a protected title, lack of standardised remuneration for midwives and varying scopes of midwifery practice in different parts of the world. The separation of midwifery from nursing is a perpetual legal issue that has made it difficult for midwives to stand up and be counted autonomous professionals. In many countries, midwifery is subsumed in nursing, despite the global acknowledgement of the value of a midwife in saving the lives of women and newborns. Without effective regulation, it is difficult to exercise professional autonomy, to claim professionalism (Chapter 10) and to delineate the midwifery scope of practice. Neither is it possible to negotiate professional boundaries, midwifery specialist roles and a career framework for midwifery.

The International Confederation of Midwives' midwifery regulation toolkit supports governments in developing regulation for midwifery services in their countries (ICM 2016). This has had some effect where it has been used but the ICM's (2017) records demonstrates that very few countries have midwifery regulation. As a result, the education and practice of midwives remains unregulated, leading to gaps in the standard of education, scope of practice and professional title. Hence, midwifery remains conflated with other cadres who also provide midwifery care (The Lancet 2014).

Moving forward, the tools developed by the ICM and the WHO (Chapters 6 and 16) make it possible to begin the process of harmonising midwifery globally. The essential competencies for basic midwifery practice (ICM 2019a, b), the Global standards for midwifery education (ICM 2013), Midwifery Educator Competencies (WHO 2014) and the Global Midwifery Education Accreditation Programme (ICM 2019a, b) are now available to guide curriculum development, midwifery teacher education and assessment of the quality of midwifery education globally. The Global Standards for Midwifery Regulation (ICM 2016)   and the Midwifery Regulation Toolkit (ICM 2018) can support governments to develop separate national midwifery regulation. The Lancet series of five papers on Midwifery (2014), a great resource for countries wishing to strengthen their regulation of midwifery, identified the different aspects of midwifery and all the factors, including legal issues, impacting on it. Once harmonised, it will be possible for midwifery to claim and assume the professional autonomy, accountability and responsibility it deserves.

Midwifery trade unions and professional associations have a role in leading the process of redefining midwifery and midwifery professionalism. They should advocate for countries to have legislation which mandates the existence of midwifery as a separate profession as well as regulation which controls the education and practice of midwives. The development and recognition of midwifery as a profession have been discussed in Chapter 10 and remain a dynamic and evolutionary process supported within a critical legal framework.

17.2.6 Environmental Factors

In this section, two meanings are applied to the term environment. Firstly, the surroundings or conditions in which midwifery is practised. This environment encompasses the legal, regulatory and policy frameworks, the physical infrastructure and space where midwifery can be practised as an autonomous profession providing dignified respectful, quality care. Secondly, the environment is defined as the natural world, how it impacts on midwifery and how midwives and maternity care reciprocally affect the planetary environment.

The surroundings in which midwifery is practised have largely been explored in the previous sections of this PESTLE analysis. In summary, disabling policy frameworks (Kennedy et al. 2018) deprive a nation of the best of midwifery and inhibit women's right of access to high-quality, respectful maternity care from Midwives.

With regard to the planetary environment, Chapter 13 described how the impact of natural hazards, such as earthquakes, tsunamis, floods and wild fires, are exacerbated by climate change and population growth. The interaction between natural hazards, conflict and vulnerability is the cause of most humanitarian disasters, laying bare inequality and discrimination. Humanitarian crises take a disproportionate toll on women and girls, and midwives too may become victims of a crisis. In some situations the work environment poses life-threatening risks to midwives and other care-providers due to epidemics such as Ebola, malaria and Zika viruses, and pandemics such as COVID-19. Women and their families have the right to quality midwifery care, even in crises; midwives also have rights to a safe working environment and protection from harm. Emergency preparedness and response planning are essential in disaster-prone areas, and midwives must be allowed to take their place in this at the highest of levels and to provide technical guidance.

Midwifery has been able to lessen reduce its carbon footprint by reducing local, national and international travel for the purposes of education and replacing this with remote learning technologies (Chapters 4 and 9). Global midwifery partnerships can also be supported and maintained through internet communication, reducing the number of international travellers (Chapter 15).

The results of the PESTLE analysis are summarised in Table 17.1.

The PESTLE analysis has demonstrated that there are multiple factors that have impacted on midwifery globally. Some have posed opportunities; some have revealed weaknesses and strengths, and others have led to the awareness of threats to the profession. The next section presents a SWOT analysis of the profession in the global context.

Table 17.1 Summary of the PESTLE analysis results of global midwifery

Political factors	Economic factors
• The global health agenda—Safe Motherhood Initiative, Millennium Development Goals and Sustainable Development Goals and the related strategies made midwifery and its value visible • Support from global bodies (UN agencies, international NGOs and global healthcare professions associations) • Disparities in midwifery practices and models of care in different countries • Desire to meet global indicators led to development of multiple cadres with the title Midwife, multiple pathways to entry and differing levels of education, which blurred midwives' identity • Multiple cadres all being called midwives with different levels of education and pathways to entering midwifery as governments wished to meet the indicators for global initiatives blurring the identity of midwifery • Governments' political impatience and inability to resource the education of midwives to global standard (3 years perceived as too long) • Midwifery has to work within weak health systems in many countries • Midwives' lack of political power and weak leadership, thus not represented in policy- and decision-making • National political strategies such as road maps for SRMNCH make midwifery relevant • Weak midwifery leadership led to lack of advocacy on critical issues	• Midwifery is cost-effective and efficient • Poor remuneration for midwives leading to migration and unscrupulous practices and poor quality of care • Migration led to the economic exploitation of midwives in their host countries • Some countries were not able to afford educating midwives at global standard • Midwifery underfunded globally • Distribution of wealth in different countries and sometimes within countries led to the increase of medicalisation of childbirth especially amongst the rich • Some governments lacked appreciation of the economic value of midwifery—the 16-fold return on investment in midwifery in lives saved

Table 17.1 (continued)

Technological factors	Social
• Technology has made information accessible to midwives, women and their families, enhancing care planning, coordination, monitoring and reporting as well as clinical decision-making and treatment • Women's access to information enhances choice and behoves midwives to remain current and open-minded • 'Infodemic' leading to confusion due to too much information • Use of artificial intelligence in midwifery education and practice, making it possible to educate many more midwives away from campus • Use of technological applications to provide information to women and conduct remote screening such as foetal heart monitoring whilst they are in their homes • Technological divide between the rich and the poor but addressed by the production of equally effective low fidelity models for low income settings by companies like Laerdal Global Health and their collaborating partners • Use of technology in some instances leading to the deskilling of midwives • The fear that technology might be preferred in place of the human touch of the midwife	• Midwifery empowers women leading to societal transformation • Population movements cause demographic societal change, impacting midwifery practice and demanding clear leadership • Civil unrest leads to the collapse of health systems. Women and newborn are most vulnerable. Midwives have to step in • Civil unrest and population displacements lead to poor mental health, substance abuse and midwives are not immune to these • Midwives need to be prepared to address the complications of unacceptable socio-cultural practices such as FGM and lead initiatives to counter these • The status of midwives in some countries is the same as that of the women. Therefore, midwives suffer the same marginalisation that women experience in that society leading to lack of recognition
Environmental factors	Legal
• Inhibitive legislative, regulatory and policy frameworks in some countries denying women access to quality midwifery care. • Lack of clear scope of practice leads to poor quality of care, disrespectful care and lack of accountability and responsibility amongst midwives • In some instances, the work environment poses a risk to the midwives' lives, e.g. in epidemics like Ebola, malaria, Zika and pandemics like COVID-19 • Midwives must be educated and enabled to respond to increasing humanitarian crises and population movements which disproportionately affect women and children • Natural disasters and massive population movements have increased the demand for midwifery to be op to date in disaster preparedness since it is usually women and newborn who are most badly affected • Midwifery can lessen its carbon footprint through less travel, more remote learning, less use of paper, improved use of technology and virtual partnerships • Technology has made it possible for midwifery to reduce its carbon footprint by using less paper, flying less to colleges as they can learn from home and write on screen without use of paper and also to maintain international partnerships despite inability to travel for whatever reason	• Weak or absent regulation of midwifery in many countries • Many countries have no legislation mandating the existence of midwifery as a separate profession, leading to midwives' lack of professional identity, recognition and autonomy. • Absent legislation that mandates the existence of midwifery in many countries leading to lack of identity, lack of recognition and lack of professional autonomy. Difficulty in being recognised as a separate profession • Lack of legislation and regulation makes it difficult to demand appropriate remuneration for midwives and to delineate the scope of practice and for midwives to practise their full scope according to their education • Midwifery often conflated with nursing further compromising the identity of the profession • Global tools exist for the development of midwifery regulation in different countries, i.e. the Global Standards for Midwifery Regulation (ICM 2016) and the Midwifery Regulation Toolkit (ICM 2018) • Tool available for the assessment of the quality of midwifery education—the Midwifery Education Accreditation Programme (ICM 2019a, b) • Midwifery trade unions and midwives' associations can take on leadership advocating for the harmonisation of midwifery globally using all available tools available

17.3 SWOT Analysis: Strengths, Weaknesses Opportunities and Threats to Midwifery Globally

The PESTLE analysis above has broadly defined issues explored in this book in a thematic fashion for readers. This is followed by a short SWOT analysis, drawing these themes together to summarise the internal and external resources available for strengthening midwifery globally and the potential internal and external barriers to this. Strengths and weaknesses tend to be in the present; opportunities and threats tend to be in the future (Businessballs 2020). These are explored briefly below and then presented in Table 17.2.

17.3.1 Strengths

Strengths identify the unique contribution of midwives to global health and development. This includes the growing body of evidence that mid-

wives save lives and improve over 50 other outcomes for women and their families. Investing in midwives represents good value for money and leads to gender empowerment. Midwives are geographically close to women, are required in every setting in every country and have a broad skill set to care for women throughout their life course.

17.3.2 Weaknesses

Identifying weakness allows midwives to understand factors internal to the midwifery profession that may hinder progress. This includes the lack of clarity about what midwives are and what they do, the conflation of midwifery with nursing and the development of substitute cadres that lead to confusion amongst service users and policymakers, weak leadership and representation of midwifery at the highest levels, lack of sufficient legal and regulatory frameworks for midwifery in many countries and insufficient opportunities for career progression.

Table 17.2 Strengths, weaknesses, opportunities and threats to global midwifery

Strengths	Weaknesses

• Evidence for the life-saving impact of midwives and the value of high-quality midwifery care (Nove et al 2020, Lancet 2014)
 • Strong current global policy context that recognises midwives unique contribution to achieving global goals
 • Support for midwifery from global bodies such as WHO, UNFPA, international NGOs, global professional organisations
 • Evidence for the cost-effectiveness and efficiency of midwives
 • Midwives are everywhere and work closest to where women and their families live
 • Midwives provide the full continuum of care through a woman's life
 • Midwifery enables gender empowerment, for clients and for midwives
 • The effectiveness of midwifery services with minimal use of technology
	• In many countries there is/are still:
	   - Insufficient numbers and distribution of midwives
	   - Disabling regulatory and policy frameworks
	   - Prevalence of poor quality, disrespectful midwifery care resulting from poor quality midwifery education
	   - Too many substitute cadres causing confusion about role and identity of midwives
	   - Lack of professional and public esteem for midwives
	   - Conflation of midwifery with nursing
	   - Different pathways and educational entry requirements for midwifery education
	   - Absent career pathway and poor remuneration for midwives
	   - Lack of midwifery-specific regulation and legislation
	   - Weak midwifery leadership and and lack of representation at policy- and decision- making level
	   - Midwives not able to perform their full scope of practice
	   - Poor transport links
	   - Insufficient equipment and supplies
	 • Enabling environment for midwives not clearly defined
	 • Globally midwives are not prepared for their role in humanitarian and other crisis situations
	 • Midwives do not always speak with one voice

Table 17.2 (continued)

Opportunities	Threats
• Opportunity to avert 41% of maternal deaths, 39% of newborn deaths and 26% of stillbirths equating to 2.2 million deaths averted by 2035 through scaling up of midwifery (Nove et al 2020) • New State of the World's Midwifery Report expected in 2021 • Availability of tools to harmonise midwifery globally • Global initiatives emphasising the importance of midwives and midwifery services • Technological advances present new opportunities for learning, collaboration and practice development	• Global health crises such as pandemics and epidemics • Conflict, climate change, disasters and human migration • Impact of colonial past on regulation, education and practice of midwifery • Global economic downturn following COVID-19 pandemic may turn focus away from investing in midwives • The rise in medicalisation of birth in both low- and high- income countries • Not protecting the title midwife leading to continued short-term staff solutions for shortage of midwives

17.3.3 Opportunities

Opportunities usually arise from situations outside an organisation (Mindtools 2020), for example trends that can offer an advantage. Strengths can also be turned into opportunities. Midwives have an opportunity in the current positive policy framework which is supporting the development of global midwifery, for example the WHO's commitment to strengthening midwifery and global policies such as 'Survive, Thrive, Transform' (WHO 2018b) that place midwives at the centre-stage in sexual, reproductive, maternal, newborn and adolescent health. Other opportunities lie in the availability of data, such as that in the State of the World's Midwifery reports, that strengthens the evidence for the effectiveness of midwives, and technology that supports new ways of communicating, learning and improving practice.

17.3.4 Threats

Threats are those factors that can negatively impact growth; it is important to identify them and take appropriate action to prevent becoming victim to them (Mindtools 2020). Threats to global midwifery include global population movements (including migration of midwives), increasing medicalisation of birth and short-term human resource solutions such as task-shifting and task-sharing. Lack of enabling environments for midwives also threaten progress.

17.4   The Leading Principles, Policy and Practice Issues Emerging from the Text

The PESTLE and SWOT analyses in this final chapter have provided an overview of the themes running through the six different sections of the book: midwifery on the global scene, the three pillars of midwifery, the profession of midwifery, midwifery across the globe and looking ahead. Bringing this comprehensive text to a conclusion, the overarching principles, policies and practice issues for global midwifery are now considered.

17.4.1 Principles

Principles are fundamental truths (Cambridge English Dictionary 2020). In this case, the fundamental truths that serve as the foundation to the beliefs and behaviours of global midwifery are summarised below.

The first principle identified is that to achieve the global agenda for sustainable development and universal health coverage, there must be a move away from the focus on mortality towards good health and well-being for all as a human right. Midwives are instrumental in promoting the reduction of preventable deaths and in demanding political commitment as a crucial component in facilitating this process. Investing adequate financial and material support in midwifery education and practice enhances the capacity of a country to enable the population not only to survive but to thrive and transform their variable situations.

Another principle is that midwifery is an autonomous profession which provides skilled, compassionate midwives' associations practitioners. To facilitate this, the professional pillars of midwifery comprise regulation to control practice, education to global standards and midwives' associations which strengthen the profession and promote an adequate and appropriate workforce. In this context, persons interested in practising midwifery should be those educated as skilled practitioners, thus maximising resources.

Principles identified from historical evidence can be used as a basis to promote continuing progress across the globe. So too, principles of harmonisation used elsewhere can be adapted to harmonise midwifery globally. In contrast to standardisation, the principle of harmonisation respects country-specific needs whilst promoting quality care in line with global standards.

Quality Maternal and Newborn Care (QMNC) is evident where midwifery exists within an environment of mutual respect and cooperation. If countries intend to provide quality care for all, then models of midwifery practice should be developed within a philosophy of woman-centred, safe and satisfying care for the provision of Sexual, Reproductive, Maternal and Neonatal Health (SRMNH) at every level.

The principle of listening to midwives, who are closest to women not only in their geographical location but also in understanding their needs and desires, should be observed by policymakers and managers, so that policy and practice are relevant, realistic and respectful, saving lives and promoting health. The principle of a supportive policy environment is also needed encourage the implementation of innovation in midwifery education and practice. The humanitarian community must also hear the voice of midwives and afford them every support in times of crisis.

The principle of professionalisation is a constantly evolving process. Whilst leadership and leadership styles take culture and other characteristics of followers into consideration, a further principle is that reliable research should provide the foundation for evidence-based midwifery practice across the globe.

Just as successful midwifery partnerships depend upon power-sharing and equity, sharing values and commitment, so too other forms of cross-cultural exchange must be nurtured within an enabling philosophy, aiming to provide mutual benefits to both parties and framed within an atmosphere of reciprocal respect for people and planet.

It is upon these principles that the foundation of a skilled global midwifery workforce rests. This dynamic process needs to continue to develop offering safety, security and satisfaction for all women and their families at that precious time surrounding birth, ensuring that 'no-one is left behind'.

17.4.2 Policy

Policy is defined as a set of ideas, or a plan, agreed officially by a group of people, a business organisation, a government or a political party (Cambridge English Dictionary 2020). In this book, the 'group of people' are the policymakers in maternal, newborn and child health. This includes UN Agencies, governments, Ministries of Health and all other leaders in the healthcare provision and decision-making arena. In general, policies are binding to the people governed by them. As a result, policies can either enable or inhibit principles becoming practice and are therefore a crucial component in any process. Political commitment is a critical component in preventing avoidable deaths and disability and in promoting a healthy population through the provision of effective midwifery care. Midwives are in an unparalleled position to advocate for enabling policies at each level and across every strata of society and must be enabled and empowered to function if global reproductive health targets are to be achieved. The policy of listening to midwives who are closest to women not only in their geographical location but also in understanding their needs and desires should be observed by decision-makers and managers, so that practice is relevant, realistic and respectful, saving lives and promoting health. A supportive policy environment is also needed to encourage the implementation of innovation in midwifery education and practice. Without doubt, maternal and neonatal healthcare policies must be enshrined in and propagate the human rights agenda. Therefore, policies that promote and facilitate a woman's right to choose as well as a midwife's right to practise in enabling clinical and political environments are vital. Similarly, policy at local, national and global levels should promote evidence-based practice and should be reviewed constantly in line with current advances in research undertaken for and by midwives.

Midwives must be represented at decision-making tables for a country to continue to develop and improve its midwifery services. Thus, inviting and encouraging midwives to participate at these levels must become the norm, in order to achieve success.

The quality, or lack of it, of those who educate midwives has been identified across the globe. Midwives should be educated primarily by midwives. National policy needs to ensure that those identified as teachers of midwifery are specifically and formally educated, supported, and afforded opportunities for continuing professional development and maintaining their competency in clinical midwifery practice.

Complementary to the regulation of other healthcare professions with which midwives will work in the multidisciplinary team, midwifery regulation must ensure that midwifery is maintained as a separate profession and must form an integral part of all national healthcare policies.

In order to enhance quality midwifery services for women, newborns and their families, governments, development partners and key stakeholders must support the strengthening of midwives' associations.

National policy should dictate that the health system infrastructure facilitates effective and timely referrals whenever and wherever they are needed. Safety and respectful care must never be compromised, and so policies outlining strategies to afford continuity of care and of carer suited to the local culture and environment need to be in place and utilised. National, local and institutional policies should uphold the principles contained in the AAAQ Framework in order to promote quality care.

Social innovation and novel approaches to partnership across different sectors are to be encouraged, but these will require sufficient funding and support from global markets. Unarguably, innovation is needed to reach the health-related SDGs and to strengthen midwifery for the future. It is therefore essential that global health policy supports innovative approaches to developing midwifery education, regulation and practice, especially for fragile and vulnerable populations. In order to facilitate this, midwives must have a seat at policymaking tables both nationally and internationally when new approaches are designed. It becomes increasingly evident that as the midwifery profession constantly develops and diversifies, midwives must be engaged at various levels of policymaking and implementation on all issues that affect childbearing women, newborns, sexual and reproductive health care and midwifery education and practice. In order to maximise these efforts, there must be a demand that governments and key stakeholders support the development of midwifery leadership. This will assist in organising and enhancing the quality of midwifery services as well as contributing to the development and management of the health workforce.

Global and national policy should motivate national governments, donors, implementing organisations and global decision makers to mobilise around three key activities, namely greater emphasis on maternal and newborn health in vulnerable communities, maternal and newborn life-saving interventions in crisis settings and strengthening the role of communities in delivering maternal and newborn health interventions. In addition, a policy should be in place to guide selection and ensure appropriate preparation and debriefing for all who cross borders to strengthen global midwifery, whether these are professionals or students. This is essential in order to enable maximum effectiveness, minimal disruption due to cross-cultural interactions and prevention of economic exploitation and trafficking. In this context, midwifery partnerships show potential in enhancing the capacity of professional midwives' associations which in turn can improve the quality of maternity care. For this reason, such partnerships need the support of policymakers.

It has been proposed that political commitment and advocacy are critical components for harmonisation. Harmonisation can function as an enabling influence in the whole process of providing acceptable, accessible and affordable quality of maternal and newborn care for a total population. The evidence concerning the importance of midwives' contribution to achieving the SDGs in this context is convincing. Policymakers would appear to hold the key to making numerous ideals a reality through ensuring that their countries use the available global tools for harmonising midwifery such as the global competencies for midwifery practice, the global standards for midwifery education and regulation and the global midwifery accreditation programme rather than perpetuating age old barriers that threaten the 2030 Agenda.

17.4.3 Practice

Appropriate midwifery practice depends on the availability of sufficient numbers of well-educated midwives who are high skilled, respected, enabled by policy and guided by considered principles to provide evidence-based care. Without them, there is little chance of achieving the targets of SDG3 in the context of Sexual, Reproductive, Maternal and Newborn Health (SRMNH). Midwives are best placed to provide woman-centred care. Evidence-based practice provided by skilled midwives must be safe, but it should also offer support and a satisfying experience that promotes optimum maternal and newborn health and well-being. It is essential therefore that as principles provide the fundamental truths to be adhered to and policy guides as to how it should be done, midwives operationalise these in their practice. The knowledge that what they are doing is mandated by policy and is based on principle enhances the confidence with which midwives practise as they will be aware of the accepted basis on which their practice rests. Thus, integrating midwives into the health systems in every country and resourcing midwifery services adequately enables midwives to practice confidently, providing quality care.

In order to facilitate a high standard of midwifery practice, midwifery educational institutions also need to be adequately resourced and staffed by those skilled in midwifery practice as well as appropriate educational approaches.

Midwifery practice must be controlled and directed by a recognised regulatory framework if the unacceptably high global maternal and perinatal mortality and morbidity rates are to be addressed. Within such a framework, midwives should be enabled to provide skilled, respectful care. The value of midwives' associations in the context of contributing to the quality of care needs to be further evaluated, but these professional organisations appear to have considerable influence on the practice of midwives in diverse situations. All midwifery care needs to be provided by skilled midwives who have been trained to international standards. Midwives practice in collaboration with obstetricians, paediatricians and other professionals as it becomes necessary. Women, their families and their communities should be able to find the practice of every midwife acceptable and therefore be eager to seek such skilled attendance during childbirth.

Innovation has the potential to transform midwifery practice and to benefit midwives, those who work with midwives and others from different disciplines. Therefore, innovation in midwifery practice should be responsible and should target the populations, and be developed in partnership with, those who most need to benefit from it. For those with digital access, digital innovations can make high-quality midwifery care more accessible. There is potential for midwives to transform their ideas into action where this will enhance practice and promote safety and satisfaction.

Midwives have become highly skilled professionals in many parts of the world. However, they need to practice to their full capacity in political and practice environments. Hence, policy and politics should enable, rather than disable or limit, midwives so that they are accessible to every woman.

Midwifery leaders are well placed to take responsibility for quality assurance as well as ensuring that evidence-based practice is adopted and adapted.

Practising midwives must ensure they are competent to perform all the basic emergency obstetric and newborn care (BEmONC) functions as well as providing respectful maternity care. This includes crisis situations when regular health systems may be fractured. Midwives must engage with women and local communities in planning care. In addition, a systematic feedback mechanism of women's experience of care and recommendations for improvement could continue to enhance midwifery practice. Midwifery practice, whether clinical, academic or in a consultancy role, needs to place the safety, health and well-being of women and babies within a human rights framework. Similarly participating in a global midwifery partnership involves practising with similar priorities and can foster personal and professional benefit to individuals and the organisations in which midwives work.

Finally, the concept of harmonisation enhances the provision of quality midwifery services everywhere. Individual professionals will share a common philosophy and a common professional identity which will compel them to practice according to agreed professional standards. Building on these principles, facilitated by enabling policy and implemented in practice, midwives offer substantial hope for the world's women, their newborns and their families. Communities served by skilled midwives can have confidence that they will not only survive but also thrive and transform. The principles, policy and practice of global midwifery stands testimony to a brighter future, even for the most vulnerable in the twenty-first-century world in crisis.

17.5 Recommendations

1. Since it has been recognised that political commitment is a critical component in preventing avoidable deaths and disability and in promoting a healthy population through the provision of effective midwifery care, governments need to recognise or renew their commitment in this respect.

2. Since there is a good return on investment as a result of lives saved and interventions averted, global bodies and governments should increase investment in midwifery education, regulation and practice, thus enabling populations not only to survive, but to thrive and to transform their situations.

3. In order to nurture a skilled workforce, governments, development partners and key stakeholders should cooperate to facilitate the retention of midwives through continuing professional development opportunities, providing supportive supervision and ensuring that midwives receive appropriate remuneration and secure working and living conditions whether they are posted to rural or urban locations.

4. There is a need to develop strong midwifery leaders to lead and guide the profession, to advocate for midwives, women/pregnant people and newborns and to represent the profession in policy- and decision-making bodies at all levels.

5. Globally, and in each country, midwifery needs to be recognised as an autonomous profession with the title 'midwife' protected and used only by those who meet global standards of competence.

6. Midwives should be educated to global standards by those who meet the global standards for midwifery educators and are able to promote safe, respectful evidence-based care.

7. Models of midwifery practice should be developed within a philosophy of woman-centred, safe and satisfying care for the provision of Sexual, Reproductive, Maternal and Neonatal Health (SRMNH) at every level.

8. If the identified global reproductive health targets are to be achieved, midwives should be participating in the development of, and be encouraged to advocate for, enabling policies and be empowered to function within enabling political and clinical environments.

9. All agencies working in maternal and child health, governments, decision-makers and managers should listen to midwives, so that practice is relevant, realistic, dignified and respectful, saving lives and promoting health.

10. National, local and institutional policies should uphold the principles contained in the

AAAQ Framework in order to promote safe and respectful quality care.

11. Global and national policy should motivate national governments, donors, implementing organisations and global decision-makers to mobilise around three key activities, namely greater emphasis on maternal and newborn health in vulnerable communities, maternal and newborn life-saving interventions in crisis settings and strengthening the role of communities in delivering maternal and newborn health interventions.

12. In order to enable maximum effectiveness and minimal disruption due to cross-cultural interactions and prevention of economic exploitation and trafficking, policies that are acceptable at the global level need to be in place to guide selection and ensure appropriate preparation and debriefing for all who cross borders, whether these are professionals, students or participating in international partnerships.

13. It should be recognised at every level that only midwives practise midwifery and do so in collaboration with obstetricians, paediatricians and other professionals as it becomes necessary.

14. Every woman, every family and every community should be able to access the care of a skilled midwife who is enabled to provide appropriate care supported by both a policy and an infrastructure which facilitates timely referral whenever deemed necessary.

15. The weaknesses and threats to global midwifery identified in this text should be systematically addressed; the strengths should be recognised and maximised and the opportunities seized in order to move with confidence towards the 2030 agenda and beyond.

References

Alonso C (2019) Open a midwifery center: a manual for launching and operating midwifery centers in global settings. Goodbirth Network

Anderson BA, Isaacs AA (2007) Simply not there: the impact of international migration of nurses and midwives-perspectives from Guyana. J Midwifery Womens Health 52(4):392–397. https://doi.org/10.1016/j.jmwh.2007.02.021

Businessballs (2020) SWOT analysis. https://www.businessballs.com/strategy-innovation/swot-analysis/. Accessed 24 Nov 2020

Cadée F, Wikund A (2020) The decade of the midwife! Sex Reprod Healthcare. https://doi.org/10.1016/j.srhc.2020.100518

Callender E, Sidebotham M, Lindsay D et al (2020) The future of the Australian midwifery workforce—impacts of ageing and workforce exit on the number of registered midwives. Women Birth. https://doi.org/10.1016/j.wombi.2020.02.023

Camacho CK, Collins-Fulea C, Krulewitch C et al (2015) The United States midwifery, education, regulation, and association work group: what is it and what does it hope to accomplish? J Midwifery Womens Health 60(2):125–127

Cambridge English Dictionary (2020). https://dictionary.cambridge.org/dictionary/english/. Accessed 22 Aug 2020

Edwards G, Seda P (2016) Empowering midwives in the UAE. MIDIRS Midwifery Digest 26(3):387–390

Every Woman Every Child (2015) Survive, thrive, transform: the global strategy for women's, children's and adolescent's health 2016–2039. https://www.everywomaneverychild.org/global-strategy/. Accessed 18 Aug 2020

Fathalla MF (2006) Human rights aspects of safe motherhood. Best Pract Res Clin Obstetr Gynaecol 20(3):409–419

Gherrisi A, Tinsa F, Soussi S et al (2016) Teaching research methodology to student midwives through a socio-constructivist educational model: the experience of the high school for science and health techniques of Tunis. Midwifery 33:46–48

Högberg U (2004) The decline in maternal mortality in Sweden: the role of community midwifery. Am J Public Health 94(8):1312–1320. https://doi.org/10.2105/AJPH.94.8.1312

House of Commons (2019) Health and social care and LGBT communities. https://publications.parliament.uk/pa/cm201919/cmselect/cmwomeq/94/94.pdf. Accessed 17 Nov 2020

International Confederation of Midwives (2013b) Global standards for midwifery education (2010) amended in 2013. https://www.internationalmidwives.org. Accessed 14 May 2019.

International Confederation of Midwives (2014a) Core document: philosophy and model of midwifery care. https://www.internationalmidwives.org/assets/files/definitions-files/2018/06/eng-philosophy-and-model-of-midwifery-care.pdf. Accessed 23 Nov 2020

International Confederation of Midwives (2014b) Core document: international code of ethics for midwives. https://www.internationalmidwives.org/assets/files/general-files/2019/10/eng-international-code-of-ethics-for-midwives.pdf. Accessed 23 Nov 2020

International Confederation of Midwives (2016) Global standards for midwifery regulation. www.internationalmidwifery.org/regulation-resources/. Accessed 30 Mar 2020

International Confederation of Midwives (2017) Position statement human rights of lesbian, gay, bisexual, transgender and intersex (LGBTI) people. https://www.internationalmidwives.org/assets/files/statement-files/2018/04/eng-lgtbi.pdf. Accessed 23 Nov 2020

International Confederation of Midwives (2018) Midwifery regulation toolkit. https://www.internationalmidwives.org/assets/files/regulation-files/2018/04/icm_toolkit_eng.pdf. Accessed 9 Jul 2020

International Confederation of Midwives (2019a) Essential competencies for midwifery practice. https://www.internationalmidwives.org/assets/files/general-files/2018/10/icm-competencies%2D%2D-english-document_final_oct-2018.pdf. Accessed 3 Jul 2020

International Confederation of Midwives (2019b) 2019 Young Midwifery Leaders Programme. https://www.internationalmidwives.org/assets/files/project-files/2019/02/final-yml-advert%2D%2D-selection-c-and-process-document.pdf. Accessed 13 Jul 2020

International Confederation of Midwives (2020) Women's rights in childbirth must be upheld during the coronavirus pandemic. https://internationalmidwives.org/icm-news/women%E2%80%99s-rights-in-childbirth-must-be-upheld-during-the-coronavirus-pandemic.html. Accessed 21 Nov 2020

Jerie C (2014) ICM: strengthening midwifery globally. https://www.healthynewbornnetwork.org/blog/icm-strengthening-midwifery-globally/. Accessed 18 Nov 2020

Kennedy HP, Myers-Ciecko JA, Camacho Carr K et al (2018) United States model of midwifery legislation and regulation: development of consensus document. J Midwifery Womens Health 63:652–659

Koblinsky M, Campbell O, Heichelheim J (1999) Organizing delivery care: What works for safe motherhood? Bulletin of the World Health Organization 77(5):399–406

Koblinsky M (ed) (2003) Reducing maternal mortality: learning from Bolivia, China, Egypt, Honduras, Jamaica, and Zimbabwe. The World Bank, Washington, DC, p 567

Lai-Boyd B (2020) Maternity care for LGBTQ+ people—how can we do better? https://www.all4maternity.com/maternity-care-for-lgbtq-people-how-can-we-do-better/. Accessed 17 Nov 2020

Luyben A, Barger M, Avery M et al (2017) Exploring global recognition of quality midwifery education: vision or fiction? Women Birth 30:184–192

Mannava P, Durant K, Fisher J et al (2015) Attitudes and behaviours of maternal health care providers in interactions with clients: a systematic review. Glob Health 11:36. https://www.ncbi.nlm.nih.gov/pmc/articles/PMC4537564/. Accessed 22 Aug 2020

MBRRACE-UK (2019) Saving lives, improving mothers' care: lessons learned to inform maternity care from the UK and Ireland Confidential Enquiries into Maternal Deaths and Morbidity 2015–17. https://www.npeu.ox.ac.uk/assets/downloads/mbrrace-uk/reports/MBRRACE-UK%20Maternal%20Report%202019%20-%20WEB%20VERSION.pdf. Accessed 24 Nov 2020

Medway P, Digance A (2017) The politics of midwifery practice: The quest to extend the boundaries by advocating for women and midwifery through political engagement. Women Birth 30(1):40–15

Meléndez J, Ochoa J, Villanueva Y et al (1999) Investigation on Maternal Mortality and Women of Reproductive Age in Honduras: Final Report Corresponding to the Year 1997 [in Spanish]. Pan American Health Organization/World Health Organization, Tegucigalpa, Honduras/Geneva

Mindtools (2020) SWOT analysis. https://www.mindtools.com/pages/article/newTMC_05.htm. Accessed 24 Nov 2020

Nathe M (2017) 7 issues that will shape the health workforce of the future. Itra Health International. https://www.intrahealth.org/vital/7-issues-will-shape-health-workforce-future. Accessed 21 Aug 2020

Nove A, Friberg I, de Bernis L et al (2020) Potential impact of midwives in preventing and reducing maternal and neonatal mortality and stillbirths: a Lives Saved Tool modelling study, Lancet Global Health, https://doi.org/10.1016/S2214-109X(20)30397-1. Accessed 14 Dec 2020

Pathmanathan I, Liljestrand J, Martins J et al (2003) Investing in maternal health: learning from Malaysia and Sri Lanka. The World Bank, Washington, DC, p 568

Professional Academy (2020) Professional Academy's marketing theories explained—live: PESTEL analysis. https://www.professionalacademy.com/events/marketing-theories-explained-live%2D%2Dpestele-analysis. Accessed 21 Aug 2020

Ralph N, Birks M, Chapman Y et al (2014) Future-proofing nursing education: an Australian perspective. SAGE Open 4(4):1–11. https://doi.org/10.1177/2158244014556633

Royal College of Midwives (RCM) (2017) The gathering storm: England's midwifery workforce challenges. https://www.rcm.org.uk/media/2374/the-gathering-storm-england-s-midwifery-workforce-challenges.pdf. Accessed 23 Nov 2020

Royal College of Midwives (RCM) (2020a) Race Matters: a statement by the RCM. https://www.rcm.org.uk/media/4128/race-matters-a-statement-by-the-rcm.pdf. Accessed 24 Nov 2020

Royal College of Midwives (RCM) (2020b) Virtual consultations. https://www.rcm.org.uk/media/4192/virtual-consultations-v20-24-july-2020-review-24-august-2020-1.pdf. Accessed 23 Nov 2020

Shiffman J (2007) Generating political priority for maternal mortality reduction in 5 developing countries. Am J Public Health 97:796–803

Shiffman J, Smith S (2007) Generation of political priority for global health initiatives: a framework and case study of maternal mortality. Lancet 370(9595):1370–1379 ten Hoope-Bender P, de Bernis L, Campbell J et al (2014) Improvement of maternal and newborn health through midwifery. Lancet 384(994):1226–1235

The Lancet (2014) Midwifery: an executive summary for the Lancet's series. https://www.thelancet.com/series/midwifery. Accessed 17 Nov 2020

United Nations (1986) Declaration on the right to development. United Nations General Assembly. In: 97th plenary meeting, 4 December. United Nations, New York

United Nations (2000) The Millennium Declaration. United Nations General Assembly. In: 8th plenary meeting, 55/2. United Nations, New York. https://www.un.org/millennium/declaration/ares552e.htm. Accessed 30 Apr 2019

United Nations (2015) Transforming our world: the 2030 Agenda for Sustainable Development. United Nations, New York

United Nations (2016) The sustainable development goals report 2016 leaving no one behind. United Nations, New York. https://unstats.un.org/sdgs/report/2016/leaving-no-one-behind. Accessed 29 Apr 2019

United Nations (2019) About the sustainable development goals. United Nations General Assembly. In: 4th plenary meeting, 70/1. United Nations, New York

United Nations (2020a) About the sustainable development goals. https://www.un.org/sustainabledevelopment/sustainable-development-goals/. Accessed 22 Aug 2020

United Nations (2020b) Unleashing the power of youth in ending female genital mutilation. UN Volunteers https://www.unv.org/Success-stories/Unleashing-power-youth-ending-Female-Genital-Mutilation. Accessed 14 Nov 2020

United Nations Population Fund (UNFPA) (2011) State of the world's midwifery 2011: delivering health, saving lives. https://www.unfpa.org/publications/state-worlds-midwifery-2011. Accessed 21 Nov 2020

United Nations Population Fund (2014) State of the world's midwifery report. A universal pathway. A woman's right to health. UNFPA, New York

van Teijlingen E (2015) Sociology of midwifery. In: Deery R, Denny E, Letherby G (eds) Sociology for midwives. Polity Press, Cambridge, pp 2–37

Walsh D (2016) Midwives, gender equality and feminism. Pract Midwife 19(3):24–26

World Health Assembly (2013) Transforming health workforce education in support of universal health coverage, WHA 66.23, Sixty sixth World Health Assembly, 2013

World Health Organization (2008) Task shifting: global recommendations and guidelines. World Health Organization, Geneva. https://www.who.int/health-systems/TTR-TaskShifting.pdf?ua=1. Accessed 2 Oct 2019

World Health Organisation (2013) Midwife educator core competencies. https://www.who.int. Accessed 13 May 2019

World Health Organization (2014) WHO Midwifery Educator Core Competencies. https://www.who.int/hrh/nursing_midwifery/educ_core_compt_adpt_tool/en/. Accessed 14 Nov 2020

World Health Organization (2016a) Midwives' voices, midwives' realities report 2016. https://www.who.int/maternal_child_adolescent/documents/midwives-voices-realities/en/. Accessed 21 Nov 2020

World Health Organization (2016b) Midwives' voices, midwives' realities report 2016: https://www.who.int/maternal_child_adolescent/documents/midwives-voices-realities/en/#:~:text=The%20%22Midwives%20voices%2C%20midwives%20realities,women%2C%20newborns%20and%20their%20families. Accessed 14 Nov 2020

World Health Organization (2017) Strengthening quality midwifery education. WHO Meeting report July 25–26, 2016. In support of Global Strategy for Women's, Children's and Adolescents' Health 2016–2030

World Health Organization (2018a) Definition of skilled health personnel providing care during childbirth. The 2018 joint statement by WHO, UNFPA, UNICEF, ICM, ICN, FIGO, IPA. 2018. https://www.who.int/reproductivehealth/publications/statement-competent-mnh-professionals/en/. Accessed 29 Apr 2020

World Health Organization (2018b) Survive, thrive, transform global strategy for women's, children's and adolescents' health (2016–2030). https://www.who.int/life-course/partners/global-strategy/global-strategy-2018-monitoring-report.pdf. Accessed 22 Aug 2020

World Health Organization (2019) Strengthening quality midwifery education for universal health coverage 2030: a framework for action. ISBN 978–92–4-151584-9

World Health Organization (2020a) Strengthening quality midwifery education for Universal Health Coverage 2030: Framework for action: https://www.who.int/maternal_child_adolescent/topics/quality-of-care/midwifery/strengthening-midwifery-education/en/. Accessed 14 Nov 2020

World Health Organization (2020b) Women's health. https://www.who.int/health-topics/women-s-health/. Accessed 22 Nov 2020

World Health Organization (2020c) Managing the COVID-19 infodemic. https://www.who.int/news/item/23-09-2020-managing-the-covid-19-infodemic-promoting-healthy-behaviours-and-mitigating-the-harm-from-misinformation-and-disinformation. Accessed 24 Nov 2020

World Health Organization and International Bank for Reconstruction and Development/The World Bank (2017) Tracking Universal Health Coverage: 2017 Global Monitoring Report. World Health Organization and the International Bank for Reconstruction and Development/The World Bank 2017. ISBN 978–92–4-151355-5. Licence: CC BY-NC-SA 3.0 IGO

World Health Organization: SEARO (2020) Regional Strategic Directions for strengthening Midwifery in the South-East Asia Region 2020–2024

Printed in the United States
by Baker & Taylor Publisher Services